Recent Developments in Antioxidants from Natural Sources

Edited by Paz Otero Fuertes and María Fraga Corral

Published in London, United Kingdom

Recent Developments in Antioxidants from Natural Sources
http://dx.doi.org/10.5772/intechopen.104365
Edited by Paz Otero Fuertes and María Fraga Corral

Contributors
Genaro Christian Pesantes Arriola, Enrique Gustavo García Talledo, César Angel Durand Gonzales, Víctor Alexis Higinio Rubio, Carlos Enrique Chinchay Barragán, Wilmer Huamani Palomino, Kehinde Sherifdeen Sowunmi, Zeenat Kaka, Rosa Huaraca Aparco, María Del Carmen Delgado Laime, Fidelia Tapia Tadeo, Henrry Wilfredo Agreda Cerna, Edwin Mescco Cáceres, Juan Alarcón Camacho, Hans Yuri Godoy Medina, Calixto Cañari Otero, Martha Teresa Ecos Ramos, Victor Raul Ochoa Aquije, Niki Franklin Flores Pacheco, Rosa Nelida Ascue Ruiz, Grecia Valverde Mamani, Veerapandi Loganathan, Lakshmi Mohan, Marika Cordaro, Roberta Fusco, Salvatore Cuzzocrea, Rosanna Di Paola, Fouad M. F. Elshaghabee, Ahmed A. Abd El-Maksoud, Gustavo M. Ambrósio F. de Gouveia, Dennis R.A. Mans, Tarique Hussain, Wa Iba, Nur Illyin Akib, Ilham, La Ode Muhammad Jumardin, Bolo Arif, Nursainuddin, Sendry Yosalina, Jumrisnanda Asmin Andas, Nadège Ngombe Kabamba, Théophile Mbemba Fundu, Paulin Mutwale Kapepula, Jean-Paul Nzundu Mbo, Justin Mboloko Esimo, Krishna R. Gupta, Shyam W. Rangari, Milind J. Umekar, Swati N. Lade, Sushil S. Burle, Marjan Assefi, Kai-Uwe Lewandrowski, Alireza Sharafshah, Sohila Nankali

First published in London, United Kingdom, 2023 by IntechOpen
IntechOpen is the global imprint of INTECHOPEN LIMITED, registered in England and Wales, registration number: 11086078, 5 Princes Gate Court, London, SW7 2QJ, United Kingdom
Printed in Croatia

British Library Cataloguing-in-Publication Data
A catalogue record for this book is available from the British Library

Additional hard and PDF copies can be obtained from orders@intechopen.com

Recent Developments in Antioxidants from Natural Sources
Edited by Paz Otero Fuertes and María Fraga Corral
p. cm.

This title is part of the Biochemistry Book Series, Volume 41
Topic: Chemical Biology
Series Editor: Miroslav Blumenberg
Topic Editors: Şükrü Beydemir and Deniz Ekinci

Print ISBN 978-1-83768-523-3
Online ISBN 978-1-83768-524-0
eBook (PDF) ISBN 978-1-83768-525-7
ISSN 2632-0983

For EU product safety concerns:
IN TECH d.o.o., Prolaz Marije Krucifikse Kozulić 3, 51000 Rijeka, Croatia,
info@intechopen.com or visit our website at intechopen.com.

IntechOpen Book Series
Biochemistry
Volume 41

Aims and Scope of the Series

Biochemistry, the study of chemical transformations occurring within living organisms, impacts all of the life sciences, from molecular crystallography and genetics, to ecology, medicine and population biology. Biochemistry studies macromolecules - proteins, nucleic acids, carbohydrates and lipids –their building blocks, structures, functions and interactions. Much of biochemistry is devoted to enzymes, proteins that catalyze chemical reactions, enzyme structures, mechanisms of action and their roles within cells. Biochemistry also studies small signaling molecules, coenzymes, inhibitors, vitamins and hormones, which play roles in the life process. Biochemical experimentation, besides coopting the methods of classical chemistry, e.g., chromatography, adopted new techniques, e.g., X-ray diffraction, electron microscopy, NMR, radioisotopes, and developed sophisticated microbial genetic tools, e.g., auxotroph mutants and their revertants, fermentation, etc. More recently, biochemistry embraced the 'big data' omics systems. Initial biochemical studies have been exclusively analytic: dissecting, purifying and examining individual components of a biological system; in exemplary words of Efraim Racker, (1913 –1991) "Don't waste clean thinking on dirty enzymes." Today, however, biochemistry is becoming more agglomerative and comprehensive, setting out to integrate and describe fully a particular biological system. The 'big data' metabolomics can define the complement of small molecules, e.g., in a soil or biofilm sample; proteomics can distinguish all the proteins comprising e.g., serum; metagenomics can identify all the genes in a complex environment e.g., the bovine rumen.
This Biochemistry Series will address both the current research on biomolecules, and the emerging trends with great promise.

Meet the Series Editor

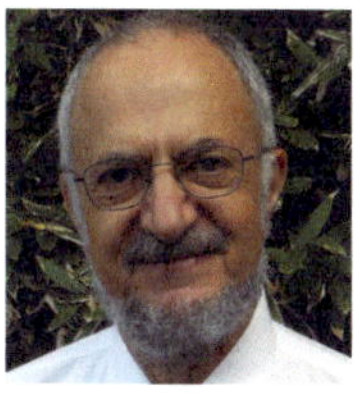

Miroslav Blumenberg, Ph.D., was born in Subotica and received his BSc in Belgrade, Yugoslavia. He completed his Ph.D. at MIT in Organic Chemistry; he followed up his Ph.D. with two postdoctoral study periods at Stanford University. Since 1983, he has been a faculty member of the RO Perelman Department of Dermatology, NYU School of Medicine, where he is codirector of a training grant in cutaneous biology. Dr. Blumenberg's research is focused on the epidermis, expression of keratin genes, transcription profiling, keratinocyte differentiation, inflammatory diseases and cancers, and most recently the effects of the microbiome on the skin. He has published more than 100 peer-reviewed research articles and graduated numerous Ph.D. and postdoctoral students.

Meet the Volume Editors

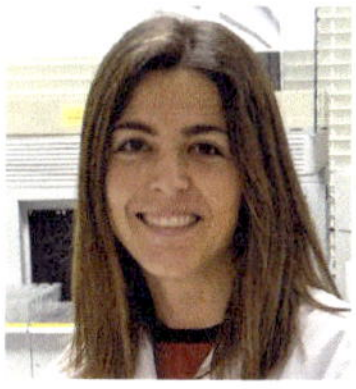

Dr. Paz Otero received her bachelor´s degree and Ph.D. in Food Science from the University of Santiago de Compostela, Spain. She has held postdoctoral research positions at Limerick Institute of Technology, Ireland (2014–2017); the Institute of Food Science Research, Autonomous University of Madrid (2017–2018); University of Vigo (2020–2022), Spain; and Mountain Research Centre, Polytechnic Institute of Bragança, Portugal (2022–2023). She has published extensively in the fields of food chemistry, toxicology, analytical chemistry, and nutrition with more than 58 research articles, 80 contributions to international congresses, 15 book chapters, and 1 edited book. Dr. Otero also serves as an invited reviewer for several research journals and guest editor for special issues.

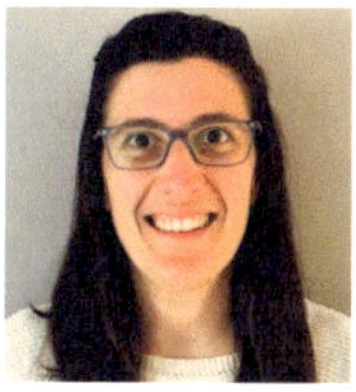

Dr. María Fraga Corral obtained a bachelor's degree in Biological Sciences in 2009, coursed two master's degrees (2009-11), and a Ph.D. in Food Safety in 2015 from the University of Santiago de Compostela, Spain. She has developed postdoctoral stages at Teagasc Food Research Centre, Agriculture and Food Development Authority, Ireland; Mountain Research Centre, Polytechnic Institute of Bragança, Portugal; and University of Vigo, Spain. She has experience in analytical detection, validation methods, and extraction techniques, which she has applied to develop different works in the fields of food safety, nutrition, and circular economy. She has published more than forty peer-reviewed articles and twenty book chapters, participated in multiple international conferences and research projects, and served as an invited reviewer for journals.

Contents

Preface

Antioxidants are compounds that inhibit oxidation, that is, they prevent free radical-induced tissue damage by avoiding the formation of radicals, scavenging them, or by promoting their decomposition. A direct link is observed between compounds with antioxidant activity and the prevention of chronic diseases like cancer or cardiovascular diseases. In this context, a variety of terrestrial plants, marine organisms, and foods are known to be rich in antioxidants, including herbs, fruits, vegetables, plants, algae, and others. Thus, it is of great importance to collect information about antioxidant molecules and their mechanisms of action and their characterization and relation to human diseases. It is also important to study sources of antioxidants and applications of antioxidants in medicine, nutraceuticals, and foods.

The book addresses recent developments in antioxidants from natural sources. Chapter 1 includes introductory concepts regarding antioxidant types and their chemical structures, whereas Chapter 2 addresses the relationship between antioxidants and the prevention of chronic diseases. Chapter 3 describes the antioxidant cellular mechanisms. Chapters 4–10 examine the sources of natural antioxidants, including some medicinal plants, foods, and microalgae. Finally, Chapters 11–13 describe some applications and practical uses of antioxidants. For example, Chapter 11 discusses the development of beverages with high anthocyanin content, Chapter 12 presents strategies for using antioxidants to improve animal reproduction, and Chapter 13 examines the uses of antioxidants in food processing.

We would like to thank our IntechOpen Commissioning Editor Ana Simcic and Author Service Manager Dolores Kuzelj for all the help and support during the publishing process. We especially appreciate and thank all authors that have contributed to the book, with a special mention to Dennis R.A. Mans from the Anton de Kom University of Suriname for contributing two chapters. Finally, we would like to thank all the authors, colleagues, and reviewers that participated in the review process of the book.

Paz Otero Fuertes and María Fraga Corral
Faculty of Science,
Department of Analytical Chemistry and Food Science,
Nutrition and Bromatology Group,
University of Vigo,
Ourense, Spain

Section 1

Introduction to Antioxidants and Their Importance in Human Health

Chapter 1

Antioxidants Sources

Marjan Assefi, Kai-Uwe Lewandrowski, Sohila Nankali and Alireza Sharafshah

Abstract

Natural antioxidants are abundant in food and medicinal plants. These natural antioxidants, particularly polyphenols and carotenoids, have numerous biological effects, including anti-inflammatory, anti-aging, anti-atherosclerosis, and anticancer properties. To examine potential cancer prevention agent sources and advance their utilization in useful food varieties, drugs, and food added substances, it is fundamental for separate cell reinforcements from food and restorative plants really and assess them suitably. This paper goes into great detail about the green extraction methods of natural antioxidants, the evaluation of antioxidant activity at the chemical and cellular levels, and their primary sources, which are food and medicinal plants.

Keywords: medicinal plants, cellular, prevention, antioxidants, natural, biological effects, anti cancer

1. Introduction

Reactive oxygen species (ROS) and reactive nitrogen species (RNS) like superoxide, hydroxyl, and nitric oxide can damage DNA and oxidize proteins and lipids in cells in a biological system. Typically, the body's cell reinforcement framework can dispose of these extremists, keeping the harmony among oxidation and against oxidation. However, environmental toxins, cigarette smoking, alcohol, radiation, or other forms of exposure can cause excessive ROS and RNS production [1]. These ROS and RNS can cause a variety of chronic and degenerative diseases because they upset the balance between oxidation and antioxidation. The increased intake of exogenous antioxidants would lessen the damage caused by oxidative stress by acting as free radical scavengers, singlet oxygen quenchers, and reducing agents. An oxidative chain reaction would not start or spread as a result of this [2, 3].

The majority of the exogenous antioxidants come from food and medicinal plants like mushrooms, beverages, flowers, spices, and traditional medicinal herbs. In addition, the industries that process agricultural by-products are potential significant natural antioxidant sources. Polyphenols (phenolic acids, flavonoids, anthocyanins, lignans, and stilbenes), carotenoids (xanthophylls, carotenes), and vitamins (vitamins E and C) are the primary natural antioxidants derived from plant materials. In general, these natural antioxidants, particularly polyphenols and carotenoids, have a wide range of biological effects, including anti-aging, anti-cancer, anti-inflammatory, and antibacterial effects [4].

Food science and nutrition are paying a lot of attention to the effective extraction methods of natural antioxidants, the appropriate evaluation of antioxidant activity, and the fact that their primary sources are food and medicinal plants. Ultrasound-assisted extraction, microwave-assisted extraction, enzyme-assisted extraction, pressurized liquid extraction, supercritical fluid extraction, high hydrostatic pressure extraction, pulsed electric field extraction, and high voltage electrical discharges extraction are just a few green non-conventional methods that have been developed to improve the efficiency with which antioxidant components are extracted from plant materials. Additionally, a variety of evaluation assays, such as the Trolox equivalence antioxidant capacity (TEAC) assay, the ferric ion reducing antioxidant power (FRAP) assay, the oxygen radical absorbance capacity (ORAC) assay, the inhibiting the oxidation of low-density lipoprotein (LDL) assay, the cellular antioxidant activity assay, and others, have been developed to further evaluate the antioxidant capacities of extracts from natural products, particularly those that These tests have been used to rank antioxidant plants and suggest the best foods for antioxidant consumption. The purpose of this review is to provide a summary of the methods used to extract natural antioxidants, methods used to evaluate antioxidant activity, and their primary sources, which are food and medicinal plants [5–7].

The type and concentration of the extraction solvent, the extraction temperature, the extraction time, and the extraction pH are just a few of the extraction factors that have a significant impact on the efficiency of the extraction. Antioxidants have been extracted from food and medicinal plants using a variety of solvents. The chemical nature and polarity of the antioxidant compounds to be extracted determine the solvent selection. The majority of the phenolics, flavanoids, and anthocyanins are antioxidants that dissolve in water. Extraction frequently makes use of polar and medium-polar solvents like water, ethanol, methanol, propanol, acetone, and their aqueous mixtures. Carotenoids are antioxidants that dissolve in lipids. For extraction, common organic solvents like mixtures of hexane with acetone, ethanol, and methanol or ethyl acetate with acetone, ethanol, and methanol have been used [8, 9].

Antioxidants can be extracted from food and medicinal plants using a variety of extraction methods, including conventional and non-conventional methods. The

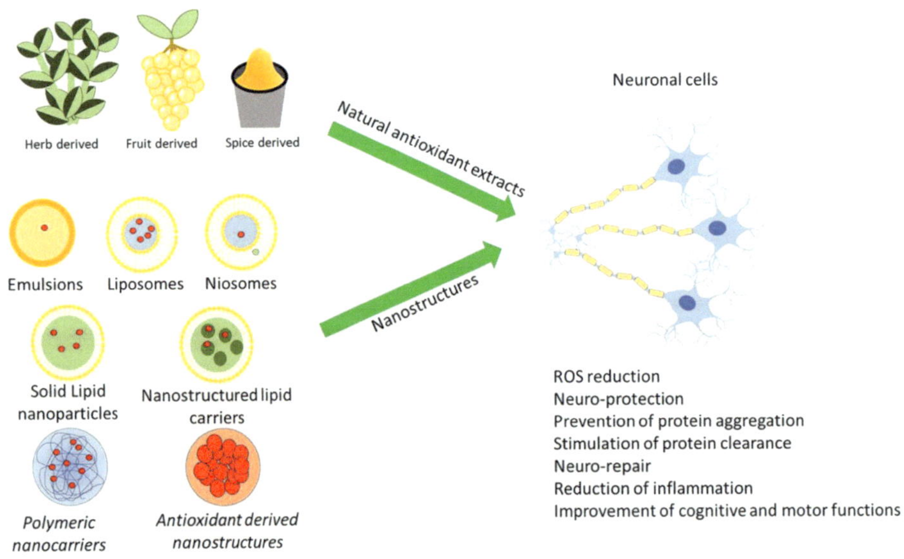

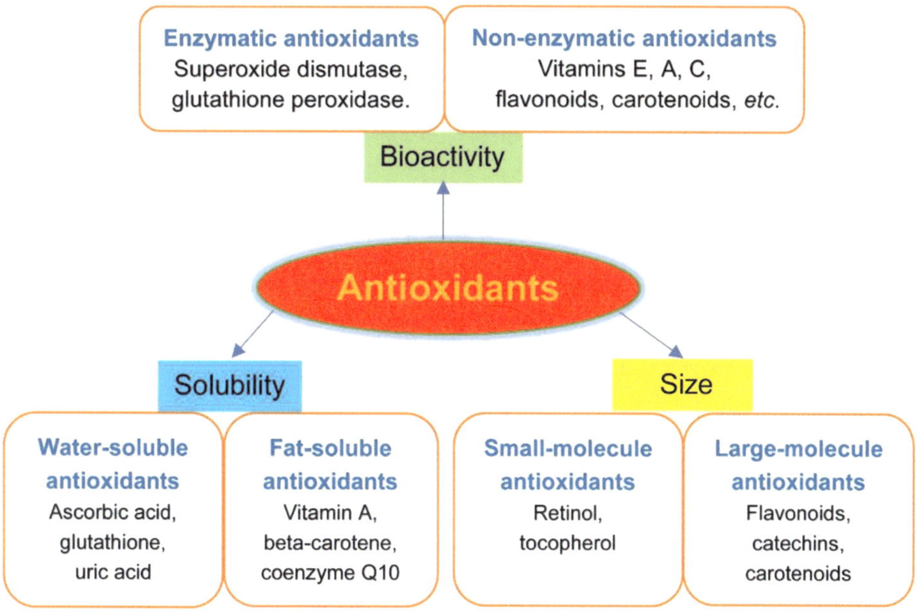

most common conventional extraction methods are hot water bath, maceration, and Soxhlet extraction. These methods take a long time, use a lot of organic solvents, and have low extraction yields. Additionally, the long heating process in hot water bath and Soxhlet extraction may cause thermolabile compounds to break down [10]. Non-conventional techniques like ultrasound, microwave, pressurized liquid, enzyme hydrolysis, supercritical fluids, high hydrostatic pressure, pulsed electric field, and high voltage electrical discharges have been investigated for the purpose of obtaining antioxidants from plants in a way that is both energy efficient and economically sustainable.

2. Main resources of natural antioxidants

The TEAC assay, which measures antioxidants' capacity to scavenge free radicals, the FRAP assay directly measures antioxidants' reducing capacity, and the total phenols assay by FCR evaluates the phenolic contents of tested samples are the primary sources of natural antioxidants [11–13]. The combination of the TEAC, FRAP, and FCR methods is frequently utilized to evaluate the antioxidant activity in order to carry out in-depth research on various aspects of antioxidants. Numerous food and medicinal plants, such as fruits, vegetables, cereal grains, edible and wild flowers, macro-fungi, medicinal plants, spices, and so on, have been widely estimated to have antioxidant properties [14]. A combination of the results from the FRAP, TEAC, and FCR assays was used to identify the varieties with strong antioxidant properties. In general, these findings demonstrated that diverse categories had a wide range of antioxidant capacities. From 0.11 0.01 to 72.11 2.19 mol Fe(II)/g, 0.84 0.03 to 80.68 2.11 mol Trolox/g, and 11.88 0.11 to 585.52 18.59 mg GAE/100 g, respectively, the FRAP, TEAC, and FCR values of 62 fruits varied. 56 vegetables had FRAP, TEAC, and FCR values ranging from 2.69 to 60.9 mol Fe(II)/g, 6.93 to 33.63 mol Trolox/g, and 4.99 to 23.27 mg GAE/g, respectively. From 5.23 0.23 to 126.19 2.91 mol Fe(II)/g, 0.62 0.14 tso 30.03 1.10 mol trolox/g, and 1.35 0.15 to 9.47 0.48 mg GAE/g, respectively, the FRAP, TEAC, and FCR values of 24 cereal grains varied. From 0.14 to 1844.85 mol Fe(II)/g, 0.99 to 1544.38 mol Trolox/g, and 0.19 to 101.33 mg GAE/g, respectively, the FRAP, TEAC, and FCR values of 223 medicinal plants varied. Clearly, medicinal plants had significantly higher antioxidant activities and total phenolic content than fruits, vegetables, and cereals among these varieties with strong antioxidant properties [11, 15, 16].

Moreover, the cancer prevention agent exercises of food and restorative plants have additionally been assessed by cell reinforcement action measures in light of various cell types. The 27 vegetables' cellular antioxidant activities ranged from not detected (tomato) to 41.9 6.2 mol of QE/100 g (beet). The 25 fruits' cellular antioxidant activities ranged from 3.15 0.21 mol of QE/100 g (banana) to 292 11 mol of QE/100 g (wild blueberry). In the two examinations, these outcomes showed that CAA values were fundamentally connected with absolute phenolic content. Surarit and others based on HL-60 cells, it was reported that the ethanolic bran extracts of 11 Thai red and purple and two non-pigmented rice varieties performed the following cellular antioxidant activities: non-pigmented rice followed by purple rice in the same order as red rice in terms of phenolic and flavonoid content in these rice extracts [17, 18].

Chemical assays cannot completely capture the sample's in vivo behavior when evaluating its antioxidant capacity. Antioxidants must be evaluated for their efficacy under more biologically relevant conditions. Although more expensive and time-consuming, animal models and human studies are more suitable for evaluation [19]. The cellular antioxidant activity (CAA) assay has been developed to evaluate antioxidant capacities as intermediate testing methods. The Dichlorofluorecin (DCFH) method is a common CAA assay that measures antioxidants' ability to prevent DCFH oxidation. In human hepatocarcinoma HepG2 cells, ABAP-generated peroxyl radicals easily convert DCFH that is trapped within the cells to fluorescent dichlorofluorescein (DCF). Fluorescence could be used to monitor DCF (exc = 485 nm, em = 538 nm). The antioxidant capacity of bioactive components is inversely proportional to the decrease in cellular fluorescence [20–23]. Human red blood cells, human endothelial EA.hy926, human colon cancer Caco-2 cells, human macrophage U937 cells, and mouse macrophage RAW264.7 cells have all been utilized for the CAA assay, with the exception of HepG2 cells. Additionally, a microfluidic cell chip-based CAA assay with arrayed microchannels has been developed to evaluate plant antioxidants. There are 48 distinct parallel array channels and 288 round cell culture micro chambers on the microfluidic chip. With this method, a multimode reader could simultaneously test eight groups of diverse samples at six distinct concentrations.

Tests of antioxidant enzyme expression, inhibition of pro-oxidant enzymes, and activation vs. repression of redox transcription factors are also included in the evaluation of antioxidant activity at the cellular level [15]. These tests are in addition to the ability to scavenge ROS/RNS. Caco-2 cells were used to test the antioxidant properties of the extracts made from five brown seaweeds. Both the activity of the antioxidant enzymes catalase (CAT) and superoxide dismutase (SOD) and the amount of glutathione (GSH) present were evaluated [24]. According to these cellular assays, *Pelvetia canaliculata* could exert its antioxidant capacity in Caco-2 cells primarily by preventing H_2O_2-mediated SOD depletion. In addition, the antioxidant enzyme activities of glutathione peroxidase (GPx) and glutathione reductase (GR) in three Argentine red wines were evaluated. Wine was found to have some protective effects on H_2O_2-exposed cells, which were attributed to the increased activity of the antioxidant enzymes GPx and GR. In addition, phenols (like curcumin) or food extracts (like blueberries) have been used to treat cultured cells, resulting in a suppression of NF-B activation as an anti-oxidant response. Curcumin treatment reduced NF-B and activator protein-1 activation as well as IL-8 release in alveolar epithelial cells, according to a study. GSH levels and mRNA expression of the glutamylcysteine ligase catalytic subunit were also higher in treated cells than in untreated ones [25–27].

The ability of antioxidants to slow down the oxidation of 2,2′-azobis-2-methylpropanimidamide, dihydrochloride, (AAPH) or 2,2′-azobis(2-amidinopropane) dihydrochloride, dihydrochloride, (ABAP) is measured using the total radical trapping antioxidant potential (TRAP) assay [28–30]. The variation in the rate of the reaction is measured using fluorometry (ex = 495 nm and e When compared to the rate before the antioxidants were added, the reaction's rate of fluorescence decay slows after they were added [31, 32]. The lag phase duration in comparison to Trolox's lag phase serves as the basis for the quantification. The assumption that antioxidants exhibit a lag phase and that the length of the lag phase is positively correlated with antioxidant capacity underpins the use of the lag phase. However, the potential of antioxidants that play a role after the lag phase is completely ignored because not every antioxidant component possesses an obvious lag phase [33–35].

As a more physiologically relevant measure of antioxidant capacity, the inhibition of induced lipid autoxidation has been developed. Free radical initiator (Cu(II) or 2,2′-azobis(2-amidinopropane) dihydrochloride (AAPH)), substrate (linoleic acid or LDL), and antioxidants are typically present in the reaction solution. Cu(II) or AAPH causes linoleic acid autoxidation, or LDL. A UV spectrometer measures conjugated dienes' peroxidation at 234 nm for the lipid components. The reaction begins when a radical initiator is present, and the accumulation of conjugated diene oxides is indicated by an increase in absorbance at 234 nm. The reaction rate slows down after antioxidants are added until the antioxidant is used up. The lag time is measured during the period and used to evaluate antioxidant capacity [36, 37].

The use of a biologically relevant substrate, which makes the results relevant to oxidative reactions in vivo, is this method's main advantage over other in vitro assays. One of the major drawbacks of this method is the variability of the LDL samples, which can vary between donors because LDL is isolated from blood samples. As a result, it is challenging to develop this approach into a high-throughput antioxidant evaluation assay that is consistent and repeatable. The results, on the other hand, would be more reproducible if linoleic acid or its methyl ester was used as an oxidation substrate rather than LDL. However, in the presence of water, linoleic acid would form micelles, and since UV absorbance cannot directly monitor the progression of the reaction in micelles, the method's accuracy may be compromised [38–40].

2.1 Natural sources of polyphenols

Polyphenols, such as phenolic acids, flavonoids, lignans, and stilbenes, are found in a lot of food and medicinal plants. Examples of phenolic acids include cinnamic acid derivatives like p-coumaric, caffeic, and ferulic, as well as benzoic acid derivatives like gallic acid and hydroxybenzoic acids. The hydroxycinnamic acids are more prevalent in edible plants than the hydroxybenzoic acids [41, 42]. The hydroxycinnamic acids are found to be abundant in fruits like blueberries, kiwis, plums, cherries, and apples (0.5–2 g hydroxycinnamic acids/kg fresh wt). While ferulic acid is the most abundant phenolic acid in cereal grains and accounts for approximately 90% of the total polyphenol content of wheat grain, caffeineic acid is the most abundant phenolic acid and accounts for 75–100% of the total hydroxycinnamic acid content in many fruits. Except for certain red fruits, black radish, and onions, edible plants typically contain very little hydroxybenzoic acid. They are not thought to be particularly nutritious due to their low content [43–45].

The majority of edible fruits and vegetables contain a lot of flavonoids. Flavonols, flavanones, catechins, flavones, anthocyanidins, and isoflavonoids are among its subclasses. Flavonoids come in a variety of forms and concentrations from various food sources. In edible plants, quercetin is typically the most abundant flavonol. Onion is the food with the most quercetin in it. Quercetin levels are relatively low in wine and tea. Kaempferol (broccoli), myricetin (berries), and isorhamnetin (onions) are additional flavonols. Citrus fruits are almost entirely devoid of flavanones. Oranges and mandarins contain the most hesperidin and narirutin flavonoids, while grapefruit contains the most naringin and narirutin flavonoids. Catechins as a rule exist as aglycones or esterified with gallic corrosive. Tea and red wine are the two foods that contain the most catechins [46–48]. Additionally, luteolin and apigenin are the most important flavones. Celery and red pepper are the primary sources for the diet. Anthocyanins like pelargonidin, cyanidin, and delphinidin are what give edible plants like plums, eggplant, and many berries their red, blue, or violet hues [49–51]. The isoflavonoids, for example, isoflavones genistein and daidzein, principally exist in vegetables. Soybean and soy products are the most abundant food source [52, 53].

Linseed, which contains low amounts of matairesinol and secoisolariciresinol (up to 3.7 g/kg dry wt), is the most abundant dietary source of lignans. These same lignans are also found in other algae, leguminous plants like lentils, cereals like wheat and triticale, fruit like pears and prunes, and certain vegetables like garlic, asparagus, and carrots. Resveratrol is a stilbene whose numerous bioactivities have been extensively studied. Resveratrol (0.3–7 mg aglycones/L and 15 mg glycosides/L) is abundant in red wine [54–56].

2.2 Natural sources of carotenoids

Natural pigments called carotenoids include -carotene, lycopene, lutein, and zeaxanthin. All beautiful palatable plants, particularly dim green and yellow-orange verdant, are the great wellsprings of carotenoids [57]. Carotenoids' absorption is primarily dependent on their preparation with oils or fats due to thesir lipid solubility. Among the carotenoids, −carotene is most frequently found in edible plants with the highest provitamin A activity, like acerola, mango, carrot, nuts, and oil palm [58, 59]. A type of red pigment is called lycopene. It almost only exists in the tissues of algae and vegetables. Tomato items like juices, soups, sauces, and ketchup, as well as their handling waste and strip are significant wellsprings of lycopene. The trans isomer accounts for the majority of the lycopene found in tomatoes (between 79 and 91%) [60–62]. The most prevalent xanthophylls found in green and dark leafy vegetables like lettuce, spinach, peas, and broccoli are lutein and zeaxanthin. Zeaxanthin, which accounts for 97.4% of all carotenoids, is also found in the red marine microalga *P. cruentum*.

3. Conclusion

In conclusion, the various nutritional functions and health benefits of antioxidants derived from food and medicinal plants have been the subject of increasing research. Natural antioxidant extraction and antioxidant activity assessment techniques, as well as their primary sources from food and medicinal plants, are summarized in this review [63–65]. Due to their reduced extraction time, energy consumption, and use of harmful organic solvents, as well as their higher extraction yields for recovering antioxidant compounds from food and medicinal plants, the aforementioned non-conventional methods have the potential to replace or enhance existing extraction methods [66]. Despite this, the majority of them are not suitable for use in industrial settings due to the complicated installation procedures and high cost of the equipment. As a result, finding a balance between cost and energy will be a crucial area of study in the future. The future development trend would be the combination of multiple extraction technologies and the automated potential of these non-conventional extraction technologies to take advantage of the various extraction methods and minimize their disadvantages [67]. The determination of total polyphenolic content by FCR, scavenging free radical ability by TEAC, metal-reducing activity by FRAP, and a kind of cellular-based assay are all suggested for assessing the antioxidant activity of plant materials. Standardizing the operating conditions of the same analysis method and the expression of results is also recommended to make it possible to compare various samples and studies [68–70].

Author details

Marjan Assefi[1]*, Kai-Uwe Lewandrowski[2], Sohila Nankali[3] and Alireza Sharafshah[4]

1 University of North Carolina at Greensboro, Greensboro, USA

2 Center for Advanced Spine Care of Southern Arizona, Tucson, USA

3 North Central University, USA

4 University of Isfahan, Isfahan, Iran

*Address all correspondence to: massefi@aggies.ncat.edu

References

[1] Fang YZ, Yang S, Wu G. Free radicals, antioxidants, and nutrition. Nutrition. 2002;**18**:872-879. DOI: 10.1016/S0899-9007(02)00916-4

[2] Peng C, Wang X, Chen J, Jiao R, Wang L, Li YM, et al. Biology of ageing and role of dietary antioxidants. BioMed Research International. 2014;**2014**:831841. DOI: 10.1155/2014/831841

[3] Li S, Tan HY, Wang N, Zhang ZJ, Lao L, Wong CW, et al. The role of oxidative stress and antioxidants in liver diseases. International Journal of Molecular Sciences. 2015;**16**:26087-26124. DOI: 10.3390/ijms161125942

[4] Wang F, Li Y, Zhang YJ, Zhou Y, Li S, Li HB. Natural products for the prevention and treatment of hangover and alcohol use disorder. Molecules. 2016;**21**:64. DOI: 10.3390/molecules21010064

[5] Zhou Y, Zheng J, Li S, Zhou T, Zhang P, Li HB. Alcoholic beverage consumption and chronic diseases. International Journal of Environmental Research and Public Health. 2016;**13**:522. DOI: 10.3390/ijerph13060522

[6] Baiano A, del Nobile MA. Antioxidant compounds from vegetable matrices: Biosynthesis, occurrence, and extraction systems. Critical Reviews in Food Science and Nutrition. 2015;**56**:2053-2068. DOI: 10.1080/10408398.2013.812059

[7] Cai YZ, Luo Q, Sun M, Corke H. Antioxidant activity and phenolic compounds of 112 traditional Chinese medicinal plants associated with anticancer. Life Sciences. 2004;**74**:2157-2184. DOI: 10.1016/j.lfs.2003.09.047

[8] Shan B, Cai YZ, Sun M, Corke H. Antioxidant capacity of 26 spice extracts and characterization of their phenolic constituents. Journal of Agricultural and Food Chemistry. 2005;**53**:7749-7759. DOI: 10.1021/jf051513y

[9] Fu L, Xu BT, Gan RY, Zhang Y, Xu XR, Xia EQ, et al. Total phenolic contents and antioxidant capacities of herbal and tea infusions. International Journal of Molecular Sciences. 2011;**12**:2112-2124. DOI: 10.3390/ijms12042112

[10] Fu L, Xu BT, Xu XR, Qin XS, Gan RY, Li HB. Antioxidant capacities and total phenolic contents of 56 wild fruits from south China. Molecules. 2010;**15**:8602-8617. DOI: 10.3390/molecules15128602

[11] Fu L, Xu BT, Xu XR, Gan RY, Zhang Y, Xia EQ, et al. Antioxidant capacities and total phenolic contents of 62 fruits. Food Chemistry. 2011;**129**:345-350. DOI: 10.1016/j.foodchem.2011.04.079

[12] Deng GF, Xu XR, Guo YJ, Xia EQ, Li S, Wu S, et al. Determination of antioxidant property and their lipophilic and hydrophilic phenolic contents in cereal grains. Journal of Functional Foods. 2012;**4**:906-914. DOI: 10.1016/j.jff.2012.06.008

[13] Guo YJ, Deng GF, Xu XR, Wu S, Li S, Xia EQ, et al. Antioxidant capacities, phenolic compounds and polysaccharide contents of 49 edible macro-fungi. Food & Function. 2012;**3**:1195-1205. DOI: 10.1039/c2fo30110e

[14] Deng GF, Lin X, Xu XR, Gao LL, Xie JF, Li HB. Antioxidant capacities and total phenolic contents of 56 vegetables. Journal of Functional Foods. 2013;**5**:260-266. DOI: 10.1016/j.jff.2012.10.015

[15] Li S, Li SK, Gan RY, Song FL, Kuang L, Li HB. Antioxidant capacities and total phenolic contents of infusions from 223 medicinal plants. Industrial Crops and Products. 2013;**51**:289-298. DOI: 10.1016/j.indcrop.2013.09.017

[16] Li AN, Li S, Li HB, Xu DP, Xu XR, Chen F. Total phenolic contents and antioxidant capacities of 51 edible and wild flowers. Journal of Functional Foods. 2014;**6**:319-330. DOI: 10.1016/j.jff.2013.10.022

[17] Li Y, Zhang JJ, Xu DP, Zhou T, Zhou Y, Li S, et al. Bioactivities and health benefits of wild fruits. International Journal of Molecular Sciences. 2016;**17**:1258. DOI: 10.3390/ijms17081258

[18] Zhang JJ, Li Y, Zhou T, Xu DP, Zhang P, Li S, et al. Bioactivities and health benefits of mushrooms mainly from China. Molecules. 2016;**21**:938. DOI: 10.3390/molecules21070938

[19] Deng GF, Shen C, Xu XR, Kuang RD, Guo YJ, Zeng LS, et al. Potential of fruit wastes as natural resources of bioactive compounds. International Journal of Molecular Sciences. 2012;**13**:8308-8323. DOI: 10.3390/ijms13078308

[20] Manach C, Scalbert A, Morand C, Remesy C, Jimenez L. Polyphenols: Food sources and bioavailability. The American Journal of Clinical Nutrition. 2004;**79**:727-747

[21] Jenab M, Riboli E, Ferrari P, Sabate J, Slimani N, Norat T, et al. Plasma and dietary vitamin C levels and risk of gastric cancer in the European prospective investigation into cancer and nutrition (EPIC-EURGAST). Carcinogenesis. 2006;**27**:2250-2257. DOI: 10.1093/carcin/bgl096

[22] Li AN, Li S, Zhang YJ, Xu XR, Chen YM, Li HB. Resources and biological activities of natural polyphenols. Nutrients. 2014;**6**:6020-6047. DOI: 10.3390/nu6126020

[23] Arathi BP, Raghavendra-Rao SP, Vijay K, Baskaran V, Lakshminarayana R. Metabolomics of carotenoids: The challenges and prospects—A review. Trends in Food Science and Technology. 2015;**45**:105-117. DOI: 10.1016/j.tifs.2015.06.003

[24] Zhang YJ, Gan RY, Li S, Zhou Y, Li AN, Xu DP, et al. Antioxidant phytochemicals for the prevention and treatment of chronic diseases. Molecules. 2015;**20**:21138-21156. DOI: 10.3390/molecules201219753

[25] Wojtunik-Kulesza KA, Oniszczuk A, Oniszczuk T, Waksmundzka-Hajnos M. The influence of common free radicals and antioxidants on development of Alzheimer's disease. Biomedicine & Pharmacotherapy. 2016;**78**:39-49. DOI: 10.1016/j.biopha.2015.12.024

[26] Balmus IM, Ciobica A, Trifan A, Stanciu C. The implications of oxidative stress and antioxidant therapies in inflammatory bowel disease: Clinical aspects and animal models. Saudi Journal of Gastroenterology. 2016;**22**:3-17. DOI: 10.4103/1319-3767.173753

[27] Prasad KN. Simultaneous activation of Nrf2 and elevation of antioxidant compounds for reducing oxidative stress and chronic inflammation in human Alzheimer's disease. Mechanisms of Ageing and Development. 2016;**153**:41-47. DOI: 10.1016/j.mad.2016.01.002

[28] Salomone F, Godos J, Zelber-Sagi S. Natural antioxidants for non-alcoholic fatty liver disease: Molecular targets and clinical perspectives. Liver International. 2016;**36**:5-20. DOI: 10.1111/liv.12975

[29] Zhou Y, Li Y, Zhou T, Zheng J, Li S, Li HB. Dietary natural products for prevention and treatment of liver cancer. Nutrients. 2016;**8**:156. DOI: 10.3390/nu8030156

[30] Zhou Y, Zheng J, Li Y, Xu DP, Li S, Chen YM, et al. Natural polyphenols for prevention and treatment of cancer. Nutrients. 2016;**8**:515. DOI: 10.3390/nu8080515

[31] Zheng J, Zhou Y, Li Y, Xu DP, Li S, Li HB. Spices for prevention and treatment of cancers. Nutrients. 2016;**8**:495. DOI: 10.3390/nu8080495

[32] De Camargo AC, Bismara Regitano-d'Arce MA, Telles Biasoto AC, Shahidi F. Enzyme-assisted extraction of phenolics from winemaking by-products: Antioxidant potential and inhibition of α-glucosidase and lipase activities. Food Chemistry. 2016;**212**:395-402. DOI: 10.1016/j.foodchem.2016.05.047

[33] Belwal T, Dhyani P, Bhatt ID, Rawal RS, Pande V. Optimization extraction conditions for improving phenolic content and antioxidant activity in Berberis asiatica fruits using response surface methodology (RSM). Food Chemistry. 2016;**207**:115-124. DOI: 10.1016/j.foodchem.2016.03.081

[34] Sharmila G, Nikitha VS, Ilaiyarasi S, Dhivya K, Rajasekar V, Kumar ANM, et al. Ultrasound assisted extraction of total phenolics from Cassia auriculata leaves and evaluation of its antioxidant activities. Industrial Crops and Products. 2016;**84**:13-21. DOI: 10.1016/j.indcrop.2016.01.010

[35] Van Tang N, Hong NTP, Bowyer MC, van Altena IA, Scarlett CJ. Influence of solvents and novel extraction methods on bioactive compounds and antioxidant capacity of Phyllanthus amarus. Chemical Papers. 2016;**70**:556-566

[36] Strati IF, Oreopoulou V. Effect of extraction parameters on the carotenoid recovery from tomato waste. International Journal of Food Science and Technology. 2011;**46**:23-29. DOI: 10.1111/j.1365-2621.2010.02496.x

[37] Ho KKHY, Ferruzzi MG, Liceaga AM, Martin-Gonzalez MFS. Microwave-assisted extraction of lycopene in tomato peels: Effect of extraction conditions on all-trans and cis-isomer yields. LWT – Food Science and Technology. 2015;**62**:160-168. DOI: 10.1016/j.lwt.2014.12.061

[38] Barba FJ, Zhu Z, Koubaa M, Sant'Ana A.S., Orlien V. Green alternative methods for the extraction of antioxidant bioactive compounds from winery wastes and by-products: A review. Trends in Food Science and Technology. 2016;**49**:96-109. DOI: 10.1016/j.tifs.2016.01.006

[39] Xu DP, Zhou Y, Zheng J, Li S, Li AN, Li HB. Optimization of ultrasound-assisted extraction of natural antioxidants from the flower of Jatropha integerrima by response surface methodology. Molecules. 2016;**21**:18. DOI: 10.3390/molecules21010018

[40] He B, Zhang LL, Yue XY, Liang J, Jiang J, Gao XL, et al. Optimization of ultrasound-assisted extraction of phenolic compounds and anthocyanins from blueberry (Vaccinium ashei) wine pomace. Food Chemistry. 2016;**204**:70-76. DOI: 10.1016/j.foodchem.2016.02.094

[41] Faidi K, Baaka N, Hammami S, El Mokni R, Mighri Z, Mhenni MF. Extraction of carotenoids from Lycium ferocissimum fruits for cotton dyeing: Optimization survey based on a central composite design method. Fibers and Polymers. 2016;**17**:36-43. DOI: 10.1007/s12221-016-5424-0

[42] Azmir J, Zaidul ISM, Rahman MM, Sharif KM, Mohamed A, Sahena F, et al. Techniques for extraction of bioactive compounds from plant materials: A review. Journal of Food Engineering. 2013;**117**:426-436. DOI: 10.1016/j.jfoodeng.2013.01.014

[43] Li AN, Li S, Xu DP, Xu XR, Chen YM, Ling WH, et al. Optimization of ultrasound-assisted extraction of lycopene from papaya processing waste by response surface methodology. Food Analytical Methods. 2015;**8**:1207-1214. DOI: 10.1007/s12161-014-9955-y

[44] Li Y, Fabiano-Tixier AS, Tomao V, Cravotto G, Chemat F. Green ultrasound-assisted extraction of carotenoids based on the bio-refinery concept using sunflower oil as an alternative solvent. Ultrasonics Sonochemistry. 2013;**20**:12-18. DOI: 10.1016/j.ultsonch.2012.07.005

[45] Milutinovic M, Radovanovic N, Corovic M, Siler-Marinkovic S, Rajilic-Stojanovic M, Dimitrijevic-Brankovic S. Optimisation of microwave-assisted extraction parameters for antioxidants from waste Achillea millefolium dust. Industrial Crops and Products. 2015;77:333-341. DOI: 10.1016/j.indcrop.2015.09.007

[46] Espada-Bellido E, Ferreiro-Gonzalez M, Carrera C, Palma M, Barroso CG, Barbero GF. Optimization of the ultrasound-assisted extraction of anthocyanins and total phenolic compounds in mulberry (Morus nigra) pulp. Food Chemistry. 2017;**219**:23-32. DOI: 10.1016/j.foodchem.2016.09.122

[47] Virot M, Tomao V, Le Bourvellec C, Renard CMCG, Chemat F. Towards the industrial production of antioxidants from food processing by-products with ultrasound-assisted extraction. Ultrasonics Sonochemistry. 2010;**17**:1066-1074. DOI: 10.1016/j.ultsonch.2009.10.015

[48] Liu CT, Wu CY, Weng YM, Tseng CY. Ultrasound-assisted extraction methodology as a tool to improve the antioxidant properties of herbal drug Xiao-chia-hu-tang. Journal of Ethnopharmacology. 2005;**99**:293-300. DOI: 10.1016/j.jep.2005.02.018

[49] Kazemi M, Karim R, Mirhosseini H, Hamid AA. Optimization of pulsed ultrasound-assisted technique for extraction of phenolics from pomegranate peel of Malas variety: Punicalagin and hydroxybenzoic acids. Food Chemistry. 2016;**206**:156-166. DOI: 10.1016/j.foodchem.2016.03.017

[50] Pan Z, Qu W, Ma H, Atungulu GG, McHugh TH. Continuous and pulsed ultrasound-assisted extractions of antioxidants from pomegranate peel. Ultrasonics Sonochemistry. 2011;**18**:1249-1257. DOI: 10.1016/j.ultsonch.2011.01.005

[51] Xu WJ, Zhai JW, Cui Q, Liu JZ, Luo M, Fu YJ, et al. Ultra-turrax based ultrasound-assisted extraction of five organic acids from honeysuckle (Lonicera japonica Thunb.) and optimization of extraction process. Separation and Purification Technology. 2016;**166**:73-82. DOI: 10.1016/j.seppur.2016.04.003

[52] Bouras M, Chadni M, Barba FJ, Grimi N, Bals O, Vorobiev E. Optimization of microwave-assisted extraction of polyphenols from Quercus bark. Industrial Crops and Products. 2015;77:590-601. DOI: 10.1016/j.indcrop.2015.09.018

[53] Tomaz I, Maslov L, Stupic D, Preiner D, Asperger D, Kontic JK. Recovery of flavonoids from grape skins by enzyme-assisted

extraction. Separation Science and Technology. 2016;**51**:255-268. DOI: 10.1080/01496395.2015.1085881

[54] Ranveer RC, Patil SN, Sahoo AK. Effect of different parameters on enzyme-assisted extraction of lycopene from tomato processing waste. Food and Bioproducts Processing. 2013;**91**:370-375. DOI: 10.1016/j.fbp.2013.01.006

[55] Kamali H, Khodaverdi E, Hadizadeh F, Ghaziaskar SH. Optimization of phenolic and flavonoid content and antioxidants capacity of pressurized liquid extraction from Dracocephalum kotschyi via circumscribed central composite. Journal of Supercritical Fluids. 2016;**107**:307-314. DOI: 10.1016/j.supflu.2015.09.028

[56] Golmakani E, Mohammadi A, Sani TA, Kamali H. Phenolic and flavonoid content and antioxidants capacity of pressurized liquid extraction and perculation method from roots of Scutellaria pinnatifida a Hamilt. Subsp alpina (Bornm) Rech. F. The Journal of Supercritical Fluids. 2014;**95**:318-324. DOI: 10.1016/j.supflu.2014.09.020

[57] Talmaciu AI, Volf I, Popa VI. A comparative analysis of the "green" techniques applied for polyphenols extraction from bioresources. Chemistry & Biodiversity. 2015;**12**:1635-1651. DOI: 10.1002/cbdv.201400415

[58] Shang YF, Kim SM, Um B. Optimisation of pressurised liquid extraction of antioxidants from black bamboo leaves. Food Chemistry. 2014;**154**:164-170. DOI: 10.1016/j.foodchem.2013.12.050

[59] Sanagi MM, See HH, Ibrahim W, Abu NA. Determination of carotene, tocopherols and tocotrienols in residue oil from palm pressed fiber using pressurized liquid extraction-normal phase liquid chromatography. Analytica Chimica Acta. 2005;**538**:71-76. DOI: 10.1016/j.aca.2005.02.028

[60] Esclapez MD, Garcia-Perez JV, Mulet A, Carcel JA. Ultrasound-assisted extraction of natural products. Food Engineering Reviews. 2011;**3**:108-120. DOI: 10.1007/s12393-011-9036-6

[61] Soria AC, Villamiel M. Effect of ultrasound on the technological properties and bioactivity of food: A review. Trends in Food Science and Technology. 2010;**21**:323-331. DOI: 10.1016/j.tifs.2010.04.003

[62] Chemat F, Zill-e-Huma KMK. Applications of ultrasound in food technology: Processing, preservation and extraction. Ultrasonics Sonochemistry. 2011;**18**:813-835. DOI: 10.1016/j.ultsonch.2010.11.023

[63] Pereira P, Cebola MJ, Oliveira MC, Bernardo-Gil MG. Supercritical fluid extraction vs. conventional extraction of myrtle leaves and berries: Comparison of antioxidant activity and identification of bioactive compounds. Journal of Supercritical Fluids. 2016;**113**:1-9. DOI: 10.1016/j.supflu.2015.09.006

[64] Kazan A, Koyu H, Turu IC, Yesil-Celiktas O. Supercritical fluid extraction of Prunus persica leaves and utilization possibilities as a source of phenolic compounds. Journal of Supercritical Fluids. 2014;**92**:55-59. DOI: 10.1016/j.supflu.2014.05.006

[65] Jimenez-Aguilar DM, Escobedo-Avellaneda Z, Martin-Belloso O, Gutierrez-Uribe J, Valdez-Fragoso A, Garcia-Garcia R, et al. Effect of high hydrostatic pressure on the content of phytochemical compounds and antioxidant activity of prickly pears (Opuntia ficus-indica) beverages. Food

Engineering Reviews. 2015;7:198-208. DOI: 10.1007/s12393-015-9111-5

[66] Lee D, Ghafoor K, Moon S, Kim SH, Kim S, Chun H, et al. Phenolic compounds and antioxidant properties of high hydrostatic pressure and conventionally treated ginseng (Panax ginseng) products. Quality Assurance and Safety of Crops & Foods. 2015;7:493-500. DOI: 10.3920/QAS2014.0416

[67] Rosello-Soto E, Barba FJ, Parniakov O, Galanakis CM, Lebovka N, Grimi N, et al. High voltage electrical discharges, pulsed electric field, and ultrasound assisted extraction of protein and phenolic compounds from olive kernel. Food and Bioprocess Technology. 2015;**8**:885-894. DOI: 10.1007/s11947-014-1456-x

[68] Teh S, Niven BE, Bekhit AEA, Carne A, Birch EJ. Microwave and pulsed electric field assisted extractions of polyphenols from defatted canola seed cake. International Journal of Food Science and Technology. 2015;**50**:1109-1115. DOI: 10.1111/ijfs.12749

[69] Segovia FJ, Luengo E, Corral-Perez JJ, Raso J, Pilar AM. Improvements in the aqueous extraction of polyphenols from borage (*Borago officinalis* L.) leaves by pulsed electric fields: Pulsed electric fields (PEF) applications. Industrial Crops and Products. 2015;**65**:390-396. DOI: 10.1016/j.indcrop.2014.11.010

[70] Luengo E, Alvarez I, Raso J. Improving the pressing extraction of polyphenols of orange peel by pulsed electric fields. Innovative Food Science and Emerging Technologies. 2013;**17**:79-84. DOI: 10.1016/j.ifset.2012.10.005

Chapter 2

Dietary Regulation of Keap1/Nrf2/ARE Pathway: Focus on Acai Berries and Pistachios and Cashews as Natural Food Sources

Rosanna Di Paola, Salvatore Cuzzocrea, Roberta Fusco and Marika Cordaro

Abstract

Inflammation is a biological reaction to oxidative stress in which cell starts producing proteins, enzymes, and other substances to restore homeostasis, while oxidative stress could be intrinsically a biochemical imbalance of the physiologically redox status of the intracellular environment. The nuclear factor erythroid 2-related factor 2 (Nrf2)/antioxidant response element (ARE) pathway, which controls the transcription of numerous antioxidant genes that protect cellular homeostasis and detoxification genes that process and eliminate all toxic compounds and substances before they can cause damage. The Nrf2 pathway is the heart of the daily biological response to oxidative stress. Transient activation of Nrf2 by diet can upregulate antioxidant enzymes to protect cells against oxidative stress inducers. In this chapter, we summarize the effects of some novel foods in the regulation of the Nrf2/ARE pathway and its cellular mechanisms.

Keywords: food, oxidative stress, inflammation, diet, Nrf2

1. Introduction

A diet rich in fruits and vegetables has numerous positive effects on the body. In fact, in recent years, research has turned its attention to substances of natural origin: these are rich in essential nutrients with potential therapeutic actions. Nutrients include mainly: vitamins, minerals, fiber, fatty acids, flavonoids, anthocyanins, and carotenoids; the presence of these mainly gives it antioxidant, anti-inflammatory, antimicrobial, antiproliferative, hypoglycemic, cholesterol-lowering, neuroprotective, and cardioprotective action [1]. Recently, the consumption of dried fruits and by-products has gained special attention, among them we can mention in these chapter Cashews, Acai berries, and Pistachios. These components give it anti-inflammatory, antioxidant, antimicrobial, antiproliferative, and astringent actions thanks to the presence of nutrients and substances with different therapeutic actions that give them mainly action against inflammation and oxidative stress as demonstrated in several studies both in vivo and in vitro. Additionally, we briefly discuss the two main molecular pathways involved: NF-E2-related factor 2 (Nrf2) for oxidative stress and NFkB for inflammation (**Figure 1**).

1.1 Nrf2

Nrf2 is one of the most important regulators that shields cells from ROS and xenobiotics that play a key role against the production of antioxidant and detoxifying enzymes [2, 3]. Nrf2 shields cells against stressors such as xenobiotics in food, radiation, reactive oxygen species (ROS), and endogenous chemicals. As a result, activating the Nrf2 pathway may be a viable chemoprevention method [4]. ROS act as a second messenger in cellular communication, but they can alter natural components as lipids, proteins, and DNA, having a detrimental effect on the biological system [5]. Nrf2 is a member of basic leucine zipper genes (bZIP) that are universally expressed in a variety of tissues and cell types and have a conserved structural domain known as a cap'n'collar domain. The leucine zipper region basic's portion is in charge of DNA binding, whereas the acidic area is necessary for transcriptional activation. The heterodimerization of Nrf2 with other bZIP proteins is required for ARE-mediated transcriptional activation [6]. Keap1, an E3 ubiquitin ligase substrate adaptor that is redox-sensitive, controls how much Nrf2 is present inside the cell [7]. Keap1 interacts to Nrf2 in the cytoplasm when the body is not under stress, promoting ubiquitination and proteasomal destruction of Nrf2. The ubiquitin E3 ligase activity of the Keap1-Cul3 complex decreases with exposure to chemicals (typically electrophiles) or ROS, and Nrf2 is stabilized. As it builds up in the nucleus, stable Nrf2 activates the target genes [8]. Under oxidative stress, free freshly produced Nrf2 translocates to the nucleus and heterodimerizes with one of the small Maf (musculoaponeurotic fibrosarcoma oncogene homolog) proteins. The Nrf2-Keap1 association is resolved in a dose-dependent manner. The enhancer sequences known as antioxidant response elements (AREs), which are found in the regulatory regions of Nrf2 target genes. Nrf2 coordinates the expression of several genes, including not only genes encoding antioxidant enzymes but also a series of genes involved in various processes

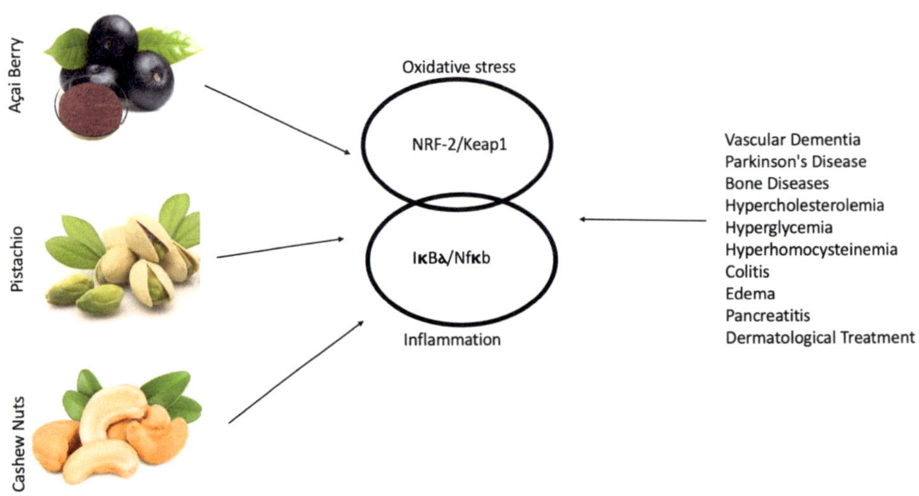

Figure 1.
Açai berry, pistachio, cashew nuts regulation of oxidative stress and inflammation.

including respiratory, cerebrovascular, and neurodegenerative diseases [9–11]. In **Figure 2**, the mechanism of action of Nrf2 is clearly demonstrated. Briefly, (1) Nrf2 is sequestered to the cytoplasm through binding with Keap1 and continually shuttled to the proteasome for degradation. (2) After a response to external stressors, Keap1 cysteine residues are oxidized and Nrf2 serine (Ser) 40 is phosphorylated by protein kinase C (PKC). (3) Nrf2 is then able to translocate into the nucleus and bind to ARE responsive genes in order to increase or decrease their expression. (4) Subsequently, a delayed response to external stressors causes the phosphorylation of GSK-3β by tyrosine (Tyr) kinases. (5) GSK-3β then activates Src kinases, allowing for their translocation into the nucleus. (6) These Src kinases phosphorylate Nrf2 Tyr568, which allows for nuclear export, (7) ubiquitination, and degradation of Nrf2. (8) However, if the insulin receptor signaling is initiated, GSK-3β activity is inhibited. (9) Keap1 is also able to regulate Nrf2 activity through sequestration with PGAM5 to the mitochondria [12].

Multiple genes are impacted by Nrf2 that encode proteins serving as redox balancing agents, detoxifying enzymes, stress response proteins, and metabolic enzymes [6]. Examples of antioxidant detoxification enzymes induced by Nrf2 include heme oxygenase 1 (HO-1) and manganese-dependent superoxide dismutase (Mn-SOD) [13]. Nuclear HO-1 interacts with Nrf2 under oxidative stress, preventing GSK3-mediated phosphorylation along with ubiquitin-proteasomal destruction and extending its accumulation in the nucleus. The preferential transcription of phase II detoxifying enzymes such NQO1 and glucose-6-phosphate dehydrogenase (G6PDH), a regulator of the pentose phosphate pathway, depends on this control of Nrf2 post-induction by nuclear HO-1 [14]. Moreover, the SODs are a family of antioxidant enzymes that catalyze the dismutation of superoxide free radical anions, which are generated during a variety of metabolic activities and lead to the creation of oxygen and hydrogen peroxide molecules. Copper-zinc SOD (Cu, Zn-SOD) and MnSOD, the two primary forms of SODs, are located in the cytoplasm and mitochondria, respectively [15]. It was demonstrated that Nrf2-mediated upregulation of antioxidant

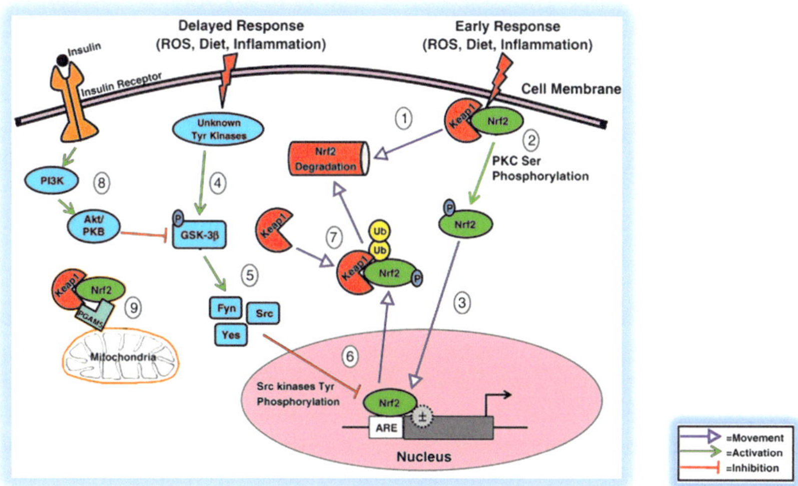

Figure 2.
Schematic diagram of Nrf2 regulation.

Class	Source	Mechanisms of Nrf2 induction	Reference
Isothiocyanates	Cruciferous vegetables	• Keap1-cys151 • Activation of ERK1/2 and Akt kinase • Acceleration of Nrf2 protein synthesis • De-methylation of Nrf2 promoter	[22–27]
Phenols	Ginger	• De-methylation of Nrf2 promoter • Binding with cysteine residue of Keap1	[28–30]
Organosulfur	Garlic	• Keap1- Cys288 • Inducing ROS production • Activation PI3K/Akt/Nrf2	[29–31]
Polyphenol	Tea	• Activation of the p38 MAPK and the ERK1/2 signaling pathways • Dissociation of Nrf2 from Keap1 and Increasing the nuclear translocation Activation of ERK1/2 and PI3K/Akt	[32–35]
Isoflavone	Lupin, fava beans, soybeans, kudzu, coffee and psoralea	• Increasing keap1 S-nitrosylation and enhancing DNA-binding activity of Nrf2 • Increasing PI3K activity	[36, 37]

Table 1.
Selected Nrf2 activators present in diet.

enzymes as GSTs and MnSOD would act to minimize oxidative-stress-induced damage [16].

1.2 Nrf2 and NF-κB

To maintain the physiological balance of cellular redox state and to control the cellular response to stress and inflammation, it is hypothesized that Nrf2 and NF-κB signaling pathways work in concert. NF-κB is a complex protein system constituted by transcription factors that regulate the expression of genes influencing innate and adaptive immunity, inflammation, oxidative stress responses, and B-cell development. NF-κB proteins can be divided into two classes according to whether they include or lack a transactivation domain. Since p50 and p52 lack the transactivation domains that RelA (p65), RelB, and c-Rel possess. Heterodimerization with the Rel proteins is necessary for them to activate transcription [17]. Nrf2/ARE signaling plays a crucial role in the protection against oxidative stress and is responsible for the maintenance of homeostasis and redox balance in cells and tissues. In contrast, NF-κB is also a redox-regulated transcription factor, which regulates inflammatory responses and cellular injury [18]. Firstly, Nrf2 inhibits oxidative-stress-mediated NF-κB activation by decreasing the intracellular ROS levels. Furthermore, Nrf2 prevents the IκB-α proteasomal degradation and inhibits nuclear translocation of NF-κB [19]. Studies suggest that Nrf2 counteracts the NF-κB-driven inflammatory response by competing with transcription co-activator cAMP response element (CREB) binding protein (CBP) [20, 21]. Histones are acetylated by the CBP-p300 complex, which also makes DNA accessible for the construction of the transcriptional machinery.

Additionally, the Nrf2 and p65 non-histone proteins, as well as others, have their lysine residues acetylated by the CBP-p300 complex. Since, CBP also preferentially interacts with p65, the overexpression of p65 limits the availability of CBP for Nrf2 interaction; accordingly, knockdown of p65 promotes Nrf2 complex formation with CBP (**Table 1**) [38].

2. Açai berry

The Açaí berry is a little, spherical fruit (about the size of a grape) that is green while immature and turns dark purple when it is fully developed. It comes from the Açaí palm, a native of Central and South America that also thrives in marshes and flood plains in addition to the Amazon region. Açaí berries are eaten fresh or juiced as food. The juice can be used as a natural food colorant and is commercially employed in jelly, syrup, ice cream, liquors, energy drinks, and a range of other beverages [39]. Açaí juice is viscous and contains 5.9% fats and 2.4% protein. The apple pulp has 12% fats and 4% protein. Vitamins A, C, and E, calcium, phosphorus, iron, and thiamine are among the nutrients. The Açaí berries of the *Euterpe oleracea* plant are thought to be a source of bioactive substances, particularly anthocyanins and unsaturated fatty acids, which are known to have health-promoting properties. These berries may help to reduce metabolic stress and inflammation while enhancing antioxidant protection. Orientin, isoorientin, vanillic acid, as well as the anthocyanins cyanidin-3-glucoside and cyanidin-3-rutinoside, are only a few of the polyphenolic components having antioxidant capabilities found in acai extracts. Acai pulp is rich in proanthocyanins and total phenolics, but also contains trace amounts of anthocyanins. Industrially processed samples have a significant percentage of proanthocyanidins, but naturally occurring anthocyanins are significantly enriched (20 times more). The unprocessed Açai pulp extracts reduced the expression of pro-inflammatory genes such as interleukin-1, cyclooxygenase-2, nitric oxide synthase, and interleukin-6 and dramatically inhibited the generation of nitric oxide, which has been linked to proanthocyanidins in the initial inflammatory response [40]. These chemicals' existence is mostly associated with their anti-inflammatory, antiproliferative, antioxidant, and cardioprotective properties [41]. Açai can be used to treat certain diseases due to its anti-inflammatory and antioxidant effects, acting at the level of the Nrf2 pathway. It has also been shown that Açai may act on different pathways; for example, according to some studies, it goes to act on peroxisome proliferator-activated receptors (PPARs) α and γ, going to decrease the transcription of various genes, including pro-inflammatory, pro-oxidants, and those affecting lipid metabolism genes. Another pathway that goes to modulate is that of Nf-kB, going to decrease the production of pro-inflammatory cytokines. For example, the fruit has been used to treat Vascular Dementia (VaD), which is the secondary most frequent reason for inherited biological cognitive impairment [42]. VaD is caused by an oxidative stress increase, which might cause cognitive decline brought on by aging and neurological diseases. Since oxidative and inflammatory stressors may reduce synaptic plasticity and memory by resulting in dendritic modification and cell death, important brain regions such as the hippocampus should be more susceptible to these situations. Additionally, the expression of microtubule-associated protein 2 (MAP-2) and α-Tubulin, two significant neuronal markers of well-being, is altered in the brain of VaD patients [43, 44]. Furthermore, it has been demonstrated that impaired autophagy alters protein "quality control," accumulates unwanted proteins and organelles in brain cells [45]. In this study, Açai Berry was useful to conteract VaD alterations in the brain. Açaí berries can also mitigate Parkinson's disease progression, which is the second most prevalent neurological condition in people over 65 [46]. Recent studies have revealed that the Nrf2/ARE signaling cascade is the most likely target for therapeutic therapy, despite advancements in our understanding of the pathophysiology of PD [47]. The oral administration of Açaí berries has shown an important decrease of ROS and an increase of Nrf2 expression. Also, in this study, the authors observed a significantly improvement in both motor and non-motor deficits, histological alteration, pro-inflammatory cytokine release, neutrophilic infiltration, and lipid peroxidation limiting dopaminergic neuronal death [48]. Some studies, additionally, have shown Açai berries' anti-inflammatory properties in a model of co-culture between Caco-2 and RAW 264.7 macrophages, which has the potential to prevent intestinal inflammatory diseases, due to anthocyanin improved Tight Junction barrier integrity and reduce gastrointestinal inflammation by preventing the expression of cytokines, especially IL-6, IL-8, and PGE2 through inhibition of COX-2 [49]. Açai barriers can also be used for anti-inflammatory treatment of bone diseases such as periodontal disease are triggered by chronic inflammation causing the upregulation of osteoclastogenesis. This in turn shifts the bone remodeling process toward increased bone resorption [50]. Inflammatory cytokines have been associated with bone destruction, having a role in the regulation of the expression of the receptor activator of nuclear factor kappa B (RANK) and receptor activator of nuclear factor kappa B ligand (RANKL), which is a vital step in the activation of osteoclastogenesis [51]. Açai-berry extract (ABE) on the reduction of osteoclast formation and resorptive activity of RANKL-induced osteoclast precursor cells. Moreover, ABE also modulated the secretion of several inflammatory cytokines during osteoclastogenesis and osteoclast activity [52]. Açai seeds, according to some studies, regulate NF-κB and Nrf2/ARE pathways protecting lung against acute and chronic inflammation [53]. Moreover, studies have shown the cytotoxic effect of Açai seeds against the MCF-7 breast cancer cell line. This effect is given by the ability to induce ROS synthesis inside these cells. But also, it induces morphological changes and reduces cells viability, due to flavonoids content [54]. In high-fat mice, Açai seed extract reduces the activation of the renin-angiotensin system, oxidative stress, and inflammation in the white adipose tissue [55]. Acai seed prevented the body weight rise brought on by the heart failure diet, which was correlated with the diminution of adipocyte area and the accumulation of visceral fat, indicating that the diminution of adipose mass may contribute to the acai seed-mediated decrease in body weight. These advantageous effects of acai seed were also connected to a significant decrease in the serum levels of total cholesterol (TC), triglycerides (TG), very low-density lipoprotein (VLDL), and low-density lipoprotein (LDL), indicating a favorable impact of Açai seed on the altered lipid profile [56]. The pulp of Açai can be used, for example, to mitigate colitis-associated colon carcinogenesis, which is one of the most common cancers in the modern world. A lesion caused by acute inflammation was characterized microscopically by a coagulative necrosis process and had macroscopic signs of necrosis. According to the phytochemical tests, the lyophilized acai pulp (AP) utilized in the in vivo trial included significant amounts of the phytonutrients cyanidin 3-rutinoside (C3R) and cyanidin 3-glusoside (C3G). Additionally, the concentration of anthocyanins may range between açai samples utilized in various research. Cells' ability to move slightly less after receiving acai pulp treatment [57, 58].

3. Pistachios

Pistachios originate in West Asia and are traded in the Mediterranean, Europe, and the East. The only species that produces edible nuts is *Pistacia Vera* L. (Pistacio), which is a member of the Anacardiaceae family [59]. The fact that pistachio plants can grow in a variety of soil types and survive dryness is crucial for sustainability because semi-arid regions require vital water consumption. The pistachio fruit is an edible drupe with a thin, soft coating. The endocarp, which is covered with a fleshy, thin hull that is light green in color with red undertones, is inedible. In comparison to other nuts, pistachios contain a high concentration of compounds that have antioxidant and anti-inflammatory properties [60]. Nuts have positive health effects on a variety of metabolic conditions, including hypercholesterolemia, hyperglycemia, hyperhomocysteinemia, and everything else that goes along with them. Pistachios has a high nutritional content and is consumed frequently over the world because it has significant nutritional properties and offers many health advantages [60]. One of the foods that must be included in a nutritious and balanced diet is the eating of nuts. Protein, fiber, monounsaturated fatty acids, minerals, and vitamins are all present in excellent amounts in pistachios, but they are also a good source of carotenoids, phenolic acids, flavonoids, and anthocyanins (**Table 2**).

Lutein, zeaxanthin, and a variety of other bioactive phenolic compounds found in pistachios help to improve endothelial function, glycemic management, and antioxidant and anti-inflammatory activity. The highest concentrations of potassium, tocoferol, and phytosteroids can be found in citrus fruits [61, 62]. Lipophilic extracts from the peel and kernel of raw shelled pistachios contain fatty acids, phytosterols, and tocopherols, according to phytochemical study. These polyphenols in pistachios have strong antioxidant action. Gallic acid and other phenolic chemicals, such as phenol acids, flavonoids, stylibenes, and tannins, have one or more aromatic rings and hydroxyl groups [63–65]. As a great source of phenolic compounds, pistachios have strong antioxidant properties that can block ROS, preventing the oxidation of biological macromolecules [66]. The activity of the various pistachio nut components was evaluated in a number of in vitro and in vivo investigations, and the various lipophilic (carotenoids, tocopherols, and chlorophyll) and hydrophilic extracts were

Macronutrient and energy content	g/100 g
Protein	20.2
Total lipid	45.3
Saturated fatty acids	5.9
Monounsatured fatty acids	23.3
Polyunsaturated fatty acids	14.4
Carbohydrate, by difference	27.2
Fiber, total dietary	10.6
Sugars, total	7.66
Starch	1.67
Energy	2340 kJ

Table 2.
Macronutrients content in 100 g of Pistacio. Source: U.S. Department of Agriculture Food Data Central 2019.

compared [67]. The hydrophilic extract exhibits higher antioxidant activity than the lipophilic components in the kernel, and this activity has been observed to block the metal-dependent and independent lipid oxidation of bovine liver microsomes in a dose-dependent manner [68]. Human low-density lipoprotein (LDL) has also been shown to oxidize less when exposed to copper [60]. Compared with the kernel, the tegument of the pistachio contains a higher level of antioxidant activity. By combining lipophilic and hydrophilic extracts with macrophages that have been stimulated by lipopolysaccharide (LPS), this was proven [69]. The hydrophilic tegument extracts shows stronger inhibition by subsequently reducing nitric oxide (NO) production. The extracts markedly decreased ROS formation. According to the findings of this in vitro study, the tegument extract had a higher concentration of phenolic compounds and hence had more antioxidant activity. In mature adipocytes, these fractions greatly decreased lipid accumulation. Additionally, it has been proposed that the antiproliferative properties of pistachios contribute to their anticancer properties. The growth of LT97 colon adenoma cells has been shown to be inhibited by pistachio fermentation supernatants in vitro in a dose-dependent manner [66]. Additionally, pistachio fermentation supernatants have been shown to increase antioxidant activity, which promotes the expression of catalase (CAT), which lessens DNA damage brought on by hydrogen peroxide (H_2O_2) [70]. According to the findings of these investigations, roasting pistachios may alter their phytochemical composition and improve biological activity [71]. The gut microbiota, a complex ecology that varies according to anatomical location, is another crucial area of study in science. Obesity, type 2 diabetes, and other illnesses can sometimes cause the microbiota to become out of balance and enter a state of dysbiosis [72, 73]. Diet also plays a significant part in this. According to a study comparing the intake of almonds and pistachios on treated volunteers, the consumption of pistachios was able to change the microbiota's composition more than almonds [74]. According to studies on the microbiome, eating pistachios in moderation can help the body's microbiota get back into balance by boosting the population of helpful bacteria and lowering acute inflammatory conditions. In fact, pistachio supplementation has been found to repair the intestinal microbiota in diabetic rats on a high-fat diet. Drug resistance is a widespread issue, and novel treatments are the focus of current research. Because they include bioactive substances that can be employed as antimicrobials and antivirals, plant extracts play a significant role in medicine. Bactericide properties of raw, salted, roasted pistachios have been demonstrated. Additionally, the effectiveness of a Pistacia Vera metabolic extract against staphylococcal infections has been demonstrated. Pistachios contain polyphenols, which can be extracted alone or combined with other medications to make a potent alternative to antibiotics [75]. Additionally, polyphenols have antiviral properties. Pistachios contain polyphenols, which can be extracted alone or combined with other medications to make a potent alternative to antibiotics. Additionally, polyphenols have antiviral properties. This has been shown to prevent replication of Herpes Simplex Virus Type 1 (HSV-1). Pure polyphenol extracts were used to treat the condition, which inhibited the expression of many viral proteins and the creation of viral DNA [76]. It is important to keep in mind that pistachio component quantities can differ depending on genotype, pre- and post-harvest circumstances, and storage [77]. Numerous experimental models have been used to examine the anti-inflammatory properties of pistachio components in acute inflammatory states such paw edema [78–81], LPS inflammation [69], and chronic inflammation models such as colitis [82]. By contrasting raw, shelled pistachios with salted and roasted pistachios, the therapeutic effects of pistachios were discovered in an experimental animal model of paw edema generated in rats. In contrast to roasting, which results in a 60% drop-in antioxidant activity, eating raw shelled natural pistachios has been shown to result in reduced nitrate protein production [68, 82, 83]. A diet with a balanced intake of pistachios has been demonstrated to enhance serum concentrations of tocopherol, lutein, and carotene. In addition, pistachio consumption has been proven to decrease oxidized LDL concentrations in randomized trials of healthy patients and hypercholesterolemic subjects [84]. Malondialdehyde (MDA), a by-product of lipid peroxidation, was reduced, and blood antioxidant potential was improved by eating pistachios [85]. Numerous studies have demonstrated the critical role played by bioactive components in mastic oil produced from Pistachio Lentiscus in the treatment of ulcerative colitis, where inflammation and oxidative stress play a significant role. Myeloperoxidase (MPO) activity was dramatically decreased by flavonoids and other bioactive substances [86]. Mastic oil therapy reduces the inflammatory response of ulcerative colitis, which is mediated by cytokines such as TNF- and IL-6. These research studies sought to emphasize the critical function of the pistachio's bioactive components and the potential significance of including them in a nutritious, well-balanced diet [87, 88]. In particular, Nrf2 pathway plays a significant role in antioxidant activity. When there is a redox imbalance, this pathway becomes less active, which depletes the body's supply of antioxidant enzymes. The release of pro-inflammatory cytokines can also activate the NF-B signaling pathway, which results in decreased Nrf2 pathway activity and oxidative stress conditions. Inflammatory response and oxidative stress are modulated, according to a study done after the extraction of polysaccharides from *Pistacia vera* L. Pistachio polysaccharides decreased inflammation and oxidative stress by boosting antioxidant production through the Nrf2 pathway and attenuating the NF-kB pathway [89, 90]. The positive effects of bioactive substances are dose-dependent, it should be noted. Additionally, research has been done on the therapeutic effects of pistachios in experimental models of neurodegenerative diseases for cognitive problems [91]. In particular, lutein and zeaxanthin improved cellular communication required for light processing and the growth of neural circuits in the visual system, which helped improve memory and motor performance when pistachios were supplemented [92]. The anti-inflammatory and antioxidant properties of pistachio bioactive components are dose-dependent, it should be noted. By preventing the cellular aging phenomenon brought on by inflammation and oxidative stress, their balanced consumption in the diet might enhance quality of life.

4. Cashew

Cashew (*Anacardium occidentale L.*) is a tree that originates in Brazil, but with the exploration has also spread to Asia and Africa. Cashew is a perennial plant belonging to the family of the Anacardiaceae: these plants have a considerable height, the trunk is irregular and short, the leaves evergreen elliptical oblate, while flowers are small with sepals and petals gathered in a panicle. The cashew fruit consists of an accessory fruit and a true fruit. The accessory fruit is called cashew apple and, when it reaches full maturity, is a kidney-shaped drupe, inside of which is the cashew nut surrounded by a double shell. From the cultivation of this plant, the fruit is used: both cashew apple and cashew nut; but more recently also a by-product, the cashew nut shell liquid [93–95]. The cashew nut has remarkable nutritional properties due to its various components: lipids including polyunsaturated and monounsaturated fatty acids; amino acids including glutamic acid, aspartic acid and leucine; minerals such as calcium, potassium, and magnesium. Cashew apple is rich in sugars and minerals; the cashew nut shell liquid is rich in phenols and has antimicrobial properties. In addition, cashew by-products have several properties: the cashew skin extract is a good antioxidant; instead, the bark is rich in tannins and has astringent, anti-inflammatory, hypoglycemic, antibacterial, and antimutagenic properties. Also in cashews other molecules with possible therapeutic effects are: saponins, catenins, tannins, carotenoids, and anthocyanins. With regard to the therapeutic applications of cashew, several studies have shown that its molecules grant it different actions reason why different therapeutic effects are being evaluated recently. Foremost among them, the anacardic acid is an antimicrobical agent, particularly it acts against Gram-positive bacteria; another application of anacardic acid is such as antitumoral agent, in fact has been shown to act by blocking the HAT enzyme: this is an enzyme involved in the acetylation of histones [96]. Furthermore, some studies have highlighted how anacardic acid induces autophagy and apoptosis. Certainly among the most studied therapeutic applications today are the antioxidant and anti-inflammatory effects of cashew nuts [97]. The anti-inflammatory effects of cashew are due to its interaction with the transcriptional factor NFkB, specifically there is inhibition of this pathway, resulting in a decrease in proinflammatory cytokines. Antioxidant effects are due to action on several factors: the anacardic acid acts on lipid peroxidation and lipoxygenase [98]; in addition, polyphenols and flavonoids have antioxidant action as they modulate oxidative balance and also have been seen to act on the Nrf2 pathway, promoting its translocation into the nucleus resulting in the synthesis of cytoprotective enzymes such as NADPH quinone dehydrogenase NQO-1 and HO-1. Additionally, the modulation of Nrf2 pathway influences other important molecular pathways and mechanism: such as NLRP3 and apoptosis. Several studies have been conducted in recent years to evaluate the effects of cashew nut consumption, and these have yielded positive effects in the treatment of various diseases. In in vitro studies, the activity of cashew nuts on the human microbiota was evaluated: the effects obtained induce a change in metabolic activity with potential prebiotic activities [99]; the cashew apple juice contains gluco- oligosaccharides that promote the growth of the microbiota [99] . In vivo studies included different experimental protocols going to investigate various pathologies. Among neurodegenerative diseases, a study has been done on Parkinson's disease: the pathology has been induced by rotenone in male rats, and then they were treated with anacardic acid; analyses have shown that there is a decrease in oxidative stress, specifically there is modulation of mitochondrial respiration and superoxide dismutase [100]. In in vivo study was evaluated two aspects of cashew nuts: antioxidant and anti-inflammatory action in different model of inflammatory disease: such as colitis, edema, and pancreatitis. In colitis model, the pathology was induced intrarectally through injection of dinitrobenzene sulfonic acid (DNBS); subsequently, the cashews were administrated orally. Findings have shown that cashew nut consumption inhibits the inflammatory pathway NFkB and activates the expression of antioxidants such as superoxide dismutase [97]. The pancreatitis was induced in CD1 mice by cerulein; in this case, the cashew acts on Nrf2 pathway and on NRLP3 pathway: Nrf2 translocates into the nucleus by inducing the synthesis of cytoprotective enzymes such as HO-1 hemeoxygenase and superoxide dismutase; instead the cashew acts on NRLP3 reducing its levels resulting in decreased pro-inflammatory cytokines. These effects are probably due to its components such as flavonoids and polyphenols [101]. The edema was induced by carrageenan injection in male rats, and the results showed that the administration of cashew reduced edema formation and induced the endogenous antioxidants activity; and also in this study is shown the analgesic effect [102]. The antioxidant and anti-inflammatory action of cashew nuts is evaluated also in multi-organ pathology such as Hyperhomocysteinemia [103, 104]. Among the cardiovascular diseases considered was ischemia/reperfusion injury, in this model demonstrated that the consumption of cashew acts on lipid peroxidation, tissue myeloperoxidase activity, and reactive oxygen species generation: inducing a decrease of levels; also there is a decrease of pro-inflammatory cytokines and an increase of antioxidant activity. In addition, studies have shown that cashew consumption reduces the risk of cardiovascular disease: probably because of its concentration of fatty acids, which also have a hypolipidemic action [105, 106]. Other studies have shown that not only cashew nut consumption has therapeutic effects but also its derivatives such as extracts. The leaf extract of Anacardium has an anti-inflammatory and bronchodilatory action: this is shown by in vivo studies on animal model. In this case, the effects are due to a derivative present in the extract, oleamide [107]. In the dermatological field, there is some evidence to suggest a possible application of cashews as a dermatological treatment as well, but extensive studies have not yet been conducted [108]. Certainly the in vitro and in vivo studies carried out demonstrate action on inflammation and oxidative stress, particularly cashews modulate important pathways, such as Nrf2 and NFkB. The latest studies instead are also focusing on the anticancer effect, and this food might have evaluated antiproliferative action on cancer cells [109].

5. Conclusion

It has been increasingly clear in recent years how nutrition may affect the prevention and/or treatment of several chronic diseases. Based on the food ingredients that can have positive effects on health, a balanced and diverse diet is advised. For instance, antioxidant chemicals can fight free radicals directly or indirectly by boosting cellular endogenous antioxidant defenses, such as by activating Nrf2. Resveratrol, catechin, and allicin are a few chemical substances found in the human diet that have strong biological effects and may be good for cardiovascular health. They also prevent ROS damage by upregulating phase II detoxifying enzymes and raising levels of cellular glutathione. Açai berries, cashew nuts, and pistachios are some of the bioactive ingredients of the diet that are covered in this chapter. Since the majority of studies are in vitro or in animals, and it is unknown how far these doses can be extrapolated to be effective in humans, it is not yet possible to establish safe and effective doses for supplementation, taking into account all the studies that have been discussed in this chapter. The usage of food ingredients does, however, seems to have the benefits of relatively low toxicity, a wealth of resources, and low cost. Therefore, "nutritional therapy" emerges as a crucial method for preventing and/or treating a variety of diseases, enhancing the welfare of people, and trials to determine their efficacy should be carried out.

Acknowledgements

These authors want to thank Doctors Livia Interdonato, Ylenia Marino, Alessia Arangia, and Gianluca Antonio Franco for their incredible contribution.

Conflict of interest

The authors declare no conflict of interest.

Author details

Rosanna Di Paola[1], Salvatore Cuzzocrea[1], Roberta Fusco[1*] and Marika Cordaro[2]

1 Department of Chemical, Biological, Pharmaceutical and Environmental Sciences, University of Messina, Messina, Italy

2 Department of Biomedical, Dental and Morphological and Functional Imaging, University of Messina, Messina, Italy

*Address all correspondence to: rfusco@unime.it

References

[1] Chang SK, Alasalvar C, Shahidi F. Superfruits: Phytochemicals, antioxidant efficacies, and health effects - a comprehensive review. Critical Reviews in Food Science and Nutrition. 2019;**59**(10):1580-1604

[2] Genovese T et al. Açaí (Euterpe Oleraceae Mart.) seeds regulate NF-κB and Nrf2/ARE pathways protecting lung against acute and chronic inflammation. Cellular Physiology and Biochemistry: International Journal of Experimental Cellular Physiology, Biochemistry, and Pharmacology. 2022;**56**(S2):1-20

[3] Mohan S, Gupta D. Crosstalk of toll-like receptors signaling and Nrf2 pathway for regulation of inflammation. Biomedicine & Pharmacotherapy. 2018;**108**:1866-1878

[4] Huang Y et al. The complexity of the Nrf2 pathway: Beyond the antioxidant response. The Journal of Nutritional Biochemistry. 2015;**26**(12):1401-1413

[5] Panda P et al. Biomarkers of oxidative stress tethered to cardiovascular diseases. Oxidative Medicine and Cellular Longevity. 2022;**2022**:9154295

[6] Kaspar JW, Niture SK, Jaiswal AK. Nrf2: INrf2 (Keap1) signaling in oxidative stress. Free Radical Biology and Medicine. 2009;**47**(9):1304-1309

[7] Tonelli C, Chio IIC, Tuveson DA. Transcriptional regulation by Nrf2. Antioxidants & Redox Signaling. 2018;**29**(17):1727-1745

[8] Suzuki T, Yamamoto M. Molecular basis of the Keap1–Nrf2 system. Free Radical Biology and Medicine. 2015;**88**:93-100

[9] D'Amico R et al. Açai berry mitigates Parkinson's disease progression showing dopaminergic neuroprotection via Nrf2-HO1 pathways. Molecular Neurobiology. 2022;**59**:1-15

[10] D'Amico R et al. Palmitoylethanolamide/Baicalein regulates the androgen receptor signaling and NF-κB/Nrf2 pathways in benign prostatic hyperplasia. Antioxidants. 2021;**10**(7):1014

[11] D'Amico R et al. Atrazine inhalation worsen pulmonary fibrosis regulating the nuclear factor-erythroid 2-related factor (Nrf2) pathways inducing brain comorbidities. Cellular Physiology and Biochemistry. 2021;**55**:704-725

[12] Vomhof-DeKrey EE, Picklo MJ Sr. The Nrf2-antioxidant response element pathway: A target for regulating energy metabolism. The Journal of Nutritional Biochemistry. 2012;**23**(10):1201-1206

[13] Cordaro M et al. Cashew (*Anacardium occidentale L.*) nuts modulate the Nrf2 and NLRP3 pathways in pancreas and lung after induction of acute pancreatitis by cerulein. Antioxidants. 2020;**9**(10):992

[14] Biswas C et al. Nuclear heme oxygenase-1 (HO-1) modulates subcellular distribution and activation of Nrf2, impacting metabolic and anti-oxidant defenses. Journal of Biological Chemistry. 2014;**289**(39):26882-26894

[15] Fridovich I. Superoxide radical and superoxide dismutases. Annual Review of Biochemistry. 1995;**64**(1):97-112

[16] Breedon SA, Hadj-Moussa H, Storey KB. Nrf2 activates antioxidant enzymes in the anoxia-tolerant red-eared

slider turtle, Trachemys scripta elegans. Journal of Experimental Zoology Part A: Ecological and Integrative Physiology. 2021;**335**(4):426-435

[17] Gilmore TD. The Rel/NF-κB signal transduction pathway: Introduction. Oncogene. 1999;**18**(49):6842-6844

[18] Karin M, Yamamoto Y, Wang Q. The IKK NF-κB system: A treasure trove for drug development. Nature Reviews Drug Discovery. 2004;**3**(1):17-26

[19] Yerra VG et al. Potential therapeutic effects of the simultaneous targeting of the Nrf2 and NF-κB pathways in diabetic neuropathy. Redox Biology. 2013;**1**(1):394-397

[20] Brigelius-Flohé R, Flohé L. Basic principles and emerging concepts in the redox control of transcription factors. Antioxidants & Redox Signaling. 2011;**15**(8):2335-2381

[21] Sandberg M et al. NRF2-regulation in brain health and disease: Implication of cerebral inflammation. Neuropharmacology. 2014;**79**:298-306

[22] Eggler AL et al. Identification of the highly reactive cysteine 151 in the chemopreventive agent-sensor Keap1 protein is method-dependent. Chemical Research in Toxicology. 2007;**20**(12):1878-1884

[23] Hu C et al. Modification of keap1 cysteine residues by sulforaphane. Chemical Research in Toxicology. 2011;**24**(4):515-521

[24] Zhang DD, Hannink M. Distinct cysteine residues in Keap1 are required for Keap1-dependent ubiquitination of Nrf2 and for stabilization of Nrf2 by chemopreventive agents and oxidative stress. Molecular and Cellular Biology. 2003;**23**(22):8137-8151

[25] Jakubíková J et al. Role of PI3K/Akt and MEK/ERK signaling pathways in sulforaphane-and erucin-induced phase II enzymes and MRP2 transcription, G2/M arrest and cell death in Caco-2 cells. Biochemical Pharmacology. 2005;**69**(11):1543-1552

[26] Zhang C et al. Sulforaphane enhances Nrf2 expression in prostate cancer TRAMP C1 cells through epigenetic regulation. Biochemical Pharmacology. 2013;**85**(9):1398-1404

[27] Su Z-Y et al. Requirement and epigenetics reprogramming of Nrf2 in suppression of tumor promoter TPA-induced mouse skin cell transformation by SulforaphaneActivating Nrf2 blocks TPA-induced JB6 transformation by SFN. Cancer Prevention Research. 2014;**7**(3):319-329

[28] Khor TO et al. Pharmacodynamics of curcumin as DNA hypomethylation agent in restoring the expression of Nrf2 via promoter CpGs demethylation. Biochemical Pharmacology. 2011;**82**(9):1073-1078

[29] Farombi EO et al. Curcumin attenuates dimethylnitrosamine-induced liver injury in rats through Nrf2-mediated induction of heme oxygenase-1. Food and Chemical Toxicology. 2008;**46**(4):1279-1287

[30] Wu J et al. Neuroprotection by curcumin in ischemic brain injury involves the Akt/Nrf2 pathway. PLoS One. 2013;**8**(3):e59843

[31] Kim S et al. Keap1 cysteine 288 as a potential target for diallyl trisulfide-induced Nrf2 activation. PLoS One. 2014;**9**(1):e85984

[32] Kanzaki H et al. Nrf2 activation attenuates both orthodontic tooth movement and relapse. Journal of Dental Research. 2015;**94**(6):787-794

[33] Wang Y et al. Epigallocatechin-3-gallate attenuates transforming growth factor-β1 induced epithelial-mesenchymal transition via Nrf2 regulation in renal tubular epithelial cells. Biomedicine & Pharmacotherapy. 2015;**70**:260-267

[34] Yang G-Z et al. Epigallocatechin-3-gallate protects HUVECs from PM2. 5-induced oxidative stress injury by activating critical antioxidant pathways. Molecules. 2015;**20**(4):6626-6639

[35] Na H-K et al. (−)-epigallocatechin gallate induces Nrf2-mediated antioxidant enzyme expression via activation of PI3K and ERK in human mammary epithelial cells. Archives of Biochemistry and Biophysics. 2008;**476**(2):171-177

[36] Wang R et al. Genistein attenuates ischemic oxidative damage and behavioral deficits via eNOS/Nrf2/HO-1 signaling. Hippocampus. 2013;**23**(7):634-647

[37] Xi Y-D et al. Flavonoids protect cerebrovascular endothelial cells through Nrf2 and PI3K from β-amyloid peptide-induced oxidative damage. Current Neurovascular Research. 2012;**9**(1):32-41

[38] Sun Z, Chin YE, Zhang DD. Acetylation of Nrf2 by p300/CBP augments promoter-specific DNA binding of Nrf2 during the antioxidant response. Molecular and Cellular Biology. 2009;**29**(10):2658-2672

[39] Natural Medicines Comprehensive Database, 3d ed. Compiled and edited by Jellin JM, Gregory P, Batz F, Hitchen K, Burson S, Shaver K, et al. Stockton, CA: Therapeutic Research; 2000

[40] Xiong J et al. Phenolic content, anti-inflammatory properties, and dermal wound repair properties of industrially processed and non-processed acai from the Brazilian Amazon. Food & Function. 2020;**11**(6):4903-4914

[41] Yamaguchi KK et al. Amazon acai: Chemistry and biological activities: A review. Food Chemistry. 2015;**179**:137-151

[42] Orgogozo JM, Abadie E. Vascular dementia: European perspectives. Alzheimer Disease and Associated Disorders. 1999;**13**(Suppl 3):S192-S200

[43] Santiago-Mujika E et al. Tubulin and tubulin posttranslational modifications in Alzheimer's disease and vascular dementia. Frontiers in Aging Neuroscience. 2021;**13**:730107

[44] Sabbatini M et al. The hippocampus in spontaneously hypertensive rats: An animal model of vascular dementia? Mechanisms of Ageing and Development. 2002;**123**(5):547-559

[45] Poulose SM et al. Modulation of oxidative stress, inflammation, autophagy and expression of Nrf2 in hippocampus and frontal cortex of rats fed with acai-enriched diets. Nutritional Neuroscience. 2017;**20**(5):305-315

[46] Warner TT, Schapira AH. Genetic and environmental factors in the cause of Parkinson's disease. Annals of Neurology. 2003;**53**(Suppl 3):S16-S23 discussion S23-5

[47] Smith PF. Inflammation in Parkinson's disease: An update. Current Opinion in Investigational Drugs. 2008;**9**(5):478-484

[48] Gureev AP, Popov VN. Nrf2/ARE pathway as a therapeutic target for the treatment of Parkinson diseases. Neurochemical Research. 2019;**44**(10):2273-2279

[49] D'Amico R et al. Acai berry mitigates Parkinson's disease progression showing dopaminergic neuroprotection via Nrf2-HO1 pathways. Molecular Neurobiology. 2022;**59**(10):6519-6533

[50] Kim KJ et al. Acai berry extract as a regulator of intestinal inflammation pathways in a Caco-2 and RAW 264.7 co-culture model. Journal of Food Biochemistry. 2021;**564**

[51] Boyle WJ, Simonet WS, Lacey DL. Osteoclast differentiation and activation. Nature. 2003;**423**(6937):337-342

[52] Hsu H et al. Tumor necrosis factor receptor family member RANK mediates osteoclast differentiation and activation induced by osteoprotegerin ligand. Proceedings of the National Academy of Sciences of the United States of America. 1999;**96**(7):3540-3545

[53] Brito C et al. Extract of acai-berry inhibits osteoclast differentiation and activity. Archives of Oral Biology. 2016;**68**:29-34

[54] Genovese T et al. Acai (Euterpe Oleraceae Mart.) seeds regulate NF-kappaB and Nrf2/ARE pathways protecting lung against acute and chronic inflammation. Cellular Physiology and Biochemistry. 2022;**56**(S2):1-20

[55] Genovese T et al. Role of bevacizumab on vascular endothelial growth factor in Apolipoprotein E deficient mice after traumatic brain injury. International Journal of Molecular Sciences. 2022;**23**:4262

[56] Kalupahana NS, Moustaid-Moussa N. The renin-angiotensin system: A link between obesity, inflammation and insulin resistance. Obesity Reviews. 2012;**13**(2):136-149

[57] Santos IB et al. Acai seed extract prevents the renin-angiotensin system activation, oxidative stress and inflammation in white adipose tissue of high-fat diet-fed mice. Nutrition Research. 2020;**79**:35-49

[58] Ferguson L, Polito V, Kallsen C. The Pistachio tree; botany and physiology and factors that affect yield. Pistachio Production Manual. 4th ed. Davis, CA, USA: University of California Fruit & Nut Research Information Center; 2005. pp. 31-39

[59] Ferguson, L., V. Polito, and C. Kallsen, The Pistachio tree; botany and physiology and factors that affect yield. Pistachio Production Manual, 4th ed. Davis, CA, USA, University of California Fruit & Nut Research Information Center, 2005: p. 31-39.

[60] Mandalari G et al. Pistachio nuts (Pistacia vera L.): Production, nutrients, bioactives and novel health effects. Plants. 2021;**11**(1):18

[61] Food and H. Drug Administration. Food labeling: Revision of the nutrition and supplement facts labels. Final rule. Federal Register. 2016;**81**(103):33741-33999

[62] Caruso G, Barone C, Parisi S. The regulation (EC) No 1169/2011 and food packaging. New obligations and correlated consequences. World Food Regulation Review. 2015;**24**(8):26

[63] Dreher ML. Pistachio nuts: Composition and potential health benefits. Nutrition Reviews. 2012;**70**(4):234-240

[64] Bulló M et al. Nutrition attributes and health effects of pistachio nuts. British Journal of Nutrition. 2015;**113**(S2):S79-S93

[65] Liu Y, Blumberg J, Chen CY. Quantification and bioaccessibility of

California pistachio bioactives (259.1). The FASEB Journal. 2014;**28**:259.1

[66] Yuan W et al. Quantification of phytochemicals, cellular antioxidant activities and Antiproliferative activities of raw and roasted American pistachios (Pistacia vera L.). Nutrients. 2022;**14**(15):3002

[67] Mandalari G et al. Bioaccessibility of pistachio polyphenols, xanthophylls, and tocopherols during simulated human digestion. Nutrition. 2013;**29**(1):338-344

[68] Gentile C et al. Antioxidant activity of Sicilian pistachio (Pistacia vera L. var. Bronte) nut extract and its bioactive components. Journal of Agricultural and Food Chemistry. 2007;**55**(3):643-648

[69] Grace MH et al. In vitro lipolytic, antioxidant and anti-inflammatory activities of roasted pistachio kernel and skin constituents. Food & Function. 2016;**7**(10):4285-4298

[70] Glei M et al. Chemopreventive potential of raw and roasted pistachios regarding colon carcinogenesis. Nutrients. 2017;**9**(12):1368

[71] Ballistreri G, Arena E, Fallico B. Influence of ripeness and drying process on the polyphenols and tocopherols of Pistacia vera L. Molecules. 2009;**14**(11):4358-4369

[72] Chang C, Lin H. Dysbiosis in gastrointestinal disorders. Best Practice & Research Clinical Gastroenterology. 2016;**30**(1):3-15

[73] Fan Y, Pedersen O. Gut microbiota in human metabolic health and disease. Nature Reviews Microbiology. 2021;**19**(1):55-71

[74] Yanni AE et al. Functional modulation of gut microbiota in diabetic rats following dietary intervention with pistachio nuts (Pistacia vera L.). Metabolism open. 2020;**7**:100040

[75] Bisignano C et al. In vitro antimicrobial activity of pistachio (Pistacia vera L.) polyphenols. FEMS Microbiology Letters. 2013;**341**(1):62-67

[76] Musarra-Pizzo M et al. In vitro anti-HSV-1 activity of polyphenol-rich extracts and pure polyphenol compounds derived from pistachios kernels (Pistacia vera L.). Plants. 2020;**9**(2):267

[77] Bolling BW, McKay DL, Blumberg JB. The phytochemical composition and antioxidant actions of tree nuts. Asia Pacific Journal of Clinical Nutrition. 2010;**19**(1):117

[78] Ben Khedir S et al. In vivo evaluation of the anti-inflammatory effect of Pistacia lentiscus fruit oil and its effects on oxidative stress. Evidence-based Complementary and Alternative Medicine. 2016;**2016**:6108203

[79] Ahmad NS et al. Analgesic and anti-inflammatory effects of Pistacia integerrima extracts in mice. Journal of Ethnopharmacology. 2010;**129**(2):250-253

[80] Esmat A et al. Anti-inflammatory activity of Pistacia khinjuk in different experimental models: Isolation and characterization of its flavonoids and galloylated sugars. Journal of Medicinal Food. 2012;**15**(3):278-287

[81] Giner-Larza EM et al. Anti-inflammatory triterpenes from Pistacia terebinthus galls. Planta Medica. 2002;**68**(04):311-315

[82] Naouar MS et al. Preventive and curative effect of Pistacia lentiscus oil in experimental colitis. Biomedicine & Pharmacotherapy. 2016;**83**:577-583

[83] Paterniti I et al. The anti-inflammatory and antioxidant potential of pistachios (Pistacia vera L.) in vitro and in vivo. Nutrients. 2017;**9**(8):915

[84] Hernández-Alonso P et al. Beneficial effect of pistachio consumption on glucose metabolism, insulin resistance, inflammation, and related metabolic risk markers: A randomized clinical trial. Diabetes Care. 2014;**37**(11):3098-3105

[85] Kocyigit A, Koylu A, Keles H. Effects of pistachio nuts consumption on plasma lipid profile and oxidative status in healthy volunteers. Nutrition, metabolism and cardiovascular diseases. 2006;**16**(3):202-209

[86] Ostovan M et al. The anti-inflammatory effect of Pistacia lentiscus in a rat model of colitis. Journal of Inflammation Research. 2020:369-376

[87] Rahimi R et al. Efficacy of tricyclic antidepressants in irritable bowel syndrome: A meta-analysis. World Journal of Gastroenterology: WJG. 2009;**15**(13):1548

[88] Froushani SMA, Mashouri S. The beneficial effects of hypiran in ameliorating rat model of ulcerative colitis. Zahedan Journal of Research in Medical Sciences. 2018;**20**(1):e58919

[89] Khan H et al. Targeting NF-κB signaling pathway in cancer by dietary polyphenols. Critical Reviews in Food Science and Nutrition. 2020;**60**(16):2790-2800

[90] Carillon J et al. Superoxide dismutase administration, a potential therapy against oxidative stress related diseases: Several routes of supplementation and proposal of an original mechanism of action. Pharmaceutical Research. 2013;**30**(11):2718-2728

[91] Nuzzo D et al. Regular intake of pistachio mitigates the deleterious effects of a high fat-diet in the brain of obese mice. Antioxidants. 2020;**9**(4):317

[92] Zafar J et al. Biochemical and immunological implications of lutein and Zeaxanthin. International Journal of Molecular Sciences. 2021;**22**(20):10910

[93] Dendena B, Corsi S. Cashew, from seed to market: A review. Agronomy for Sustainable Development. 2014;**34**(4):753-772

[94] Oloso A, Clarke B. Some aspects of strength properties of cashew nuts. Journal of Agricultural Engineering Research. 1993;**55**(1):27-43

[95] Sharma P et al. Valorization of cashew nut processing residues for industrial applications. Industrial Crops and Products. 2020;**152**:112550

[96] Hamad FB, Mubofu EB. Potential biological applications of bio-based anacardic acids and their derivatives. International Journal of Molecular Sciences. 2015;**16**(4):8569-8590

[97] Siracusa R et al. The antioxidant and anti-inflammatory properties of *Anacardium occidentale L.* cashew nuts in a mouse model of colitis. Nutrients. 2020;**12**(3):834

[98] dos Santos AT et al. Potentialities of cashew nut (*Anacardium occidentale*) by-product for pharmaceutical applications: Extraction and purification technologies, safety, and anti-inflammatory and anti-arthritis activities. Revista Brasileira de Farmacognosia. 2020;**30**(5):652-666

[99] Menezes FNDD et al. Impact of cashew (*Anacardium occidentale L.*) by-product on composition and metabolic activity of human colonic microbiota in vitro indicates prebiotic

properties. Current Microbiology. 2021;**78**(6):2264-2274

[100] Medeiros-Linard CFB et al. Anacardic acids from cashew nuts prevent behavioral changes and oxidative stress induced by rotenone in a rat model of Parkinson's disease. Neurotoxicity Research. 2018;**34**(2):250-262

[101] Fusco R et al. The role of cashew (*Anacardium occidentale L.*) nuts on an experimental model of painful degenerative joint disease. Antioxidants. 2020;**9**(6):511

[102] Cordaro M et al. Cashew (*Anacardium occidentale L.*) nuts counteract oxidative stress and inflammation in an acute experimental model of carrageenan-induced paw edema. Antioxidants. 2020;**9**(8):660

[103] Gugliandolo E et al. Neuroprotective effect of artesunate in experimental model of traumatic brain injury. Frontiers in Neurology. 2018;**9**:590

[104] Di Paola D et al. Chronic exposure to Vinclozolin induced fibrosis, mitochondrial dysfunction, oxidative stress, and apoptosis in mice kidney. International Journal of Molecular Sciences. 2022;**23**(19):11296

[105] Fusco R et al. Consumption of *Anacardium occidentale L.*(cashew nuts) inhibits oxidative stress through modulation of the Nrf2/ HO− 1 and NF-kB pathways. Molecules. 2020;**25**(19):4426

[106] Kris-Etherton PM et al. The effects of nuts on coronary heart disease risk. Nutrition Reviews. 2001;**59**(4):103-111

[107] Olajide OA et al. Effects of Anacardium occidentale stem bark extract on in vivo inflammatory models. Journal of Ethnopharmacology. 2004;**95**(2-3):139-142

[108] Borges J. Cashew tree (*Anacardium occidentale*): Possible applications in dermatology. Clinics in Dermatology. 2021;**39**(3):493-495

[109] Al-Hazzani A et al. Formulation of cashew nut shell liquid (CSNL) nanoemulsion, a potent inhibitor of human MCF-7 breast cancer cell proliferation. Medicinal Chemistry Research. 2012;**21**(7):1384-1388

Chapter 3

Antioxidants Obtained from the Natural Sources: Importance in Human Health

Sushil S. Burle, Krishna R. Gupta, Swati N. Lade, Shyam W. Rangari and Milind J. Umekar

Abstract

Now a day the interest in natural and synthetic antioxidants is increasing very rapidly in functional food ingredients and dietary supplements. The differences between the number of free radicals and antioxidants are the main cause of the oxidative damage of lipids, proteins, and DNA. In this chapter, we are summarising the natural antioxidants which have been obtained from plants, animals, or microbial sources. Flavonoids are the most comprehensive antioxidant compounds which are obtained from natural sources. These flavonoids are reactive toward many radicals which are studied by many researchers under various experimental conditions and their structural activity relationships have been recognised. This chapter includes the various types of antioxidants obtained from natural sources and their impact on human health as pharmaceutical, nutraceutical, and phytoceuticals as well as their use in the treatment of various diseases along with the mechanism of action.

Keywords: free radical, natural antioxidants, phytoceuticals

1. Introduction

The antioxidant is defined as the any substance at very low concentration compared with that of an oxidizable substrate significantly which delays or inhibits oxidation of the substrate. According to the Halliwell and Gutteridge the antioxidants are the substance that prevents oxidative damage to a target molecules [1]. The antioxidant act as a oxidation inhibitors at very low concentration when people are using them to prevent the health damages ours due to the polluted plants and various factors which causes the illness in human beings [2]. For the survival of human beings the oxygen plays very important role under some situation it shows the deleterious effects on the human body. The negative effects of oxygen are due to the formation and activity of number of chemical compounds it knows as the reactive oxygen species (ROS). These ROS is collectively including both oxygen radicals and several non-radical oxidising agents that mostly take part in the intitation or propagation of chain reaction [3]. The reactive species are free radicals that represent a class of highly reactive intermediate chemical entities whose reactivity is derived from the presences of unpaired electron in the chemical formula structure. There are the two main major group in the living cells: enzymatic and non enzymatic antioxidants these enzymatic are again further divided into the primary and secondary enzymatic. The primary is composed of three important enzymes which prevents the formation and neutralisation of the free radicals by donating two electrons to reduces the peroxidase by forming selenols and also eliminates peroxidase as potential substrate for the fenton reaction catalase which turns hydrogen peroxide into water and molecular oxygen one of the most important and efficient antioxidants known today which turns hydrogen peroxide into water and molecular oxygen—one of the most important and efficient antioxidants known today, when just one molecule of catalase converts 6 billion molecules of hydrogen peroxide. The superoxide dismutase which changes the superoxide anions into hydrogen peroxide which is act as catalase.

1.1 Antioxidant

The antioxidant is the substances that prevent the oxidative damage in the body all the cell in the body requires the oxygen (O_2) for energy production and naturally produced free radical as a byproduct which causes damage. Antioxidants act as "free radical scavengers" and repair the damage done by free radicals. This term was used in late nineteen and early twenty centuries. The antioxidant molecules are capable of preventing the oxidation of other molecules. These are obtained from both naturally as well as synthetic source [4].

1.1.1 Types of antioxidant

Antioxidants are classified in two ways depending on their solubility one is hydrophilic which is soluble in water and other hydrophobic which is water-insoluble but soluble in lipids. The water-soluble antioxidant reacts with oxidant present in cell cytosol and blood plasma. On the other hand, the hydrophobic antioxidant prevents the cell membrane from lipid peroxidation. Traditionally these antioxidants are of two classes' primary or chain-breaking antioxidant and secondary or preventative antioxidant [5, 6].

Mechanisms of primary antioxidant as follows

$$L\bullet + AH \rightarrow LH + A\bullet \tag{1}$$

$$LO\bullet + AH \rightarrow LOH + A\bullet \tag{2}$$

$$LOO\bullet + AH \rightarrow LOOH + A\bullet \tag{3}$$

$$A\bullet + A\bullet \rightarrow AA \tag{4}$$

Where L• is a lipid radical, AH• inhibited antioxidant (**Figure 1**).

1.1.2 Use of Antioxidant

- They prevent the oxidative degradation of polymers like plastics, adhesives, and rubber which causes the loss of strength and flexibility in these materials [7].

- It used in neurodegenerative diseases like Parkinsonism, Alzheimer and amyotrophic sclerosis diseases treatment.

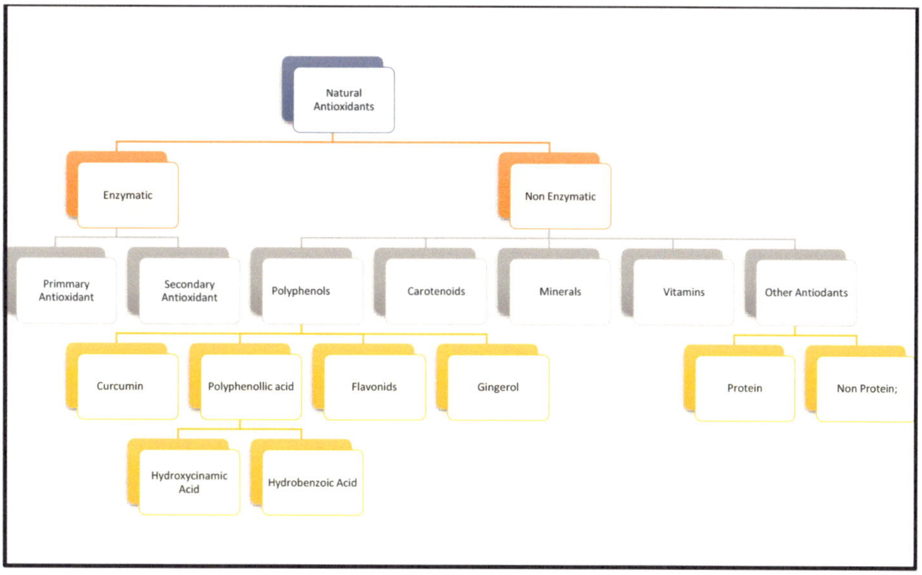

Figure 1.
Classification of antioxidants found in natural sources.

- They are used in the treatment of various brain injury, sodium thiopental, superoxide dismutase mimetic and propofol is used for the treatment of reperfusion injury and trauma.

- Vitamins like E and C also used as an antioxidant out of which Vit. E it helps for the protection of cells and tissues from lipid peroxidative damage caused due to free radicals While Vit. C used as a supplement by inactivating free radicals produced through normal cellular activity and stressors

- An antioxidant like ascorbic acid, carotenoids, amino acids, peptides, flavonoids and other phenolic compounds might also play an important role in physiological and dietary antioxidants.

2. Free radicals

These are highly reactive chemical species. These reactive oxygen species generated in phagocytosis, mitochondrial respiratory chain, fertilisation, and arachidonic acid metabolism. These free radicals are a species which contains an unpaired electron in an atomic orbital. They either donate an electron or extract an electron from other molecules. [8] Chain reactions of these radicals are dividing into three parts viz., Initiation, Propagation, and Termination.

In initiation reaction a net increase in the number of free radicals, while in propagation reaction are those reactions involving free radicals in which the total number of free radicals are same. Further in termination reaction, the net reduction in the number of free radicals takes place. Two free radicals combine to form a more stable species.

2.1 Types of free radicals

As a free radical originated from oxygen atom hence it is called as a reactive oxygen species (ROS) this ROS include a superoxide (O_2^-), Hydroxyl (OH), hydrogen peroxide (H_2O_2), peroxyl (ROO), nitric oxide (NO) and alkoxy (RO) until completely reduced to water. The large no superoxides are produced in mitochondrial and microsomal electron chain. On the other hand, the cytochrome oxidase is retained by the moderately reduced oxygen intermediated bound to its active site. All other elements of mitochondrial respiratory chain transfer the electron directly to oxygen and not preserve the reduced oxygen intermediate in the active site [9].

2.1.1 Super oxide ion

This is an oxygen molecule which contains extra electron. This free radical causes damage to DNA, Mitochondria. The body can neutralise the superoxide radical by producing Superoxide dismutase.

2.1.2 Hydroxyl radical

It produced by the reduction of an oxygen molecule in electron transport chain. These hydroxyls radical are highly reactive in nature and cannot eliminate by an enzymatic reaction. As it is more reactive it damages most of the organic molecules like DNA, Lipid, Carbohydrate, and proteins.

2.1.3 Nitrogen species

These are also called reactive nitrogen species. The metals like copper and iron have many numbers of unpaired electrons which can also act as free radicals. These metals have not strong affinity of the electron but can effortlessly accept and donate electrons.

2.1.4 Oxygen radical

The radical are mostly formed by the immune system. These generally cause the oxidation of cholesterol and LDL.

2.2 Free radical and biology

It helps for intracellular killing of bacteria by phagocyte cells such as macrophages and granulocytes.

Superoxide and Hydroxyl radical are most important radical due to their reactivity. These radicals take part in unwanted side reaction this side reaction results in cell damage. As it concentration increase it may lead to cell injury and finally death of the cell. This action is responsible for various disease conditions like myocardial infarction, stroke, cancer, diabetes etc. Few symptoms of ageing like atherosclerosis are also recognised to free radical-induced oxidation of numerous chemicals. Apart from this disease it may also involve in Parkinson's disease, senile deafness caused due to drugs, Alzheimer disease, and schizophrenia [10].

2.2.1 Sources of free radicals

The free radicals are the byproduct of cellular processes and these are produced from metal cofactors by spontaneous catalyzation. Nowadays the environmental sources act as a measured source of free radicals as the radiation is increasing largely around the city are also responsible for the radiation sources includes the mobile phone, X-ray, computer and television set etc. apart from this mental stress is also one of the sources of free radical generation [11].

3. Oxidation

The utilisation of oxygen for generation of energy by metabolism of food nutrients is most important part for survival of all living beings. This oxygen is extremely reactive atom which is useful for the destruction of singlet oxygen, hydroperoxyl radical, superoxide radical, organic peroxides, nitric oxide, peroxynitrite and triplet oxygen. The oxygen which is consumed during the breathing it produces free radical production and apart from this environmental factors such as smoke, pollutants, and certain chemicals also contribute to their formation. This leads to the starting of chain reactions in cells and it can cause damage or death to the cell [12]. The Mechanisms with antioxidant properties were purposefully included to fatty meals in order to disrupt chain processes by substituting free radical intermediates and inhibiting other oxidation reactions. Antioxidants, such as ascorbic acid, thols, and polyphenols, help to neutralise free radicals by oxidising themselves and acting as reducing agents. In the packaged food, the antioxidant is added separately to prevent the generation of free radicals and to ensure food safety.

The various properties of radicals like accepting or donating an electron from other molecules which leads to the stabilising the free radical at the beginning but stats to produces another process which leads to the damage of biological molecules like Proteins Carbohydrates lipids and DNA which leads to the homeostatic disruption [13].

3.1 Concept of oxidative stress

The Oxidative stress explain the relation between the disease and free radicals. The normal healthy human body, generates the pro-oxidants in the form of reactive nitrogen species and reactive oxygen species and reactive nitrogen species are useful for the maintains of all antioxidant level. This delicately maintained balance is shifted in favour of pro-oxidants whenever it is exposed to various environmental, physico-chemical, and pathological agents such as cigarette smoking, atmospheric pollutants, radiation UV rays, toxic chemicals, overnutrition, and advanced glycation end products (AGEs) in diabetes. It has been linked to the genesis of over 100 human illnesses as well as the ageing process [5].

3.2 Molecular damage induced by free radicals

Various biological molecules present in our body are attacked by the various free radicals which leads to the impairment of cell functions and damaged the molecules produces the diseased states.

3.3 Lipids and lipid peroxidation

The lipids present in membrane are highly susceptible to free radical damage when this lipid reacted with free radicals can undergo highly damaging chain reaction of lipid peroxidation leading to both direct and indirect effects. The lipid peroxidation mediated by the free radical process in this the intitation caused by the species attack which abstract a hydrogen atom from the methylene group which leave an unpaired electron on the carbon atom. Molecular rearrangement stabilises the resulting carbon radical to form a conjugated diene, which can then combine with an oxygen molecule to form a lipid peroxyl radical. These radicals can then extract hydrogen atoms from additional lipid molecules to generate lipid hydroperoxides, further propagating lipid peroxidation. A variety of responses can end the peroxidation process. The most important one involves the reactivity of LOO• or lipid radical (L•) with an antioxidant molecule such as vitamin E or -tocopherol (-TOH), resulting in a more stable tocopherol phenoxyl radical that is not engaged in further chain reactions. Other cellular antioxidants, such as vitamin C or GSH.

Many toxicologically interesting chemicals are produced during the lipid peroxidation process, including malondialdehyde, 4-hydroxynonenal, and other 2-alkenals. Isoprostanes are unique products of arachidonic acid lipid peroxidation, and procedures such as mass spectrometry and ELISA-assay kits have recently become available to identify isoprostanes [14, 15].

3.4 Proteins

Protein oxidation by ROS/RNS can result in the formation of both stable and reactive molecules, such as protein hydroperoxides, which can generate additional radicals when they interact with transition metal ions.

Although the majority of oxidised proteins that are functionally inactive are quickly removed, some can accumulate over time and contribute to the damage associated with ageing as well as a variety of diseases. Lipofuscin, a peroxidized lipid and protein aggregation, forms in the lysosomes of aged cells and Alzheimer's disease brain cells [16].

3.5 Carbohydrates

Many toxicologically interesting chemicals are produced during the lipid peroxidation process, including malondialdehyde, 4-hydroxynonenal, and other 2-alkenals. Isoprostanes are unique products of arachidonic acid lipid peroxidation, and procedures such as mass spectrometry and ELISA-assay kits have recently become available to identify isoprostanes [13].

3.6 DNA

The interaction of DNA with ROS or RNS causes oxidative damage to the DNA. •OH, eaq-, and H• free radicals react with DNA by adding to bases or removing hydrogen atoms from the sugar moiety. •OH attacks the C4—C5 double bond of pyrimidine, resulting in a variety of oxidative pyrimidine damage products such as thymine glycol, uracil glycol, urea residue, 5-hydroxydeoxyuridine, 5-hydroxydeoxycytidine, hydantoin, and others. Similarly, when •OH reacts with purines, it produces 8-hydroxydeoxyguanosine (8-OHdG), 8-hydroxydeoxyadenosine, formamidopyrimidines, and other unidentified purine oxidative products. Several repair pathways are involved in the repair of DNA damage [9, 17]. 8-OHdG has been linked to cancer and is regarded as a trustworthy marker for oxidative DNA damage.

3.7 Significance of antioxidants in relation to disease

Zinc is a trace element that functions as a cofactor for approximately 200 human enzymes, including the cytoplasmic antioxidant Cu-Zn SOD, an isoenzyme of SOD found mostly in the cytosol. Selenium, a trace element, also serves as a cofactor for glutathione peroxidase. Vitamin E and tocotrienols (produced from palm oil) are powerful lipid-soluble antioxidants that act as a "chain breaker" during lipid peroxidation in cell membranes and other lipid particles like LDL [18, 19].

Vitamin E is considered the "gold standard antioxidant" against which other antioxidant-containing compounds are tested, particularly in terms of biological activity and therapeutic importance. The recommended daily intake varies from 400 to 800 IU. Ascorbic acid (vitamin C) is a free radical scavenger that is water soluble. The daily suggested dose is 60 mg. Aside from these carotenoids, other carotenoids such as beta-carotene, lycopene, lutein, and others function as important antioxidants, quenching 1O2 and ROO•. Flavonoids, which are typically present in plants as colouring pigments, can act as powerful antioxidants at varying concentrations [5, 18, 19].

3.8 Antioxidants and human disease prevention

Several epidemiological studies have discovered an inverse association between established antioxidants/phytonutrient levels in tissue/blood samples and the occurrence of cardiovascular disease, cancer, or mortality from these diseases. A recent meta-analysis, however, reveals that supplementing with largely single antioxidants may not be as beneficial. A point of view that contradicts preclinical and epidemiological data on the use of antioxidant-rich foods. Based on the majority of epidemiological and casecontrol studies, recommendations for daily dietary intake of several well-known antioxidants, such as vitamin E and C, as well as others, were produced. Because of dietary variances, antioxidant requirements in India differ from those in industrialised western nations. There are also a variety of antioxidant-rich dietary supplements that have been studied for effectiveness. Many laboratories in India are researching the antioxidant impact of plant chemicals, primarily sourced from natural sources, that can protect against such damage. Carotenoids, curcumin from turmeric, flavonoids, caffeine (found in coffee, tea, and other beverages), orientin, vicenin, glabridin, glycyrrhizin, emblicanin, punigluconin, pedunculagin, 2-hydroxy-4-methoxy benzoic acid, dehydrozingerone, picroliv, withaferin, yakuchinone, gingerol, chlorogenic acid, van (a water-soluble analogue of chlorophyll) [20].

3.9 Newer therapeutic approaches using antioxidants

Over the last three decades, antioxidant-based drugs/formulations for the prevention and treatment of complicated illnesses such as atherosclerosis, stroke, diabetes, Alzheimer's disease (AD), Parkinson's disease, cancer, and others have emerged. The significance of dietary antioxidants in the prevention of numerous human illnesses, including cancer, atherosclerosis, stroke, rheumatoid arthritis, neurodegeneration, and diabetes, has been substantially influenced by free radical theory. Dietary antioxidants may offer intriguing therapeutic potential in delaying the onset of Alzheimer's disease and its associated consequences in the elderly population. There are two neuroprotective clinical studies with antioxidants available: the Deprenyl and tocopherol antioxidant treatment of Parkinson's research. India can manufacture world-class products by combining traditional knowledge and contemporary science. As a result, it has launched a fast-track effort to develop novel pharmaceuticals by expanding on established therapies and examining the country's various plant and microbial sources. This initiative is not only the world's largest undertaking of its sort in terms of scale, variety, and access to talent and resources, but it is also unique [21].

3.10 Ayurveda, antioxidants and therapeutics

Ayurvedic medications are often tailored to an individual's constitution using a unique holistic approach. Ayurvedic Indian and traditional Chinese systems are living 'great traditions,' and they play major roles in the bioprospecting of novel medications from medicinal plants, which are also high in antioxiodants. According to current estimates, around 80% of people in underdeveloped nations still rely on traditional medicine, which is mostly focused on diverse kinds of plants and animals, for their main treatment. Ayurveda is one of the most ancient and still extensively practised systems in India.

4. Sources of antioxidants, phytonutrients and functional foods

Natural substances, particularly those originating from food sources, contain a considerable amount of antioxidants. Some drinks, such as tea, are also high in antioxidants. A increasing amount of research shows that moderate tea drinking may protect against several types of cancer, cardiovascular disease, kidney stone development, bacterial infections, and dental cavities. Tea is notably high in catechins, the most abundant of which is epigallocatechin gallate (EGCG) [9, 15].

4.1 Indian medicinal plants

Aside from food sources, Indian medicinal plants contain antioxidants, such as: (with common/ayurvedic names in brackets) *Aegle marmelos* (Bengal quince, Bel), *Allium cepa* (Onion), *Allium sativum* (Garlic, Lahsuna), *Aloe vera* (Indian aloe, Ghritkumari), Amomum subulatum (Greater cardamom, Bari elachi), *Asparagus racemosus* (Shatavari), *Azadirachta indica* (Neem, Nimba) [15].

4.2 Synthetic antioxidants

Due to availability and Importance, synthetic antioxidants are commonly employed as food additives to prevent rancidification. In edible vegetable oil and cosmetics, synthetic antioxidants such as butylated hydroxyanisole, tertiary butyl hydroquinone, 2,4,5-trihydroxybutyrophenone, octyl gallate, propyl gallate, 4-hexylresorcinol and nordihydroguaiaretic acid and are utilised [22, 23]. As synthetic phenolic antioxidants, propyl gallate and butylated hydroxyanisole shown greater chemical activity in reducing chain start of unsaturated fatty acid oxidation. Although antioxidants are effective in protecting product quality during food distribution, excessive amounts of antioxidants added to food may generate toxicities or mutagenicities, putting people's health at risk. The antioxidant will be chosen based on the kind of fat and oil in the diet. Butylated hydroxyanisole and butylated hydroxytoluene dissolve in most fats and oils, however they work best in animal fats. When consumed in conjunction with other meals, it has a more favourable impact than when used alone. Propyl gallate, on the other hand, which is not easily soluble, is more effective in vegetable oils than butylated hydroxyanisole and butylated hydroxytoluene, tertiary butyl hydroquinone is the most efficient antioxidant for slowing oxidation in unsaturated fats such as vegetable oils. Lower quantities of tertiary butyl hydroquinone can achieve oxidative stability than other synthetic antioxidants [24].

4.3 Natural and synthetic antioxidants

Natural and synthetic antioxidants are utilised as food additives in the food business to help extend the shelf life and appearance of various foods. Synthetic phenolic antioxidants (butylated hydroxyanisole, propyl gallate and butylated hydroxytoluene [BHT]) substantially suppress oxidation; for example, chelating compounds like Metals can be bound by ethylene diamine tetraacetic acid (EDTA), reducing their contribution to the process. Antioxidants are also naturally contained in many foods and are essential for human health. They contain vitamins C and E, which may be found in fruits and vegetables and seeds and nuts, respectively. Antioxidants can be found in vitamins (ascorbic acid and -tocopherol), herbs and spices (rosemary, thyme, oregano, sage, basil, pepper, clove, cinnamon, and nutmeg), and plant extracts (tea and grapeseed). While synthetic antioxidants (such as butylated hydroxytoluene and butylated hydroxyanisole) are commonly used to protect the quality of ready-to-eat food items, public concern about their safety has prompted the food industry to explore natural antioxidants. Some people's health issues have been induced by synthetic antioxidants. Butylated hydroxyanisole, butylated hydroxytoluene, and tertiary butyl hydroquinone appear to be the most troublesome antioxidants, with gallates coming in second position and having been utilised in food items with certain limits since the late 1950s. TBHQ is a relatively recent addition to the list of antioxidants permitted in food; it was approved for use as an antioxidant in food in Europe in 2004. Butylated hydroxyanisole, butylated hydroxytoluene, and tertiary butyl hydroquinone are typically found in meals containing oil and fat. Their activity is comparable to that of Vitamin E, which is utilised as an alternative antioxidant in some of the same products. These antioxidants may exist alone in a diet, but they are frequently combined with other molecules that have antioxidant action, such as phosphoric acid, propyl gallate, citric acid, and ascorbic acid [17, 25].

4.4 Health concerns of synthetic antioxidants

While the bulk of studies have been conducted on animals, there is still a substantial body of research that has discovered issues with synthetic antioxidants in humans [26–28]. The **Table 1** below covers some of the human health concerns associated with butylated hydroxyanisole, butylated hydroxytoluene, and tertiary butyl hydroquinone. In one study, seven people reported symptoms such as vasomotor rhinitis, headache, flushing, asthma, conjunctival suffusion, dull retrosternal (behind the breastbone) pain radiating to the back, diaphoresis (excessive sweating), or somnolence after being exposed to butylated hydroxyanisole and butylated hydroxytoluene (sleepiness). In a subsequent trial looking for cross-reactivity with aspirin, they

Rhinitis
Angioedema
Asthma
Dermatitis
Eye Problems
Joints paints

Table 1.
Effect of butylated hydroxy anisole, butylated hydroxytoluene, and tertiary butyl hydroquinone on human health.

discovered twenty-one patients who were intolerant to butylated hydroxyanisole and butylated hydroxytoluene. A handful of persons have developed dermatitis after being exposed to these synthetic antioxidants [29]. In one investigation, tertiary butyl hydroquinone in a hair colour produced contact dermatitis, and cross sensitization with butylated hydroxyanisole and butylated hydroxytoluene was seen. According to the US Department of Health and Human Services' Carcinogens report, butylated hydroxyanisole is "reasonably expected to be a human carcinogen based on substantial evidence of carcinogenicity in experimental animals." There is also worry that "butylated hydroxytoluene. May change to other carcinogenic chemicals in the human body." One conversion product of butylated hydroxytoluene (the hydroperoxide form, for example) has been demonstrated to disrupt chemical signals conveyed from cell to cell.

5. Health issues related to the antioxidant

5.1 Neurodegenerative disorders

Because of the high amount of lipids, particularly polyunsaturated fatty acids, nervous tissue, including the brain, is very sensitive to free radical damage. Biochemical and histological investigations in Alzheimer's disease have revealed elevated levels of oxidative stress and membrane damage. Peroxidation of Lipids Changes in antioxidant enzyme levels in neurons of Alzheimer's disease patients, such as catalase and CuZn- and Mn-SOD, are associated with increasing stress. Protein oxidation, protein nitration, and lipid peroxidation have all increased. They are seen in neurofibrillary tangles and neuritic plaques. Increased levels of peroxidation products such as 4-hydroxynonenal (4-HNE) in the cerebral fluid of Alzheimer's disease patients suggest widespread lipid peroxidation. Iron ($Fe2+$) is thought to play a role in enhanced lipid peroxidation in Alzheimer's disease. Multiple pathways, including impairment of the activity of membrane ion-motive ATPases ($Na+/K+$ -ATPase and $Ca2+$ -ATPase), glucose transporters, and glutamate transporters, may contribute to neuronal mortality in Alzheimer's disease. Lipid peroxidation produces the aldehyde 4-HNE, which appears to play a key role in the neurotoxic effects of amyloid [14].

5.2 Free radicals, diabetes and ages

Experimental data suggests that free radicals have a role in the establishment of diabetes and, more crucially, the development of diabetic complications [30]. The

Free radical scavengers are useful in avoiding experimental diabetes in animal models and in type 1 (IDDM) and type 2 (NIDDM) patients, as well as in lowering the severity of diabetic sequelae. Persistent hyperglycemia in diabetic individuals causes oxidative stress due to

a. glucose autooxidation;

b. non-enzymatic glycosylation;

c. the polyol pathway.

The spontaneous reduction of molecular oxygen to superoxide and hydroxyl radicals, which are extremely reactive and interact with all biomolecules, occurs during glucose auto-oxidation. In addition, they hasten the production of advanced glycation end products (AGEs). Pyrroles and imidazoles, for example, tend to accumulate in tissue. Crosslinking AGE-protein with other macromolecules in tissues causes cell and tissue function problems. The third route by which free radicals are created in tissues is the polyol pathway [31]. This route deletes 30 lots of NADPH, which reduces the production of antioxidants like glutathione. The ability of antioxidant enzymes is also diminished as a result of protein glycation. In endothelial cells, free radicals react with nitric oxide, resulting in a reduction of vasodilation function. Long-lived structural proteins, collagen and elastin, undergo non-enzymatic crosslinking throughout life and in diabetics [32]. This abnormal protein crosslinking is mediated by AGEs generated by nonenzymatic glycosylation of proteins by glucose.

5.3 Free radical damage to DNA and cancer

DNA is a common site of free radical damage. Strand breakage (single or double strand breaks), different forms of base damage giving products such as 8-hydroxyguanosine, thymine glycol, or abasic sites, damage to deoxyribose sugar, and DNA protein cross linkages are among the numerous types of damages generated. These damages can cause heritable changes in the DNA, which can lead to cancer in somatic cells or foetal abnormalities in germ cells. The interaction of free radicals with tumour suppressor genes and proto-oncogenes suggests that they have a role in the genesis of several human malignancies [9]. Cancer occurs as a result of a series of genetic alterations. Tobacco smoking and chewing, UV rays from sunshine, radiation, viruses, chemical contaminants, and other factors can all be initiating agents. Hormones are examples of promoting agents (androgens for prostate cancer, estrogens for breast cancer and ovarian cancer). Inflammation causes the production of iNOS (inducible nitric oxide synthase), as well as COX and LOX. These are capable of initiating carcinogenesis. Experimental and epidemiological evidence show that a number of dietary components can serve as antioxidants, inhibiting cancer formation and lowering cancer risk. Vitamins A, C, E, beta-carotene, and micronutrients such as antioxidants and anticarcinogens are among them [33, 34]. The recent studied the processes behind dietary phytochemical anticancer effects. Chemopreventive phytochemicals have the ability to prevent or reverse the promotion stage of multistep carcinogenesis. They can also prevent or slow the growth of precancerous cells into malignant cells. Many of the molecular changes linked with carcinogenesis occur in cell-signalling pathways that control cell proliferation and differentiation. The family of mitogen activated protein kinases is a key component of the intracellular signalling network that maintains homeostasis (MAPKs). With the activation of the transcription factors NF-B and AP1, several intracellular signal-transduction pathways converge. These variables are prominent targets of several types of chemopreventive phytochemicals because they mediate the pleiotropic effects of both external and internal stimuli in the cellular-signalling cascades [34]. Curcumin, the active ingredient of *Curcuma longa* (Turmeric, Haldi), inhibits the production of COX2, LOX, iNOS, MMP-9, TNF, chemokines, and other cell-surface adhesion molecules, as well as cyclin D1. Human clinical studies have demonstrated that curcumin at dosages up to 10 g/day is safe and can inhibit tumour start, promotion, and metastasis. Many Long-term prospective clinical investigations are required to validate the hypothesis.

5.4 Mitochondria, oxidative protein damage and proteomics

Proteomic technologies' fast advancement and application to large-scale investigations of protein-protein interactions and protein expression patterns imply that these approaches are ideally suited to give the molecular insights required to completely comprehend oxidative harm caused by free radicals [35]. The very significant progress has been made in identifying specific proteins that are confined to the mitochondria throughout the previous two decades. Specifically, the 100 or more subunits that make up the five complexes of the electron transport chain (ETC). Several groups have recently begun to tackle the bigger task of establishing the content of complete mitochondrial proteomes from a variety of key model systems as well as human tissues, utilising contemporary mass spectrometry (MS)-based proteomic methods. Gibson and colleagues identified 684 distinct proteins from the combined peptide data acquired from over 100,000 mass spectra generated by MALDI-MS and high performance liquid chromatography (HPLC) MS/MS analysis using mitochondria isolated from human heart. These findings have been included into 'MitoProteome,' a publicly available database for the human heart mitochondrial proteome.

5.5 Free radicals and ageing

Ageing is caused by mitochondrial ROS generation and oxidative damage to mitochondrial DNA. Increased lipid peroxidation in cellular membranes as a result of oxidative stress results in fatty acid unsaturation. According to the most current study on 'free radicals and ageing, Caloric restriction (CR) is the only known experimental alteration that reduces the rate of mammalian ageing, and it has multiple beneficial impacts on rodent and likely human brains. Calorie-restricted mitochondria, like those seen in long-lived animal species, effectively inhibit ROS generation with pyruvate and malate at complex I. The oxygen consumption of the mitochondria stays same, while the free radical leak from the electron transport chain is reduced in CR. Many researchers discovered that increasing the number of oxidative stress defence systems may increase an organism's health span. Arking's group's work on artificial selection in flies resulted in organisms with much higher levels of oxidative stress tolerance and more efficient mitochondria. Indeed, lower ROS formation and increased ROS removal resulted in less oxidative damage and a later start of senescence in those flies. However, using genetic engineering techniques to introduce additional copies of these oxidative stress-resistance genes into mice did not result in a longer lifetime.

6. Conclusion

Natural ingredients are becoming increasingly popular these days. Food antioxidants and preservatives may cause lipid peroxidation and deterioration of taste and quality. Free radicals have been linked to the genesis of a wide range of important illnesses. They can cause several important biological molecules to lose shape and function. Such unfavourable alterations in the body might result in illness. Antioxidants can guard against the damage caused by free radicals at various levels of action. Plants' dietary and other components are rich in antioxidants. The link between free radicals, antioxidants, and the function of numerous organs and organ systems is extremely complicated, and the discovery of 'redox signalling' marks a watershed moment in this critical interaction. Recent research has focused on several ways for protecting vital tissues and organs from oxidative damage caused by free radicals. Many unique techniques have been developed, and substantial discoveries have been achieved in recent years. Natural antioxidants are abundant in the traditional Indian food, spices, and medicinal herbs. Increased consumption of foods with functional properties, such as high levels of antioxidants in functional foods, is one method that is gaining traction in advanced nations and is making an appearance in our country.

This chapter focuses on an overview of the potentials of numerous sources with appropriate antioxidant potential, as well as their influence on human health. Because 70–80% of the world's population cannot afford contemporary supplements and treatments, this chapter illustrates that individuals may priorities their food habits depending on the antioxidant capacity and cost-effectiveness of the accessible supply.

Conflict of interest

None.

Author details

Sushil S. Burle, Krishna R. Gupta*, Swati N. Lade, Shyam W. Rangari and Milind J. Umekar
Smt. Kishoritai Bhoyar College of Pharmacy, New Kamptee, Nagpur, India

*Address all correspondence to: krg1903@gmail.com

References

[1] Hamad AMA. Some natural antioxidants sources from foods and tree barks. International Journal of Scientific and Technology Research. 2019;**8**(6):93-98

[2] Shebis Y, Iluz D, Kinel-Tahan Y, et al. Natural antioxidants: Function and sources. FNS. 2013;**04**:643-649

[3] Shiv kumar. Free radicals and antioxidant: Human and food system. Applied Science Research. 2011;**2**: 129-135

[4] Mattill HA. Antioxidants. Annual Review of Biochemistry. 1947;**16**: 177-192. DOI: 10.1146/annurev.bi.16.070147.001141

[5] Sies H. Oxidative stress: Oxidants and antioxidants. Experimental Physiology. 1997;**82**(2):291-295. DOI: 10.1113/expphysiol.1997.sp004024

[6] Madhavi DL, Deshpande SS, Salunkhe DK. Introduction. In: Food Antioxidants: Technological, Toxicological, and Health Perspectives. New York, NY: Marcel Dekker, Inc.; 1996. pp. 1-4

[7] Melton SL. Vitamin E. In: Xiong YL, Chi-Tang H, Shahidi F, editors. Quality Attributes of Muscle Foods. Boston, MA: Springer; 1999. DOI: 10.1007/978-1-4615-4731-0_3

[8] Hemnani T, Parihar MS. Reactive oxygen species and oxidative DNA damage. Indian Journal of Physiology and Pharmacology. 1998;**42**(4):440-452

[9] Halliwell B, Gutteridge JMC. Free Radicals in Biology and Medicine. New York: Oxford University Press; 1999. pp. 1-897

[10] Tenpe CR, Aman U, Sushil B, Yeole PG. In vitro antioxidant and preliminary hepatoprotective activity of oroxylum indicum vent leaf extracts. Pharmacologyonline. 2009;**1**:35-43

[11] Gandhi V, Burle S, Kosalge S. Stem cell therapy for Parkinson's disease: A review. PharmaTutor. 2018; **6**(6):1-8

[12] Srinivasan O, Parkin KL, Fennema O, editors. Fennema's Food Chemistry. 4th ed. Boca Raton, Fla: CRC Press; 2008. p. 1144

[13] Burle S, Samanta S. Insilico design, synthesis of hybrid taurine amino acid and peptide analogues for studies on antioxidant and hepatoprotective activity. Indian Journal of Pharmaceutical Education and Research. 2017;**51**(2):S98-S109

[14] Yoshikawa T, Toyokuni S, Yamamoto Y, Naito Y, editors. Free Radicals in Chemistry Biology and Medicine. London: OICA International; 2000

[15] Devasagayam TPA, Boloor KK, Ramsarma T. Methods for estimating lipid peroxidation: Analysis of merits and demerits (minireview). Indian Journal of Biochemistry & Biophysics. 2003;**40**:300-308

[16] Stadtman ER. Protein oxidation and aging. Science. 1992;**257**(5074): 1220-1224. DOI: 10.1126/science.1355616

[17] Roman M, Jitaru P, Barbante C. Selenium biochemistry and its role for human health. Metallomics. 2014;**6**(1): 25-54

[18] Packer L, Ong ASH, editors. Biological Oxidants and Antioxidants: Molecular Mechanisms and Health Effects. Champaign: AOCS Press; 1998

[19] Kagan VE, Kisin ER, Kawai K, et al. Towards mechanism based antioxidant interventions. Annals of the New York Academy of Sciences. 2002;**959**:188-198

[20] Vivekananthan DP, Penn MS, Sapp SK, et al. Use of antioxidant vitamins for the prevention of cardiovascular disease: Metaanalysis of randomized trials. The Lancet. 2003;**361**: 2017-2023

[21] Jayaraman KS. Technology, tradition unite India's drug discovery scheme. Nature Medicine. 2003;**9**:982

[22] Guo L, Xie MY, Yan AP, Wan YQ, Wu YM. Simultaneous determination of five synthetic antioxidants in edible vegetable oil by GC–MS. Analytical and Bioanalytical Chemistry. 2006;**386**(6): 1881-1887

[23] Nazni P, Dharmaligam R. Isolation and separation of phenolic compound from coriander flowers. International Journal of Agricultural and Food Science. 2013;**4**(1):13-21

[24] Mandal S, Yadav S, Yadav S, Nema RK. Antioxidant a review. Journal of Chemical and Pharmaceutical Research. 2009;**1**(1):102-104

[25] Murthy KNC. Evaluation of antioxidant activity of pomegranate (Punicagranatum) and grapes (Vitis vinifera), [thesis] Rajeev Gandhi Univ. of Health Science, India. 2001

[26] Liu T, Stern A, Roberts LJ. The isoprostanes: Novel prostangland in-like products of the free radical catalyzed peroxidation of arachidonic acid. Journal of Biomedical Science. 1999;**6**:226-235

[27] Valko M, Leibfritz D, Moncol J, Cronin MTD, Mazur M, Telser J. Free radicals and antioxidants in normal physiological functions and human disease. The International Journal of Biochemistry and Cell Biology. 2007;**39**: 44-84

[28] Burle SS, Lade SN, Kosalge SB. Recents trends of hepatoprotective medicine. Enzyme;**1**:2

[29] Le Coz CJ, Schneider GA. Contact dermatitis from tertiary butylhydroquinone in a hair dye with cross sensitivity to BHA and BHT. Contact Dermatitis. 1987;**17**:257-258

[30] Lipinski B. Pathophysiology of oxidative stress in diabetes mellitus. Journal of Diabetes and its Complications. 2001;**15**:203-210

[31] Glugliano D, Cerriello A, Paolisso G. Diabetes mellitus, hypertension and cardiovascular disease: Which role for oxidative stress. Metabolism. 1995;**44**: 363-368

[32] Vasan S, Foiles P, Founds H. Therapeutic potential of breakers of advanced glycation end products-protein crosslinks. Archives of Biochemistry and Biophysics. 2003;**419**: 89-96

[33] Croce CM. How can we prevent cancer? Proceedings of the National Academy of Sciences of the United States of America. 2001;**98**:10986-10988

[34] Surh YJ. Cancer chemoprevention with dietary phytochemicals. Nature Reviews. Cancer. 2003;**3**:768-780

[35] Gibson BW. Exploiting proteomics in the discovery of drugs that target oxidative damage. Science. 2004;**304**: 176-177

Section 2

Sources of Natural Antioxidants

Chapter 4

Congolese Traditional Foods as Sources of Antioxidant Nutrients for Disease Prevention

Théophile Mbemba Fundu, Paulin Mutwale Kapepula, Jean Paul Nzundu Mbo, Justin Mboloko Esimo and Nadège Ngombe Kabamba

Abstract

Oxidative stress, characterized by excessive production of reactive species, is involved in several chronic diseases such as cardiovascular, chronic obstructive pulmonary, sickle cell, chronic kidney, neurodegenerative, and cancer. The negative impact of ROS and RNS, produced by endogenous and exogenous processes, is neutralized by antioxidant defenses. Given the importance of oxidative stress to human health, the use of antioxidants as therapy directs medical research toward the specificity of antioxidants causing each disease. Fruits and vegetables contain antioxidants, such as nutraceuticals, pharmaceuticals, and phytoceuticals, the consumption of which reduces the risk of developing chronic diseases. Flora of African countries is endowed with plant species that would make a putative source for new antioxidants. This article reports antioxidant activities of traditional foods from Democratic Republic of the Congo. Further studies are needed to ensure mechanisms of their functionality in the human body.

Keywords: antioxidants, Congolese diet, insects, oxidative stress, phytochemicals, reactive oxygen species, selenium, vegetables

1. Introduction

Oxygen metabolism, physiologically and regularly, produces small amounts of reactive oxygen species (ROS) to serve as an essential signaling mechanism for the maintenance of homeostasis and redox reactions in the cell [1]. Highly reactive ROS, associated with inflammation, cause tissue damage against which the cells of the human body protect themselves by various free radical defense mechanisms. However, when ROS levels are high due to an imbalance between their production and antioxidant defense mechanisms, oxidative stress occurs [2]; a situation where the cell no longer controls the excessive presence of radical's toxic oxygen, responsible for genomic and metabolic modifications, which favor the development of several diseases, in particular diabetes, cardiovascular diseases, cancer, respiratory and rheumatic diseases, and endometriosis [3]. Endogenous antioxidants and the wide

IntechOpen

variety of antioxidants in the diet, once present in all compartments of the organism, are involved in the protection of membranes and intra and extracellular environments against free radicals, and therefore against the diseases for which they are responsible. The objective of this review was to provide the therapeutic potential of Congolese traditional foods with antioxidant capacities useful in the management of various pathologies associated with oxidative damage.

2. Oxygen and ROS

Oxygen, essential for life, can also become a source of toxicity and cell degeneration. Indeed, at the level of the electron transport chain, oxygen undergoes a tetravalent reduction, which transforms it into water-generating ATP. During this process, 2% of the oxygen escapes and undergoes a monovalent reduction of one electron at ubiquinone producing the superoxide radical ($\bullet O_2^-$) with an unpaired electron on the outer shell, which is seeking to return immediately to a stable state by donating an electron or taking one from another molecule, finds itself in an energy instability that gives it its particular reactivity with respect to other atoms or molecules [4]. O_2^- can also be produced from NADH-dehydrogenase located in the inner mitochondrial membrane or from NADPH oxidase present in vascular endothelial cells [5]; it can also result from the auto-oxidation of neurotransmitters such as adrenaline, noradrenaline, dopamine, cysteine thiols, and reduced coenzymes, such as FADH2, as well as the detoxification of toxic pollutants and drugs, by the system of cytochromes P450 present in the endoplasmic reticulum [6]. The neutrophil respiratory burst and xanthine oxidase, NO synthase, and eicosanoids are also cellular sources of superoxide anion production [7]. Having a certain toxicity and being at a low concentration, the superoxide radical is eliminated by superoxyde dismutase (SOD), generating hydrogen peroxide (H_2O_2), which can also be produced by a bielectronic reduction of oxygen in the presence of oxidases of peroxisomes or by oxidative deamination of certain amines of the outer mitochondrial membrane. In the presence of metal cations, such as Fe^{2+} [8] or Cu [9], hydrogen peroxide generates, through the Fenton reaction, the hydroxyl radical ($^{\bullet}OH$), which is particularly harmful to biological tissues.

Other oxygen free radicals such as the perhydroxyl radical (HO_2), the peroxyl radical (RO), and the alkoxyl radical (RO_2) can also be formed during cellular metabolism. Another radical species is nitric oxide, which is produced by the various NO synthases (or NOS) of endothelial cells or macrophages for neuron-mediated purposes [7]. Inflammation is also an important source of oxygenated radicals produced directly by activated phagocytic cells, which are the site of a phenomenon called oxidative explosion consisting of the activation of the NADPH oxidase complex, an enzyme capable of using molecular oxygen to produce large amounts of superoxide anions at the cell membrane. This mechanism, when controlled, is essential in the fight against infection because it allows the phagocytosis of bacteria and foreign bodies. Radiation can generate free radicals, either by splitting the water molecule in the case of ionizing X or γ rays or by activating photosensitizing molecules in the case of ultraviolet rays [10, 11].

In general, ROSs include free radicals of oxygen itself as well as singlet oxygen ($^1O_2$) and non-radical reactive oxygen species, such as hydrogen peroxide (H_2O_2), RO_2H, peroxynitrite ($ONOO^-$), and HOCl, whose toxicity is significant [12].

Due to their reactivity, ROSs participate in phagocytosis, cell signaling, activating fertilization, improving muscle glucose uptake, and replenishing muscle glycogen stores [13–15] and have a bactericidal effect [16]. In addition, ROSs regulate most of the physiological functions of the body, in particular transcription factors, which activate protective genes for the cell contributing to the processes of cell repair and regeneration as well as the phenomenon of apoptosis [17].

To have a level of ROS beneficial for cellular life, it is necessary to maintain a balance inside the cell between the systems that generate free radicals and the nonenzymatic antioxidant systems [18, 19].

3. Oxidative stress

Present in excess in the body, ROS create an imbalance between prooxidant sources and antioxidant systems, generating "oxidative stress." This oxidative stress, resulting from the excessive presence of toxic oxygen radicals, causes oxidative damage to lipids, DNA, or proteins, which is the basis of many cellular dysfunctions, and the activation of the expression of genes coding for pro-inflammatory cytokines or adhesion proteins, phenomena that are partly responsible for a large number of diseases such as cancer, cardiovascular disorders, and neurodegenerative diseases [20, 21].

This disruption of the antioxidant/prooxidant balance in favor of the prooxidants can come from heavy metal poisoning; irradiation, a nutritional deficiency in one or more of the antioxidants such as vitamins or trace elements, abnormalities genetics responsible for poor coding of a protein either enzymatically antioxidant, synthesizing an antioxidant, regenerating an antioxidant, coupling defense to energy, or of a promoter of these same genes that the mutation will render unable of reacting to an excess of radicals or ischemia/repercussions following thrombosis [22–24]. In general, oxidative stress is the result of several of these factors and occurs singularly in a specific tissue and cell type, and not throughout the body.

4. Physiological and pathological oxidative stress

Oxidative stress, resulting from high levels of toxic ROS and RNS, while having a physiological role, constitutes a favorable ground for the development of various pathologies. Generated in small quantities under normal conditions, ROSs play a role of capable secondary messengers, especially in regulating the phenomenon of apoptosis or of activating transcription factors as well as in maintaining cellular homeostasis [25]. During the process of fertilization, the sperm cells secrete large amounts of ROS to pierce the membrane wall of the egg [26]. Free radical nitric oxide or $NO^{•}$, synthesized by endothelial cells, has regulatory effects for the maintenance of vascular tone, neurotransmission, renal function, and other physiological functions.

However, in the event of oxidative stress, the strong reactivity of ROS with respect to biological substrates can induce deleterious oxidative damage, which promotes the appearance of several diseases and the complications associated with them. The oxidation of lipids, for example, is a factor favoring the occurrence of cardiovascular diseases, while that of DNA is found in various stages that lead to the development of cancers [27].

The development of molecular biology has also clarified the important physiological role of ROSs, which, at high levels in the body, activate the expression of genes coding for pro-inflammatory cytokines or proteins adhesion, thus, becoming pathological. By reacting with DNA and the memory of all the biochemical composition of living beings, ROSs induce five main classes of oxidative damage, namely, oxidized bases, abasic sites, intra-strand adducts, strand breaks, and DNA-protein bridges. If these structural alterations are not "repaired," they will disrupt the DNA replication mechanisms and lead either to reading and synthesis errors by unfaithful translesional DNA polymerases resulting in a point mutation in the genome, or an impossibility of DNA copying, which will result in the initiation of the programmed suicide of the cells by a mechanism called apoptosis [28]. Not only smoking, alcoholism, obesity, and intense physical exercise but also our bad eating habits abnormally increase the production of AOEs in our bodies [29]. A diet low in fruits and vegetables and rich in antioxidants (vitamins C and E, carotenoids, polyphenols) promotes a drop in antioxidant capacity. For the sake of prevention, having effective tools to properly assess the status of oxidative stress, in an individual, in order to make the necessary corrections to their antioxidant defenses and reduce the oxidative damage induced by ROSs at the DNA level, proteins, and lipids is an imperative necessity.

5. Oxidative stress and associated diseases

Oxidative stress is implicated in the occurrence of several acute and chronic pathologies [30]. Under physiological conditions, glucose, in the presence of metallic traces, can oxidize, releasing ketoaldehydes, H_2O_2, and $^{\bullet}OH$, which will lead to the cleavage of proteins or their glycation by attachment of the ketoaldehyde, forming an AGE derivative. This phenomenon of glycosylation, very important in diabetics, contributes to the fragility of their vascular walls and their elasticity [31]. Reactive oxygen species also attack mucopolysaccharides and, in particular, cartilage proteoglycans. By altering Krebs cycle enzymes, oxidative stress negatively influences oxidative phosphorylation, promoting acidosis and early fatigue. ROSs readily react with aromatic and sulfur amino acids, altering the functions of proteins that they constitute as well as their ability to properly bind to a receptor or specifically bind a ligand, which alters cell signaling [32]. The attack on membrane lipid double bonds induces peroxidation reactions that alter membrane exchange, barrier, and information functions, modify membrane fluidity and the functioning of numerous receptors and transporters and signal transduction; that of circulating lipids lead to the formation of oxidized LDL, which, captured by specific macrophage receptors, promotes the secretion of pro-inflammatory cytokines [33] and forms the lipid deposit of the atherosclerotic plaque of cardiovascular disease. Damage to lysosome membranes promotes the release of proteases into the cytosol [34], which will aggravate protein destruction and induce muscle catabolism, responsible for the onset of atrophy or even cachexia. The human brain is very sensitive to oxidative damage due to its richness in polyunsaturated fatty acids, its high oxygen consumption, and the presence of metals with active redox potential such as copper and iron [35]. As oxidative stress increases with age, it is considered a primary etiological factor in age-related degenerative pathologies such as Alzheimer's and Parkinson's diseases. Oxidative stress also plays a crucial role in the occurrence of other neurodegenerative pathologies of toxic-nutritional origin such as konzo, tropical ataxic neuropathy, and neurolathyrism [36]. In general, oxidative damage compromises cell viability or induces other cellular responses *via* secondary reactive species leading to apoptosis or cell necrosis. The most concerning pathologies are cardiovascular diseases, cancers, diabetes, neurodegenerative diseases, and endometriosis. The biological consequences of oxidative stress vary according to the dose and the cell type. If light stresses increase cell proliferation and the expression of adhesion proteins, medium stresses facilitate apoptosis, and strong stresses cause necrosis, while violent stresses disorganize the cell membrane, leading to immediate lysis. The amplitude of oxidative stress promotes the induction of cell death processes: apoptosis and/or necrosis [37].

6. Antioxidants

Antioxidants are molecules capable of neutralizing oxidative species and preventing their oxidative damage. In a healthy individual, reactive species and antioxidant defenses are in balance, although there may be a slow accumulation of oxidative damage with age [38]. This imbalance also occurs when there is a significant decrease in antioxidant levels without necessarily an increase in ROS production. Studies on the involvement of GSH during the aging of human embryo fibroblasts in culture have reported that the activity of the antioxidant enzyme glutathione peroxidase, as well as that of glutathione reductase, constantly decreases during aging cells until reaching a drastic low level in old cells [39]. To counteract the harmful effects of ROS following excessive ROS production, living cells and tissues are equipped with enzymatic systems, endogenous molecules, and antioxidants whose essential role is to destroy these intermediates before their deleterious action and to restore the redox balance [39]. According to their mode of action, we distinguish stoichiometric antioxidants and catalytic antioxidants. The stœchiométric antioxidants are vitamins, reduced glutathione (GSH), uric acid, N-acetylcysteine, nonsteroidal anti-inflammatory drugs, certain antibiotics, polyphenols, etc. capable of neutralizing one or even a few ROSs, mainly free radicals. The catalytic antioxidants have two subgroups [40]. The first are antioxidant enzymes with direct catalytic activity, such as superoxide dismutase (SOD) and glutathione peroxidase (GPx), and the second, with indirect catalytic activity, is represented by cofactors of antioxidant enzymes such as NADPH, GSH, and selenium or reducing enzymes involved in the repair of oxidation processes such as GSH reductase, thioredoxin reductase, and also ferritin, transferrin, and desferrioxamine. By neutralizing an oxidizing enzyme molecule or activating an antioxidant enzyme, hundreds or even thousands of ROS will be eliminated by the action of a single antioxidant molecule, hence their qualification as catalytic antioxidants. According to their nature, antioxidants are enzymatic and nonenzymatic. The enzymatic group includes the primary defense enzymes that directly neutralize free radicals or prevent their formation [38], such as superoxide dismutase, catalase, and glutathione peroxidase, while the secondary are glutathione reductase and glucose-6-phospho-dehydrogenase [41]. Nonenzymatic antioxidants are mainly exogenous molecules of food origins such as polyphenols, vitamins, carotenoids, sulfur molecules, and mineral elements.

7. Micronutrients, polyphenols, and phytochemicals as natural plant antioxidants

Phytochemicals are secondary metabolites, suchas polyphenols, terpenes, nitrogen/sulfur-containing compounds, and alkaloids, found in algae, fungi, plants, and some insects such as caterpillars, not directly involved in basic life processes but constitute compounds with multiple nutritional and therapeutic beneficial effects for humans [42]. During the overflow of the body's defense system following multiple attacks due to a poor lifestyle, there is a loss of activity of antioxidant enzymes, leading to sometimes irreversible cellular disorganizations going so far as to cause cell death. Under these conditions, the presence of natural antioxidants such as micronutrients, carotenoids, and polyphenols is essential to limit oxidative damage. The best carotenoid known is β-carotene, which is the precursor of vitamin A. Recent studies showed beneficial effects of glucosinolates, including regulatory functions in inflammation, stress response, phase I metabolism, and antioxidant activities [43]. The polyphenols, according to their antioxidant, antimicrobial, and anti-inflammatory properties, have demonstrated remarkable effects in many chronic diseases such as neurodegenerative diseases, diabetes, and cardiovascular diseases. It has been reported that phenolic and flavonoid compounds act as antioxidants to exert antiallergic, anti-inflammatory, antidiabetic, antimicrobial, antipathogenic, antiviral, antithrombotic, immunomodulatory, and vasodilatory effects, and prevent diseases such as cancer, heart problems, cataracts, eye disorders, and Alzheimer's [44].

Currently, a wide variety of polyphenols showed immunomodulatory activity by altering the formation of nitric oxide and eicosanoid proteins and by inhibiting pro-inflammatory cytokines and gene expression [45]. The polyphenols are found in plants, from the roots to the fruits. In this group, we have phenolic acids (caffeic, chrolorogenic acids…), anthocyanins, anthraquinones, catechins, coumarins, flavonoids (quercetin, kaempferol, rutin…), and tannins.

About micronutrients, essential components of the diet, studies on their supplementation that might improve health status have gained immense popularity. Fruits and vegetables, such as grapes, oranges, pomegranates, apples, plums, fresh garlic, carrots, and spinach from nature, have micronutrients and are rich in molecules with high antioxidant power, including tocopherols and polyphenols, which have ammunition to fight against free radicals and stop their chain oxidation reaction [46].

8. Traditional foods as potential sources of antioxidants, nutraceuticals, pharmaceuticals, and phytoceuticals

Traditional foods, eaten and prepared by groups of people who share a common religion, language, culture, or heritage, are an expression of the culture, history, and lifestyle of a people [47, 48]. The Democratic Republic of Congo (DRC) with the largest biodiversity in Africa and a variety of ecosystems: including nearly half the African rainforests, forest-savannah ecotones, savannahs, afro -mountainous forests, large and small lakes, rivers, and swampy forests [49], and lived by most than 450 ethnic groups, has more types of cuisines, rich in traditional dietary diversity from vegetables, fruits, herbal teas, legumes, nuts, seeds, mushrooms, and insects. In three of the twenty-six provinces of the DRC, Mbemba et al. have listed 163 different vegetables, 85 species of mushrooms, 35 kinds of roots and tubers as well as 64 species of fruits, nuts, and seeds, several of which are rich in proteins of good biological value: in lipids with unsaturated fatty acids, in vitamins, and in minerals [41]. The results of our studies on the phytochemicals, micronutrient contents, and antioxidant activities of traditional foods are reported in the table below.

Vegetables represent an important part of the diet of Congolese's population. Apart from conventional vegetables originating from other countries, there are traditional vegetables specific to each ethnic group. These vegetables are rich in nutrients such as proteins, lipids, vitamins, and minerals. Studies on several vegetables have shown their richness in various secondary metabolites (**Table 1**) with therapeutic properties that would justify their use in the management of certain diseases.

Scientific names	Vernacular names	Antioxidant nutrients	Total Polyphenol (mgGAE/g DW)	Total flavonoids (mgQE/g)	Antioxidant activity IC50 (μg/mL) *		References
					ABTS	DPPH	
Abelmoshus esculentus	*Dongo dongo*	Catechines, isoquercitrin, rutin, kaempferol, myricétine, quercétin	32.94 ± 0.93	-	86.27 ± 9.2	nd	[50, 51]
Abelmoshus moshatus	*Dongo*	Myricetin	36.32 ± 1.05	-	52.36 ± 2.1	71.45 ± 14.44	[50]
Entada gigas	*Futi, Nzembo futi*	Polyphenols	54.74 ± 0,49	37.08 ± 1,02	35.4 ± 0,96	45.5 ± 0,97	[52]
Hibiscus acetosella	*Ngai*	caffeoyl-hydroxycitric acid chlorogenic acid, quercetin-3-ga- lactoside	89.05 ± 11.92	-	44.98 ± 0.87	73.79 ± 17.20	[50, 51]
Hibiscus cannabinus	*Ngai ya nseke bakai*	quercetin-3-glucoside, kaempferol-rhamnoside, neochlorogenic acid	82.97 ± 3.27	-	64.72 ± 6.17	86.04 ± 4.32	[50]
Ipomoea batatas	*Kimbondji*	Cyanidin, chlorogénic acid, ferulic acid, quercetin	76.78 ± 3.20	-	47.76 ± 3.25	233.35 ± 63.53	[50, 51]
Manihot esculenta	*Saka*	Rutin, kaempferol-3-O-rutinoside, amentoflavone	86.4 ± 2.99	-	15.10 ± 1.13	20.15 ± 1.07	[50, 51]
Manihot glaziovii	*Sakasaka*	Rutin, kaempferol-3-O-rutinoside, amentoflavone, ferulic acid	107.71 ± 7.80	-	12.42 ± 2.08	20.5 ± 1.06	[50, 51]
Megaphrynium macrostachum	*Mikungu*	Flavonoids, Phenolic acids	32.69 ± 3.65	-	79.25 ± 10.29	503.5 ± 10.29	[50, 51]
Phytolacca dodecandra	*Tidi*	Glutamic acid, Cysteine, polyphenols, terpenoids, alkaloids	4.1 ± 0.65	0.32 ± 0.05	38.37 ± 7.98	62.23 ± 12.59	[53]
Psophocarpus scandens	*Kikalakasa*	Flavonoids, phenolic acids, manganese, magnesium	64.2 ± 0,58	40.78 ± 1,11	53.2 ± 0,97	62.81 ± 0,97	[52, 54]

Scientific names	Vernacular names	Antioxidant nutrients	Total Polyphenol (mgGAE/g DW)	Total flavonoids (mgQE/g)	Antioxidant activity IC50 (µg/mL) *		References
					ABTS	DPPH	
Rungia congoensis	*Kuinini*	Polyphenols, Terpenoids	69.16 ± 5.56		18.19 ± 1.8	42.76 ± 15.72	[55]
Salacia pynaerti	*Mbondi*	Polyphenols, anthocyanes, zinc, manganese, selenium	508.34 ± 14,42	31.62 ± 2.17	2.11 ± 0.48	9.48 ± 0.61	[52]
Sesamum angustifolium auct.	*Mundjingu*	Verbascoside, Flavonoids	63.76 ± 3.76	-	31.19 ± 1.07	48.3 ± 1.02	[50, 51]
Solanum aethiopicum	*Muteta*	Chlorogénic acid, tanins	32.24 ± 4.13	-	123.89 ± 16.15	282.49 ± 27.81	[50]
Solanum gilo	*Njiyo*	Flavonoids, tanins,	72.04 ± 1.70	-	29.51 ± 0.94	163.68 ± 30.41	[50, 51]
Tetrorchirdium congolense	*Nkelekete*	Flavonoids, tanins, Terpenes	241.54 ± 2,18	21.36 ± 0,65	3.65 ± 1.03	7.13 ± 2.14	[52]

(*) Antioxidant activities were evaluated using gallic acid and quercetin as controls. (IC50 Gallic acid: 0.71 ± 0.08 and 1.07 ± 0.10; Quercetin: 1.42 ± 0.04 and 3.21 ± 0.99 in ABTS and DPPH tests, respectively).
(-) not determined

Table 1.
Antioxidant activities of Congolese traditional vegetables.

From the results obtained, it appears that traditional vegetables contain polyphenolic compounds and flavonoids, which would give them antioxidant activities that are likely to fight against free radicals to attenuate oxidative damage to cells in the human body and spare it from chronic diseases. In order of importance, we align *Salacia pynaerti, Tetrorchirdium congolense, Manihot glaziovii, Manihot esculenta, Rungia congoensis, Sesamum angustifolium, Phytolacca dodecandra, Entada gigas, Hibiscus acetosella, Ipomoea batatas, Psophocarpus scandens* etc. In addition, the leaves of *Salacia pynaerti* contain calcium, zinc, manganese as well as glutamic, methionine, and cysteine, which participate in the synthesis of glutathione [54].

Spices are an integral part of the Congolese diet. Several traditional spices have been identified in the culinary habits of the Congolese people, often unrecognized and unexploited. Spice plants and vegetables, as well as their essential oils, are important sources of antioxidants phytochemicals and micronutrients including phenolics, terpenoids, and alkaloids. Consumption of these spices in diets would reduce the occurrence of nutritional deficiencies and health problems (**Table 2**).

Spice data indicate high polyphenol content in *Curcuma longa* rhizomes and high antioxidant activity from *Piper nigrum*. Studies have reported that the consumption of turmeric longa, mixed with black pepper, slows down or even decreases the proliferation of cancer cells [57]

Mushrooms are the second most common traditional food available to the Congolese rural population after vegetables. Although they are available periodically,

Scientific names	Vernacular names	Antioxidant nutrients	Total Polyphenol (mgGAE/g DW)	Total flavonoids (mgQE/g)	Antioxidant activity IC50 (µg/mL) *		References
					ABTS	DPPH	
Aeollanthus suaveolens Mart. ex Spreng.	*Dinkombo, Ngondi longo*	Phenolic acid, Flavonoids, Terpenes	26.30 ± 3.72	-	41.82 ± 3.99	61.12 ± 7.39	[50]
Curcuma longa	*Kinginingoni, mandjano, manga*	Terpenes, Polyphenols	204.96 ± 0.019	101.3 ± 0.004	72.95 ± 16.06	338.84 ± 80.61	[56]
Monodora myristica	*Mpeya*	Terpenes, Polyphenols	7.90 ± 0,22	0.92 ± 0.04	58.34 ± 1.63	102.33 ± 0,7	[55]
Ocimum basilicum L.	*Mazulu*	Phenolic acid, Terpenes	6.52 ± 0.18	-	38.37 ± 3.13	136.77 ± 15.64	[50]
Piper nigrum	*Ketchu*	Terpenes, Polyphenols	-	-	1.4 ± 0.13	11.64 ± 4.03	[56]
Raphia sese De Wild	*Bankulu*	Chlorogenic acid	10.08 ± 0.51	-	40.71 ± 1.05	518.8 ± 95.16	[50]

(*) Antioxidant activities were evaluated using gallic acid and quercetin as controls. (IC50 Gallic acid: 0.71 ± 0.08 and 1.07 ± 0.10; Quercetin: 1.42 ± 0.04 and 3.21 ± 0.99 in ABTS and DPPH tests, respectively).
(-) not determined

Table 2.
Antioxidant activities of Congolese traditional spices.

some species are sold dried throughout the year, such as *Auricularia delicata, Lactifluus edulis,* and *Schizophyllum commune* (**Table 3**). Mushrooms are a significant source of lipophilic compounds, phenolic and indole derivatives as well as carotenoids, and some vitamins having considerable antioxidant properties.

Despite low levels of polyphenols, mushrooms contain terpenoids as well as trace of elements such as zinc and selenium, and have appreciable antioxidant activity. *Auricularia delicata, Cantharellus symoensii*, *Lactarius ssp, Lactarius tenellus,* and *Marasmius collybia* have the best antioxidant activities.

Yams are an alternative for cereals and tubers with a moderate glycemic index, close to that of corn but lower than that of rice and cassava. Congolese yams are mainly represented by *Dioscorea* species. Numerous studies have reported the high nutritional value of *Diosocorea,* particularly as an alternative source of starch and some important micronutrients. Bioactivities and health benefits of yams such as Dioscorea extracts and other preparations have been related to the presence of phytochemicals, which possess antioxidant properties. Antioxidant activities are related mainly to radical scavenging capacity and positive effects on the cell's endogenous antioxidant system. Bukatuka et al. (2016) studied five Congolese edible Dioscorea and showed that the phytochemical screening revealed the presence of polyphenols, alkaloids, and terpenoids and they have shown a good antioxidant and anti-hyperglycemic activities (55), (**Table 4**).

Dioscorea alata, Dioscorea praehensilis, and *Dioscorea bulbifera* are endowed with useful antioxidant activities. Studies have reported that *D. bulbifera* and *D. praehensilis* have a hypoglycemic and antihyperglycemic effects [59].

Scientific names	Vernacular names	Antioxidant nutrients	Total Polyphenol (mgGAE/g DW)	Antioxidant activity IC50 (µg/mL) *		References
				ABTS	DPPH	
Amanita loosic Beeli	*Walenda*	Phenolic acid, terpenes	8.82 ± 0.01	45.65 ± 1.00	1862.1 ± 425	[50]
Auricularia delicata (Mont.) Henn. 1893	*Tshilebu*	Phenolic acid, terpenes	9.53 ± 0.12	39.31 ± 1.04	252.4 ± 15.5	[50, 58]
Cantharellus rufopunctatus var ochraceus Heinem.	*Upombo*	Phenolic acid, terpenes	4.73 ± 0.02	220.3 ± 17.40	1717.09 ± 522	[50]
Cantharellus sp	*Nahoto*	Selenium, Phenolic acids, Glutamic acid, cysteine, Lycopene	6.4 ± 0.02	144.9 ± 21.80	1367.73 ± 364	[50]
Cantharellus symoensii Heinem.	*Katshondjo*	Phenolic acid, terpenes	10.32 ± 1.09	41.1 ± 1.02	1815.52 ± 418	[50]
Lactarius ssp.	Bupeshele	Phenolic acid, terpenes	7.84 ± 0.03	46.77 ± 3.58	132.13 ± 16.47	[54]
Lactarius tenellus Verbeken & Walleyn, Persoonia	*Kafuka*	Phenolic acid, terpenes	5.96 ± 1.47	43.51 ± 1.04	1603.25 ± 294	[50]
Lactifluus edulis Verbeken & Buyck	*Wundje*	Phenolic acid, terpenes	5.12 ± 0.11	262.4 ± 20.74	1318.3 ± 259	[50]
Lentinus cf cladopus	*Bupup*	Polyphenols, Terpenoids, Zinc	22.79 ± 0.21	112.95 ± 0.98	291.07 ± 0.98	[58]
Marasmius buzungolo	Bututulu	Phenolic acid, terpenes	10.32 ± 0.08	82.79 ± 3.11	145.55 ± 27.3	[54]
Marasmius collybia	Nsudi ya Babakala	Phenolic acid, terpenes	9.43 ± 0.19	62.37 ± 2.49	109.65 ± 7.3	[54]
Pleurotus tuber-regium	*Butondi*	Polyphenols, Zinc	23.37 ± 8.16	153.82 ± 1,01	281.19 ± 0.95	[58]
Schizophyllum commune Fr.	*Tshikolokoto*	Flavonoids, Phenolic acids, lycopene, Vitamin C	9.77 ± 0.40	169.8 ± 23.80	307.61 ± 25.05	[50, 58]

(*) Antioxidant activities were evaluated using gallic acid and quercetin as controls. (IC50 Gallic acid: 0.71 ± 0.08 and 1.07 ± 0.10; Quercetin: 1.42 ± 0.04 and 3.21 ± 0.99 in ABTS and DPPH tests, respectively).

Table 3.
Antioxidant activities of Congolese traditional mushrooms.

The spontaneous flora of the DRC is very rich in food fruits called wild fruits and seeds, which unfortunately are little valued by the population. These fruits are rich in polysaccharides, micronutrients (vitamins, minerals), and secondary metabolites, such as polyphenols, whose therapeutic benefits are well known (**Table 5**).

Scientific names	Vernacular names	Antioxidant nutrients	Total Polyphenol (mgGAE/g DW)	Total flavonoids (mgQE/g)	Antioxidant activity IC50 (µg/mL) *		References
					ABTS	DPPH	
Dioscorea bulbifera	*Mukadi*	Polyphenols, Vitamin C	51.12 ± 0.5	3.33 ± 0.23	93.11 ± 11.21	109.65 ± 8.81	[59]
Dioscorea domentorum	*Bisadi*	Polyphenols	30.07 ± 0.3	-	1164.13 ± 28.32	916.22 ± 65.74	[59]
Dioscorea alata	*Mboma*	Polyphenols	9.85 ± 0.09	-	35.32 ± 1.34	283.14 ± 0.04	[59]
Dioscorea bulkiliana	*Bisadi*	Polyphenols	16.58 ± 0.16	2.6 ± 0.02	97.5 ± 9.4	510.51 ± 45.97	[59]
Dioscorea praehensilis	*Bisadi*	Polyphenols	13.35 ± 0.13	2.58 ± 0.3	83.34 ± 8.74	115.88 ± 10.93	[59]

(*) Antioxidant activities were evaluated using gallic acid and quercetin as controls. (IC50 Gallic acid: 0.71 ± 0.08 and 1.07 ± 0.10; Quercetin: 1.42 ± 0.04 and 3.21 ± 0.99 in ABTS and DPPH tests, respectively).
(-) not determined

Table 4.
Antioxidant activities of Congolese edible yams.

Scientific names	Vernacular names	Antioxidant nutrients	Total Polyphenol (mgGAE/g DW)	Total flavonoids (mgQE/g)	Antioxidant activity IC50 (µg/mL) *		References
					ABTS	DPPH	
Afromomum melegueta	Tundu ya nseke	Polyphenols, terpenes	158.28 ± 0.017	2.27 ± 0,03	17.38 ± 2.34	32.71 ± 6.73	[54]
Bombacopsis glabra	Nguba mputu	Polyphenols, flavonoids, terpenes	28.45 ± 1.34	0.52 ± 0.04	77.98 ± 2.56	85.31 ± 4.64	[54]

Table 5.
Antioxidant activities of fruits and seeds.

Afromum melegueta contains a high content of polyphenols and the best antioxidant activity. Their content in gingerol, shogaol, paradole, and oleanolic acid would be responsible for their hypocholesterolemic, antitumor, anti-inflammatory, antimicrobial, and antidiabetic properties [60].

Entomophagy is remarkably ingrained in food habits in DRC, seeing that edible insects are considered a valuable traditional food for long and a sustainable source of proteins and vitamins. Study by Nsevolo et al (2021) listed 148 Congolese edible insects identified at species (100 genera, 31 families, and 9 orders dominated by the orders Lepidoptera, Orthoptera, Coleoptera, and Hymenoptera). Insects are part of the regular diet of more than two billion people around the world are delicacies [61]. In the Democratic Republic of the Congo (DRC), caterpillars are the most consumed insects, and they are consumed by more than 70% of the population throughout the year **Table 6**.

Insects are not only valuable sources of lipids, polysaccharides, proteins, and micronutrients but also are sources of bioactive compounds such as phytochemicals with numerous therapeutic properties. Anti-inflammatory, antioxidant, anticancer,

Scientific names	Vernacular names	Antioxidant nutrients	Total Polyphenol (mgGAE/g DW)	Total flavonoids (mgQE/g)	Antioxidant activity IC50 (μg/mL) *		References
					ABTS	DPPH	
Cinabra hyperbius	*Binkubala*	Rutin, Phenolic acid, selenium, Zinc	1.77 ± 0.02	0.13 ± 0.06	10.7 ± 1.4	26.6 ± 2.0	[62]
Cirina forda	*Masese*	Flavonoids, Gallic acid, Zinc	0.22 ± 0.03	5.36 ± 0.56	15.8 ± 1.7	57.0 ± 5.9	[62]
Cirina forda	*Makoso*	Phenolic acid, selenium, Zinc	0.05 ± 0.01	1.38 ± 0.15	16.6 ± 1.4	78.5 ± 1.3	[62]
Cirina forda	*Mingolo*	Phenolic acid, Zinc, Terpenes	0.81 ± 0.09	4.31 ± 0.75	20.7 ± 2.3	68.8 ± 10.4	[62]
Cirina forda	*Massamba*	Phenolic acid, terpenes	0.91 ± 0.09	1.38 ± 0.15	36.4 ± 3.8	73.6 ± 8.6	[62]
Gonimbrasia belina	*Binkubala*	Flavonoids, rutin Phenolic acid, selenium, Zinc	0.23 ± 0.03	2.78 ± 0.24	14.6 ± 1.0	54.3 ± 3.1	[62]
Imbrasia epimethea	*Benkenzo*	Phenolic acid, Zinc, terpenes	0.75 ± 0.07	0.13 ± 0.06	16.6 ± 1.6	43.5 ± 2.1	[62]
Imbrasia sp	*Mboyo*	Phenolic acid, Zinc, terpenoids	1.75 ± 0.07	3.31 ± 0.55	10.8 ± 1.2	21.7 ± 2.4	[62]
Imbrasia runcate	*Mbinzo*	Phenolic acid, Terpenes	1.99 ± 0.05	1.36 ± 0.26	12.1 ± 0.8	52.3 ± 2.7	[62]
Imbrasia runcate	*Mbinzo*	Phenolic acid, Zinc, Terpenoids	2.39 ± 0.05	1.11 ± 0.45	13.3 ± 1.5	26.6 ± 3.0	[62]

Table 6.
Antioxidant activities of insects.

and antimicrobial activities have been reported for the major phenolic compounds found in insects like kaempferol and quercetin when they are directly extracted from plants [62].

9. Conclusion

Oxidative stress, characterized by excessive production of reactive species, is involved in several chronic diseases such as cardiovascular, chronic obstructive pulmonary, sickle cell, chronic kidney, neurodegenerative, and cancer. The data reported in the tables above clearly showed that traditional foods from the biodiversity of the Democratic Republic of Congo are often unvalued, and constitute a potential source of new natural antioxidants. Indeed, the vegetables, mushrooms, yams, nuts, and fruits studied contain polyphenolic compounds, terpenes, and micronutrients, responsible for their antioxidant activities. As Congolese diets, particularly in rural areas, are based on vegetables, such as mushrooms, yams, nuts, and herbs as drinks, there is reason to consider that Congolese traditional foods are a rich source of antioxidant phytonutrients, which brings several health benefits for the population, including the prevention or management of cardiovascular diseases, neurodegenerative disorders, cancer, autoimmune diseases, and diabetes. Considering the importance of oxidative stress on human health, promoting research with a view to valuing the natural antioxidants of biodiversity in Africa, could pave the way toward the discovery of specific natural antioxidant to prevent or treat such and other chronic diseases not transmissible.

Author details

Théophile Mbemba Fundu[1], Paulin Mutwale Kapepula[2]*, Jean Paul Nzundu Mbo[1], Justin Mboloko Esimo[3] and Nadège Ngombe Kabamba[2]

1 Faculty of Sciences, Laboratoire d'analyses et de Recherches sur les Aliments et la Nutrition (LARAN), Department of Biology, University of Kinshasa, Kinshasa, Democratic Republic of Congo

2 Faculty of Pharmaceutical Sciences, Centre d'Etudes des Substances Naturelles d'Origine Végétale (CESNOV), University of Kinshasa, Kinshasa, Democratic Republic of Congo

3 Faculty of Medicine, University of Kinshasa, Democratic Republic of Congo

*Address all correspondence to: garaphmutwal@yahoo.fr

References

[1] Liguori I, Russo G, Curcio F, Bulli G, Aran L, Della-Morte D, et al. Oxidative stress, aging, and diseases. Clinical Interventions in Aging. 2018;**13**:757-772

[2] Di Giulio RT, Meyer JN. Reactive oxygen species and oxidative stress. Toxicology Fishes. 2008;**170**:273-324

[3] Kruk J, Aboul-Enein HY, Kładna A, Bowser JE. Oxidative stress in biological systems and its relation with pathophysiological functions: The effect of physical activity on cellular redox homeostasis. Free Radical Research. 2019;**53**(5):497-521

[4] Turrens JF. Mitochondrial formation of reactive oxygen species. The Journal of Physiology. 2003;**552**(2):335-344

[5] Dikalov S. Cross talk between mitochondria and NADPH oxidases. Free Radical Biology & Medicine. 2011;**51**(7):1289-1301. Available from: http://dx.doi.org/10.1016/j.freeradbiomed.2011.06.033

[6] Kwon D, Kim SM, Correia MA. Cytochrome P450 endoplasmic reticulum-associated degradation (ERAD): Therapeutic and pathophysiological implications. Acta Pharm Sin B. 2020;**10**(1):42-60. Available from: : https://doi.org/10.1016/j.apsb.2019.11.002

[7] Förstermann U, Sessa WC. Nitric oxide synthases: Regulation and function. European Heart Journal. 2012;**33**(7):829-837

[8] Velayutham M, Hemann C, Zweier JL. Removal of H_2O_2 and generation of superoxide radical: Role of cytochrome c and NADH. Free Radical Biology & Medicine. 2011;**51**(1):160-170. Available from: http://dx.doi.org/10.1016/j.freeradbiomed.2011.04.007

[9] Zhao Z. Iron and oxidizing species in oxidative stress and Alzheimer's disease. Aging Medicine. 2019;**2**(2):82-87

[10] Reisz JA, Bansal N, Qian J, Zhao W, Furdui CM. Effects of ionizing radiation on biological molecules - mechanisms of damage and emerging methods of detection. Antioxidants & Redox Signaling. 2014;**21**(2):260-292

[11] Azzam EI, Jay-Gerin JP, Pain D. Ionizing radiation-induced metabolic oxidative stress and prolonged cell injury. Cancer Letters. 2012;**327**(1-2):48-60. Available from: http://dx.doi.org/10.1016/j.canlet.2011.12.012

[12] Nakai K, Tsuruta D. What are reactive oxygen species, free radicals, and oxidative stress in skin diseases? International Journal of Molecular Science. 2021;**22**(19):1-16

[13] Slauch JM. How does the oxidative burst of macrophages kill bacteria? Still an open question. Molecular Microbiology. 2011;**80**(3):580-583

[14] Agarwal A, Virk G, Ong C, du Plessis SS. Effect of oxidative stress on male reproduction. World Journal of Mens Health. 2014;**32**(1):1

[15] Higaki Y, Mikami T, Fujii N, Hirshman MF, Koyama K, Seino T, et al. Oxidative stress stimulates skeletal muscle glucose uptake through a phosphatidylinositol 3-kinase-dependent pathway. American Journal of Physiology. Endocrinology and Metabolism. 2008;**294**(5):889-897

[16] Mourenza Á, Gil JA, Mateos LM, Letek M. Oxidative stress-generating

antimicrobials, a novel strategy to overcome antibacterial resistance. Antioxidants. 2020;**9**(5):1-16

[17] Macdonald J, Galley HF, Webster NR. Oxidative stress and gene expression in sepsis. British Journal of Anaesthesia. 2003;**90**(2):221-232. Available from: http://dx.doi.org/10.1093/bja/aeg034

[18] Espinosa-Diez C, Miguel V, Mennerich D, Kietzmann T, Sánchez-Pérez P, Cadenas S, et al. Antioxidant responses and cellular adjustments to oxidative stress. Redox Biology. 2015;**6**:183-197. Available from: http://dx.doi.org/10.1016/j.redox.2015.07.008

[19] Kurutas EB. The importance of antioxidants which play the role in cellular response against oxidative/nitrosative stress: Current state. Nutrition Journal. 2016;**15**(1):1-22. Available from: http://dx.doi.org/10.1186/s12937-016-0186-5

[20] Rea IM, Gibson DS, McGilligan V, McNerlan SE, Denis Alexander H, Ross OA. Age and age-related diseases: Role of inflammation triggers and cytokines. Frontiers in Immunology. 2018;**9**(APR):1-28

[21] Bachmann MC, Bellalta S, Basoalto R, Gómez-Valenzuela F, Jalil Y, Lépez M, et al. The challenge by multiple environmental and biological factors induce inflammation in aging: Their role in the promotion of chronic disease. Frontiers in Immunology. 2020;**11**(October):1-19

[22] Sun MS, Jin H, Sun X, Huang S, Zhang FL, Guo ZN, et al. Free radical damage in ischemia-reperfusion injury: An obstacle in acute ischemic stroke after revascularization therapy. Oxidative Medicine and Cellular Longevity. 2018;**2018**:1-17

[23] Previtali E, Bucciarelli P, Passamonti SM, Martinelli I. Risk factors for venous and arterial thrombosis. Blood Transfusion. 2011;**9**(2):120-138

[24] Lagouge M, Larsson NG. The role of mitochondrial DNA mutations and free radicals in disease and ageing. Journal of Internal Medicine. 2013;**273**(6):529-543

[25] Dröge W. Free radicals in the physiological control of cell function. Physiological Reviews. 2002;**82**(1):47-95

[26] Sanocka D, Kurpisz M. Reactive oxygen species and sperm cells. Reproductive Biology and Endocrinology. 2004;**2**(2):1-7

[27] Long J, Zhang C-J, Zhu N, Du K, Yin Y-F, Tan X, et al. Lipid metabolism and carcinogenesis, cancer development. American Journal of Cancer Research. 2018;**8**(5):778-791. Available from: http://www.ncbi.nlm.nih.gov/pubmed/29888102%0Ahttp://www.pubmedcentral.nih.gov/articlerender.fcgi?artid=PMC5992506

[28] Gardner AM, Xu FH, Fady C, Jacoby FJ, Duffey DC, Tu Y, et al. Apoptotic vs. nonapoptotic cytotoxicity induced by hydrogen peroxide. Free Radical Biology & Medicine. 1997;**22**(1-2):73-83

[29] Diggs DL, Huderson AC, Harris KL, Myers JN, Banks LD, Rekhadevi PV, et al. Polycyclic aromatic hydrocarbons and digestive tract cancers: A perspective. Journal of Environmental Science Health. 2011;**29**(4):324-357

[30] Pizzino G, Irrera N, Cucinotta M, Pallio G, Mannino F, Arcoraci V, et al. Oxidative stress: Harms and benefits for human health. Oxidative Medicine and Cellular Longevity. 2017;**2017**:1-13

[31] Hanus J, Zhang H, Wang Z, Liu Q, Zhou Q, Wang S. Induction of necrotic

cell death by oxidative stress in retinal pigment epithelial cells. Cell Death & Disease. 2013;**4**(12):1-11

[32] Valley CC, Cembran A, Perlmutter JD, Lewis AK, Labello NP, Gao J, et al. The methionine-aromatic motif plays a unique role in stabilizing protein structure. The Journal of Biological Chemistry. 2012;**287**(42):34979-34991

[33] Chen C, Khismatullin DB. Oxidized low-density lipoprotein contributes to atherogenesis via co-activation of macrophages and mast cells. PLoS One. 2015;**10**(3):1-20

[34] Machado ER, Annunziata I, van de Vlekkert D, Grosveld GC, d'Azzo A. Lysosomes and cancer progression: A malignant liaison. Frontiers in Cell Developmental Biology. 2021;**9**:1-19

[35] Cobley JN, Fiorello ML, Bailey DM. 13 reasons why the brain is susceptible to oxidative stress. Redox Biology. 2018;**15**(January):490-503. Available from: https://doi.org/10.1016/j.redox.2018.01.008

[36] Singh A, Kukreti R, Saso L, Kukreti S. Oxidative stress: A key modulator in neurodegenerative diseases. Molecules. 2019;**24**(8):1-20

[37] Nita M, Grzybowski A. The role of the reactive oxygen species and oxidative stress in the pathomechanism of the age-related ocular diseases and other pathologies of the anterior and posterior eye segments in adults. Oxidative Medicine and Cellular Longevity. 2016;**2016**:1-23

[38] Birben E, Sahiner UM, Sackesen C, Erzurum S, Kalayci O. Oxidative stress and antioxidant defense. World Allergy Organization Journal. Jan 2012;**2012**:9-19

[39] Mbemba F, Houbion A, Raes M, Remacle J. Subcellular localization and modification with ageing of glutathione, glutathione peroxidase and glutathione reductase activities in human fibroblasts. Biochimica et Biophysica Acta. 1985;**838**:211-220

[40] Mcelroy CS, Min E, Huang J, Loader JE, Hendry-hofer TB, Garlick RB, et al. Catalytic antioxidant rescue of inhaled sulfur mustard toxicity. 2016;**154**(2):341-353

[41] Remacle J, Michiels C, Raes M. The importance of antioxidant enzymes in cellular aging and degeneration. Free Radicals and Aging. 1992;**62**:1-11

[42] Behla T, Kumara K, Briscb C, Rusb M, Nistor-Cseppentoc DC, Bustead C, et al. Exploring the multifocal role of phytochemicals as immunomodulators. Biomedicine Pharmacotherapy. 2021;**133**:1-18

[43] Kaboré DS, Hema A, Koala M, Somé K, Palé E, Somé IT, et al. Evaluation des teneurs en antioxydants et micronutriments des feuilles de onze variétés de Ipomoea batatas à chairs orange et pourpre produites au Burkina Faso. Journal de la Société Ouest-Africaine de Chimie. 2021;**2022**:1-10

[44] Pot F, Santi D, Spaggiari G, Zimetti F. Polyphenol health effects on cardiovascular and neurodegenerative disorders: A review and meta-analysis. International Journal of Molecular Sciences. 2019;**20**(2):1-26

[45] Behl T, Kaur G, Sehgal A, Bhardwaj S, Singh S, Buhas C. Multifaceted role of matrix metalloproteinases in neurodegenerative diseases: Pathophysiological and therapeutic perspectives. International Journal of Molecular Sciences. 2021;**2021**:1-26

[46] Rolland Y, Sud LC. Antioxydants naturels végétaux. OCL-Journal. 2004;**2004**:419-424

[47] Trichopoulou A, Soukara S, Vasilopoulou E. Traditional foods: A science and society perspective Related papers. Trends in Food Science Technology. 2007;**18**:420-427

[48] Sproesser G, Ruby MB, Arbit N, Akotia CS, Alvarenga S, Bhangaokar R, et al. Understanding traditional and modern eating: The TEP10 framework. BMC Public Health. 2019;**2019**:1-14

[49] Inogwabini BI, Ilambu O, Gbanzi MA. Protected areas of the Democratic Republic of Congo. Conservation Biology. 2005;**19**(1):15-22

[50] Kapepula PM, Ngombe NK, Mumba DN, Katumbay DT, Frédérich M. Traditional foods as putative sources of antioxidants with health beneits in Konzo. In: Antioxidants in Foods and Its Applications. London, UK. 2018. p. 182

[51] Kapepula PM. Capacités antioxydantes et analyse phytochimique des aliments tradi- tionnels de Kahemba: Perspectives de valorisation pour la prévention du konzo. Liège: University of Liège; 2017

[52] BahatiL M, Kapepula PM, Kabamba NK, Moni B, Kafuti GM, Mungitshi M, et al. Microscopic features, chro- matographic ingerprints and antioxidant property of some unconventional green leafy vegetables consumed in Bandundu, DR Congo. Pharmacognosy Communications. 2017;7(4):158-163

[53] Iteku JB, Mbayi O, Bongo GN, Kapepula PM, Wambale JM, Lengbiye E, etal.PhytochemicalAnalysisandAssessment of Antibacterial and Antioxidant Activities of Phytolacca dodecandra L. Herit Leaf Extracts (Phytolaccaceae). International Journal of Biomedical Engineering and Clinical Science. 2019;**5**:31-39

[54] Mbemba TF. Alimentation et prevention des maladies Diabete, maladies cardiovasculaires, cancer et osteoporose. L'Harmattan RDC. 2020;**2020**:218

[55] Kapepula PM, Baku PN, Kasongo MK, Duki AM, Franck T, Mouithys-Mickalad A, et al. Anti-inflammatory and antioxidant activities of Rungia congoensis, a traditional vegetable consumed by Yombe people from Kongo Central area (DR. Congo). Natural Product Research. 2018;**2018**:1650-1654

[56] Mbemba TF. Face à la Covid, quelle alimentation adopter en RDC? L'Harmattan RDC. 2020;**2020**:1-100

[57] Prasad S, Aggarwal BB. Turmeric, the golden spice: From traditional medicine to modern medicine. In: Herbal Medicine: Biomolecular and Clinical Aspects. Second ed. Thames, Oxfordshire, UK: CRC Press; 2011. pp. 263-288

[58] Kabuyi MK, Kapepula PM, Kabengele JK, Moni B, Makengo G, Mungitshi MP, et al. Selenium content and antioxidant potential of some edible wild mushrooms from Bandundu area, DR Congo. Natural Resources. 2017;**8**:103-113

[59] Bukatuka F, Ngombe K, Mutwale K, Moni B, Makengo K, Pambu L, et al. Bioactivity and nutritional values of some Dioscorea species traditionally used as medicinal foods in Bandundu, DR Congo. European Journal of Medicinal Plants. 2016;**14**(1):1-11

[60] Mohammed A, Awolola Gbonjubola V, Anthony Koorbanally N, Shahidul IM. Inhibition of key enzymes linked to type 2 diabetes by compounds isolated from Aframomum melegueta fruit. Pharmaceutical Biology. 2017;**55**(1):1010-1016

[61] Nsevolo MP et al. Reviewing entomophagy in the Democratic Republic of Congo: Species and host

plant diversity, seasonality, patterns of consumption and challenges of the edible insect sector. Journal of Insects as Food and Feed. 2022:1-20

[62] Kapepula PM, Luzayana HW, Mukundi DL, Franck T, Lokole PB, Mbemba TF, et al. Congolese edible caterpillars, valuable sources of bioactive compounds with human health benefits. Journal of Insects as Food and Feed. 2022:1-12

Chapter 5

Recent Development in Antioxidant of Milk and Its Products

Fouad M.F. Elshaghabee, Ahmed A. Abd El-Maksoud and Gustavo M. Ambrósio F. de Gouveia

Abstract

Free radicals are produced in humans through natural metabolism or the external environment, such as diet. These free radicals are neutralized by the antioxidant system, whereas enzymes, for example, catalase, superoxide dismutase, and glutathione peroxidase, play an important role in preventing excessive free radicals. Food antioxidants give a good hand in enhancing the human antioxidant system; high consumption of a diet rich in natural antioxidants protects against the risk of diseases such as cardiovascular, cancer, diabetes, and obesity. Milk and its products are popular for a wide range of consumers. Milk contains casein, whey protein, lactoferrin, milk lipid and phospholipids, vitamins, and microelements, for example, selenium (Se), which have antioxidant properties. Furthermore, probiotication of milk either sweet or fermented could enhance the antioxidant capacity of milk. This chapter focuses on presenting recent review data on milk components with antioxidant activity and their health benefits, probiotics as antioxidant agents, and methods for enhancing the antioxidant capacity of dairy products. The key aim of this chapter is to focus on major strategies for enhancing the antioxidant capacity of milk and its products.

Keywords: essential oils, plant extracts, probiotication, dietary management, metabolic diseases, antioxidant capacity of milk

1. Introduction

Reactive species are formed during different cellular process, especially during mitochondrial respiratory chain. Reactive oxygen species (ROS) and reactive nitrogen species (RNS) are major reactive species that act as second messengers to regulate biological processes. However, they could cause oxidative stress and protein and DNA damage, which may cause different diseases such as atherosclerosis, diabetes, accelerated aging, and cardiovascular diseases [1].

Milk as a natural product is the first food for humans, and dairy products represent approximately 25–30% of an individual's diet. It also contains different components with antioxidant activity such as casein, whey protein, sulfur-containing amino acids cysteine, conjugated linoleic acid, and catalase that could restore the antioxidant system of the host [2]. Supplementation of milk with natural sources represents a dietary strategy in order to enhance the antioxidant capacity of milk and its products. Essential oils (EO) are volatile hydrophobic liquids that are extracted from a wide range of plants. They also possess different therapeutic effects, for example, anti-inflammatory and anti-microbial activities [3]. Supplementation of butter oil/ghee with different concentrations of essential oils (glove, garden cress, and jojoba) enhances its antioxidant capacity and shelf life [4, 5]. Furthermore, addition of ethanol extraction of pomegranate peels to ghee enhances the oxidative stability [6].

Probiotication means addition of probiotics (beneficial microbes for the host) to food products. It was considered as a dietary strategy for enhancing the antioxidant capacity of different fermented milk products through the ability of different probiotic strains, for example, *Lb. casei* shirota strain, to produce different metabolites from lactose fermentation or milk protein hydrolysis [7, 8]. This chapter aims to present the recent knowledge on the antioxidant potential of milk and major methods for enhancing the antioxidant capacity of dairy products.

2. Milk component with antioxidant activities: an overview

The antioxidant components in milk could be classified as non-enzymatic compounds, for example, milk proteins, and enzymatic antioxidants, for example, superoxide dismutase (SOD). **Figure 1** shows both selected antioxidant categories in milk. Casein is a major milk protein, accounting for 80% of the total protein in cow milk, and it presents in macromolecule aggregates because of the phosphorus content of casein [9]. Furthermore, the primary structure of casein has free radical scavenging activity [10]. Casein-derived phospho-peptide and phosphoserine residues can bind the non-heme iron [11]. Results obtained by Çekiç et al. [12] showed that β-casein fraction exhibited high antioxidant activity due to the presence of proline residues.

Whey protein as an antioxidant agent was used for inhibiting lipid peroxidation. The antioxidant activity of whey protein is due to its content of sulfur-containing amino acids. Addition of whey protein to soybean and salmon oils increased the oxidative stability of these products [13, 14]. The antioxidant activity of lactoferrin is due to iron-chelating activity and inhibits pro-oxidant effect and release of ROS by leucocytes [15, 16].

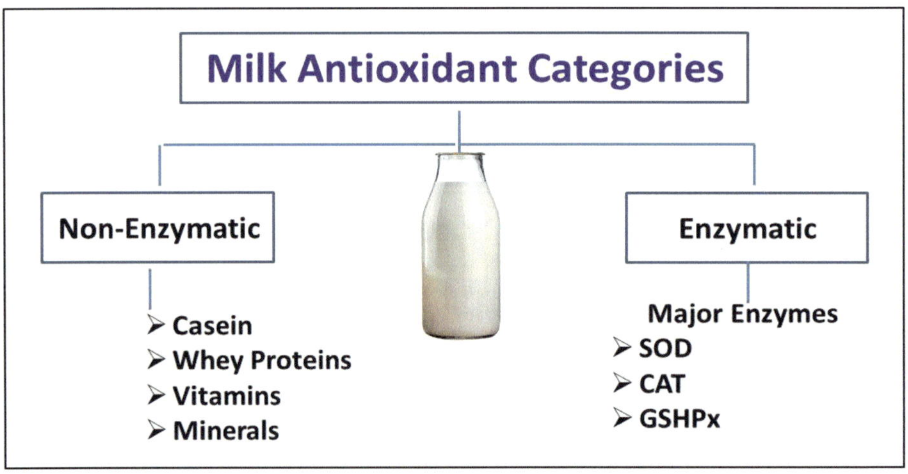

Figure 1.
The major two antioxidant categories in milk. SOD: super oxide dismutase, CAT: catalase, GSHPx: glutathione peroxidase.

Vitamins (soluble in either milk fat or milk serum) and minerals play an essential role as antioxidant factors. The antioxidant capacity of vitamins E (α-tocopherol), A, and C (ascorbic acid) as well as carotenoids is due to their ability to scavenge free radicals (mainly oxygen, hydroxyl, and peroxyl radicals), inhibit lipid peroxidation, and protect DNA from damage [17, 18]. Supplementation of milk with ascorbic acid in light-exposed milk enhanced the antioxidant capacity of milk and inhibited the degradation of riboflavin [19]. Moreover, fortification of cheddar cheese with vitamin E and selenium (Se) enhanced the oxidative stability of cheddar cheese and its shelf life [20].

Feeding strategies of dairy animals has a potential impact on levels of polyphenols, changes in amino/fatty acid composition in milk, and its overall antioxidant capacity [21]. In this respect, feeding dairy cow with carrot results in increased levels of β-carotene and α-tocopherol in milk [22]. Also, supplementation of animal feeds with fish oil and grazing improved the antioxidant capacity of cow and sheep milk, respectively [23, 24]. Recently, supplementation of grazing with tannin for dairy cow has enhanced the status of antioxidant capacity of blood plasma and cheese [25].

Enzymatic antioxidant in milk includes super oxide dismutase (SOD), glutathione peroxidase (GSHPx), and catalase (CAT). SOD safeguards cells from superoxide free radicals and lipid peroxidation [26]. Levels of SOD in cow milk range from 0.15 to 2.4 mg/L. However, the content of SOD in human milk is higher than (2.0–2.3 times) in cow milk [27]. GSHPx (Se encompassing enzyme) plays an important role in protection from lipid peroxidation [28]. Also, human milk has a higher concentration of GSHPx than caprine and cow milk [29]. A decrease in levels of selenium content and antioxidant activity could be detected with the progression of lactation [30]. Catalase (CAT: heme protein with molecular weight = 200KDa) has a dismutation effect against hydrogen peroxide [31]. The concentration of CAT in human milk is 10 times more than in cow milk, whereas the content of CAT in cow milk is approximately 1.95 U/mL [32].

3. Natural plant extracts for enhancing the antioxidant capacity of milk and its products

In recent years, there has been high focus toward the field of antioxidants and the reduction of free radicals. Milk and dairy products are essential components of human nutrition, and they are considered the carriers of several bioactive compounds that are important for a variety of biochemical and physiological functions. Milk and dairy products (yogurt and cheese), accounting for approximately 25–30% of the average human diet, are undoubtedly a rich source of compounds exhibiting antioxidant properties. Additionally, it is worth emphasizing that regular consumption of natural dairy antioxidants minimizes the risk of development of civilization diseases (e.g., cardiovascular disease, cancer, or diabetes). It also slows down the aging process in the organisms [33].

On the other hand, the consumption of natural antioxidant-rich foods improves an organism's antioxidant status by protecting it from oxidative stress and damage. Consumption of food products that are rich in natural antioxidants improves the antioxidant status of an organism through protection against oxidative stress and damage [34]. The antioxidant status of milk and dairy products can be improved with the use of natural additives in animal nutrition or at the stage of milk processing. Herbal mixtures, seeds, fruits, and waste from the fruit and vegetable industry are used most commonly [35]. Commercially, cheddar cheese was fortified by chili and red pepper by Monterey Jack Co., California, USA. Also, Khaled Khoshala for industry and trading Co., Obour city, Egypt, manufactured Egyptian soft cheese (Gebna Bida) and processed cheese fortified with green and red pepper that enhanced the shelf life of final products.

Numerous studies have tried to enhance antioxidant activities of foods by mixing them with phenolic components [36, 37]. Examples constitute the non-covalent complexes of polyphenols and proteins in foods [38, 39]. However, these types of interactions have been shown to alter the structure, function, stability, and nutritional properties of the complex [40, 41]. Though these methods are relatively cheaper, they are largely ineffective due to the reversible nature of the interactions between proteins

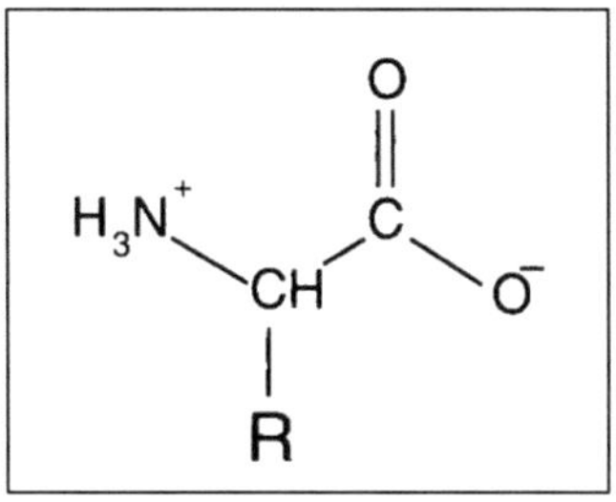

Figure 2.
Individual amino acids consist of a primary amine, a carboxylic acid group, and a unique side-chain structure (R).

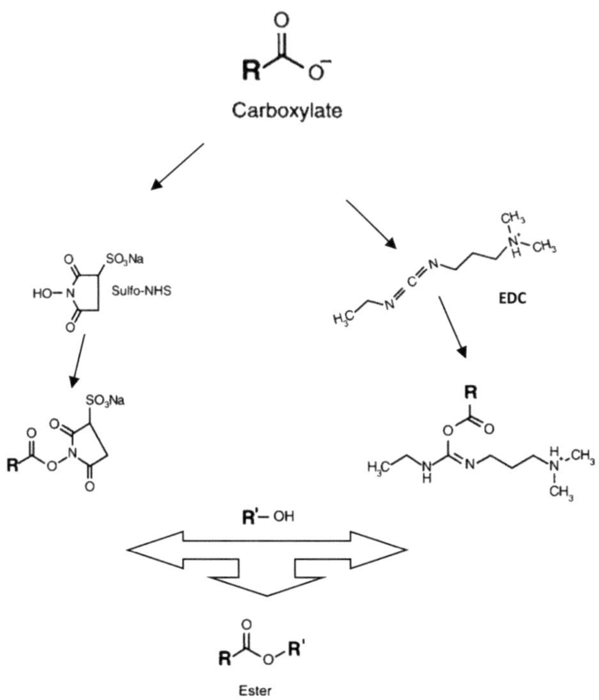

Figure 3.
Derivatives of carboxylic acids can be interacted through the use of active intermediates that react with target functional groups, NHS: N-hydroxysuccinimide; EDC: N-(3-imethylaminopropyl)-N′-ethylcarbodiimide hydrochloride.

and phenolic acids, which leads to an unstable complex for food processing conditions. Thus, covalently linking phenolic acids to proteins might be a way to generate a more stable antioxidant for food [42].

Bioconjugation involves the linking of two or more molecules to form a novel complex having the combined properties of its individual components. Natural or synthetic compounds with their individual activities can be chemically combined to produce unique substances possessing multifunctional characteristics. A protein that can bind discretely to a target molecule through the functional groups (**Figure 2**) within a complex mixture can thus be crosslinked with another detectable molecule to form a traceable conjugate. The conjugation techniques are dependent on the functional groups present on the target macromolecules to be modified. Protein molecules are the most common targets for modification with natural antioxidants such as phenolic acids (**Figure 3**) [43, 44].

4. Dairy products fortified with essential oils as antioxidant promoters

The control of free radicals, prooxidants, and oxidation intermediates is used to protect the protein and lipid components of food from oxidation [45]. In addition to oxidative damage and death of cells, tissue damage and various pathological conditions may be the consequence of oxidative stress. Deleterious changes in dairy products caused by lipid oxidation include not only flavor loss or the development of off-flavors but also color loss, nutrient value loss, and the accumulation of compounds that may be harmful to consumers' health. One of the most effective ways of reducing the lipid oxidation in dairy products is to incorporate antioxidants [46].

Free radical scavengers (FRS) inhibit lipid oxidation by reacting faster than unsaturated fatty acids with free radicals. Synthetic antioxidants such as butylated hydroxytoluene (BHT) and butylated hydroxyanisole (BHA) are widely used to prevent lipid oxidation (BHA). However, large amounts of these synthetic ingredients have been linked to carcinogenic and cytotoxic effects. Therefore, the focus has shifted toward the use of natural antioxidants such as essential oils and phenolic acids [43]. Essential oils are liquid aromatic substance, and they are extracted from plants that have been proven to be good sources of bioactive compounds with antioxidative and antimicrobial properties. Essential oils play a high role as good free radical scavengers. Also, natural essential oils have to be given a lot of interest for enhancing overall well-being, in the prevention of diseases and in the incorporation of health-promoting substances into the diet [47]. Additionally, the use of essential oils as natural antioxidants in dairy products can reduce the rate of lipid oxidation and hydrolysis and may be beneficial in increasing the shelf life of these products [46]. Marjoram, frankincense, thyme, myrtle, lemon, oregano, and lavender essential oils are commonly used as food additives. These supplementations will move the dairy products into the functional food area as healthy dairy products.

Different essential oils extracted from plant sources such as cumin, rosemary, and thyme and their mixtures have been studied for their effect on physicochemical, microbial, rheological, and sensorial attributes of ultra-filtrated (UF)-soft cheese. The results revealed that the different essential oils had remarkable antimicrobial effect on the growth of pathogenic bacteria (i.e., *Escherichia coli*, *Salmonella typhimurium*, *Staphylococcus aureus*, *Bacillus subtilis*, *Bacillus cereus*, and *Aspergillus niger*) [48].

5. Impact of probiotication of dairy foods on enhancement of their antioxidant capacity

Probiotics are *live microorganisms, which when administered in adequate amounts confer health benefits to the host* [49]. A recent definition of probiotics by Elshaghabee [50] was probiotics are live microbial strains with health impact on host when they consumed daily with enough amounts (not less than 10^6–10^8 CFU/g) and incorporated into the gut micro-biome. The main two genera of probiotics are *Lactobacillus* (*Lb.*) and *Bifidobacterium*. Different studies had led to a renewed interest in probiotics as antioxidant agents. Isolated *Lb. fermentum* from GIT mucosa could scavenge free radicals using *in vitro* model and enhance the antioxidant status and health of pigs [51]. Probiotic yeast *Sacch. cerevisiae* DSMZ strain had higher antioxidant capacity than *Lb. casei* 01 and bifidobacteria B-12 in either viable or non-viable form [52].

A mixture of probiotic bacteria containing *Lb. acidophilus* W70, *Lb. casei* W56, *Lb. salivarius* W24, *Lactococcus lactis* W58, *Bifidobacterium* (Bif.) *bifidum* W23, and *Bif. lactis* W52 enhanced de novo synthesis of GSH under severe acute pancreatitis in a rat model [53]. Furthermore, Spyropoulos et al. [54] reviewed that several probiotic species, for example, *L. lactis* and *Lb. plantarum*, could produce SOD, resulting in a protective effect against radiation-induced enteritis and colitis. Also, some species of probiotic bacteria could produce folate, which could enhance the antioxidant capacity [55].

Feeding mice with engineered *Lb. casei* BL23-producing SOD could significantly decrease the intestinal inflammation in mice with Crohn's disease [56]. Feeding boiler with spore-forming probiotics *Bacillus coagulans* could enhance the antioxidant capacity, immunity, and gut function [57]. In a human experiment, the status of total antioxidant capacity of type 2 diabetic patients was enhanced when they received yogurt containing *Lb. acidophilus* La 5 and *Bif. lactis* Bb-12 [58]. All health benefits of spore-forming probiotics with their future prospects were reviewed by Elshaghabee et al. [59].

Gut microbiota, including probiotics, has a protective effect against pathogens by competitive exclusion [60]. Imbalance in the composition of gut microbiota resulted in increased levels of ROS and could affect redox homeostatic in the host [61]. Probiotics can regulate positively the composition of gut microbiota through different mechanisms, for example, producing a wide range of organic acids, mainly lactic and acetic. Propionic and butyric acids produced from cross feeding of lactate by other gut microbiota resulting in lowered the pH of colon and inhibiting the growth of a wide range of pathogens as well as other harmful bacteria [62, 63].

Probiotic *Lb. johnsonii* BS15 could attenuate high fat diet that induced oxidative stress and modulated the ratio of *Firmicutes*/*Bacteroidetes* in mice model [64]. Also, supplementation of probiotic ABT-fermented milk with heat-treated *Sacch. cerevisiae* could significantly enhance the antioxidant capacity of the product [65]. Recently, lased-treated *Lb. casei* had higher free radical scavenging activity than non-treated cells [66, 67].

Akkermansia (A.) muciniphila represents a new generation of probiotics; it is an intestinal mucin-degrading bacterium, and it could regulate blood pressure, and it could release the endogenous hydrogen sulfide (H2S), which has been considered a potential regulator of vascular homeostasis, possibly through the regulation of vascular tone and inflammation, antioxidant mechanism, vascular cell proliferation, and apoptosis [68]. Data in **Figure 4** conclude different possible mechanisms of antioxidant activity of different probiotic genera.

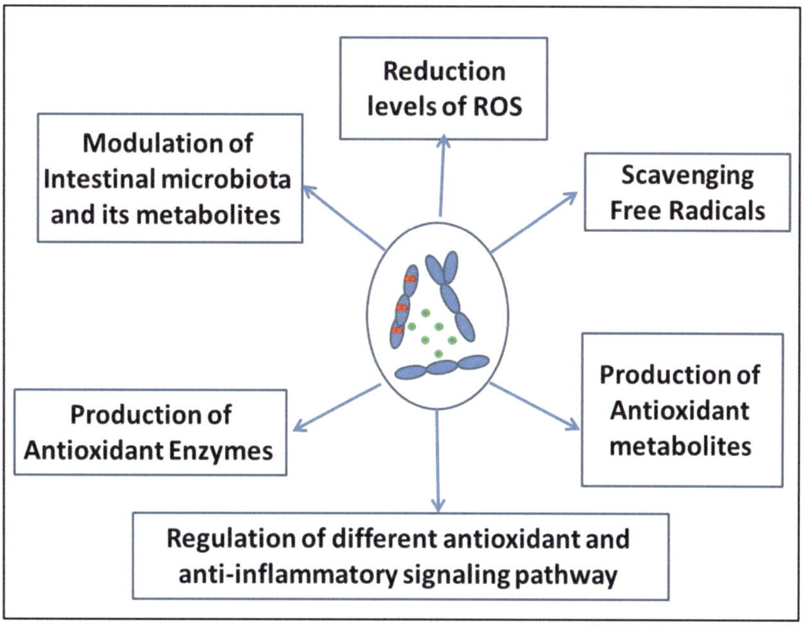

Figure 4.
Selected different possible mechanisms of probiotics as antioxidant food supplements.

6. Conclusion

In the past few years, there has been an increasing demand for natural products with antioxidant activity as well as dairy foods. Milk is the first food for mammalians. It contains different antioxidant components that cleared in this chapter. The use of different plants or herbs has been was in practice from the ancient time. Fortification of different dairy products with either plant extracts or essential oils enhanced the antioxidant capacity and quality parameters including shelf life of these products. Recently, different species of probiotics could be used also for enhancing the antioxidant capacity of fermented milks. This chapter reveals that consumers could use different methods for enhancing the antioxidant status of dairy products resulting in an enhancement the health status of consumers which serve the sustainable development goals SDG 3 (good health and wellbeing).

Author details

Fouad M.F. Elshaghabee[1]*, Ahmed A. Abd El-Maksoud[1]
and Gustavo M. Ambrósio F. de Gouveia[2]

1 Dairy Science Department, Faculty of Agriculture, Cairo University, Giza, Egypt

2 LEAF - Linking Landscape, Environment Agriculture and Food, Instituto Superior de Agronomia da Universidada de Lisboa, Lisboa, Portugal

*Address all correspondence to: elshaghabee@agr.cu.edu.eg

References

[1] Schieber M, Chandel N. ROS function in redox signaling and oxidative stress. Current Biology. 2014;**24**:453-462

[2] Richmond HD. Dairy Chemistry: A Practical Handbook for Dairy Chemists and Others Having Control of Dairies. USA: Cole Press; 2007

[3] Worwood VA. The Complete Book of Essential Oils and Aroma Therapy, Revised and Expanded: Over 800 Natural, Nontoxic, and Fragrant Recipes to Create Health, Beauty, and Safe Home and Work Environments. USA: New World Library; 2016

[4] Shende S, Shriyash P, Sumit A, Sharma V. Oxidative stability of ghee incorporated with clove extracts and bha at elevated temperatures. International Journal of Food Properties. 2014;**17**:1599-1611

[5] Taha SH, Abdel Hamid M, Awad AA, Elshaghabee FMF. Extending the shelf life of ghee using garden cress and jojoba oils as alternatives of synthetic antioxidants. Egyptian Journal of Chemistry. 2022;**65**:315-322

[6] El-Shourbagy GA, El-Zahar KM. Oxidative stability of ghee as affected by natural antioxidants extracted from food processing wastes. Annals of Agricultural Science. 2016;**59**:213-220

[7] Liu M, Bayjanov JR, Renckens B, Nauta A, Siezen RJ. The proteolytic system of lactic acid bacteria revisited: A genomic comparison. BMC Genomics. 2010;**15**:36

[8] Güler Z, Gürsoy-Balcı AC. Evaluation of volatile compounds and free fatty acids in set types yogurts made of ewes', goats' milk and their mixture using two different commercial starter cultures during refrigerated storage. Food Chemistry. 2011;**127**:1065-1071

[9] Cervato G, Cazzola R, Cestaro B. Studies on the antioxidant activity of milk caseins. International Journal of Food Sciences and Nutrition. 1999;**50**:291-296

[10] Suetsuna K, Ukeda H, Ochi H. Isolation and characterization of free radical scavenging activities peptides derived from casein. The Journal of Nutritional Biochemistry. 2000;**11**:128-131

[11] Kitts DD. Antioxidant properties of casein phosphopeptides. Trends in Food Science and Technology. 2005;**16**:549-554

[12] Çekiç SD, Demir A, Baskan KS, Tütem E, Apak R. Determination of total antioxidant capacity of milk by CUPRAC and ABTS methods with separate characterisation of milk protein fractions. The Journal of Dairy Research. 2015;**82**:177-184

[13] Tong LM, Sasaki S, McClements DJ, Decker EA. Antioxidant activity of whey in a salmon oil emulsion. Journal of Food Science. 2001;**8**:1325-1329

[14] Erel Ö. A novel automated method to measure total antioxidant capacity using a new generation, more stable ABTS radical cation. Clinical Biochemistry. 2004;**7**:277-285

[15] Rastogi N, Singh A, Singh PK, Tyagi TK, Pandey S, Shin K, et al. Structure of iron saturated Clobe of bovine lactoferrin at pH 6.8 indicates a weakening of iron coordination. Proteins. 2016;**84**:591-599

[16] Cutone A, Rosa L, Ianiro G, Lepanto MS, Bonaccorsi di Patti M, Calenti P, et al. Lactoferrin's anti-cancer properties: Safety, selectivity, and wide range of action. Biomolecules. 2020;**10**:456

[17] Mann S, Shandilya UK, Sodhi M, Kumar P, Bharti VK, Verma P, et al. Determination of antioxidant capacity and free radical scavenging activity of milk from native cows (*Bos indicus*), exotic cows (*Bos taurus*), and riverine buffaloes (*Bubalus bubalis*) across different lactation stages. International Journal of Dairy Science. 2016;**3**:66-70

[18] Cichosz G, Czeczot H, Ambroziak A, Bielecka MM. Natural antioxidants in milk and dairy products. International Journal of Dairy Technology. 2017;**70**:165-178

[19] Hagemeier J, Ramanathan M, Schweser F, Dwyer MG, Lin F, Bergsland N, et al. Iron-related gene variants and brain iron in multiple sclerosis and healthy individuals. NeuroImage: Clinical. 2018;**17**:530-540

[20] Batool M, Nadeem M, Imran M, Gulzar N, Shahid MQ, Shahbaz M, et al. Impact of vitamin E and selenium on antioxidant capacity and lipid oxidation of cheddar cheese in accelerated ripening. Lipids in Health and Disease. 2018;**17**:79

[21] Tufarelli V, Khan RU, Laudadio V. Evaluating the suitability of field beans as a substitute for soybean meal in early-lactating dairy cow: Production and metabolic responses. Animal Science Journal. 2012;**83**:136-140

[22] De Ondarza M, Wilson J, Engstrom M. Case study: Effect of supplemental β-carotene on yield of milk and milk components and on reproduction of dairy cows. The Professional Animal Scientists. 2009;**25**(4):510-516

[23] De Renobales M, Amores G, Arran J, Virto M, Barrón LJR, Bustamante MA, et al. Part-time grazing improves sheep milk production and its nutritional characteristics. Food Chemistry. 2012;**130**:90-96

[24] Puppel K, Kuczyńska B, Nałęcz-Tarwacka T, Grodzki H. Influence of linseed variety on fatty acid profile in cow's milk. Journal of the Science of Food and Agriculture. 2013;**93**:2276-2280

[25] Santillo A, Ciliberti MG, Ciampi F, Luciano G, Natalello A, Menci R, et al. Feeding tannins to dairy cows in different seasons improves the oxidative status of blood plasma and the antioxidant capacity of cheese. Journal of Dairy Science. 2022;**105**:22256-22268

[26] Matés JM, Pérez-Gómez C, Núñez de Castro I. Antioxidant enzymes and human diseases. Clinical Biochemistry. 1999;**32**:595-603

[27] Fang YZ, Yang S, Wu G. Free radicals, antioxidants and nutrition. Nutrition. 2002;**18**:872-879

[28] Kendall A, Woolcock A, Brooks A, Moore GE. Glutathione peroxidase activity, plasma total antioxidant capacity, and urinary f2-isoprostanes as markers of oxidative stress in anemic dogs. Journal of Veterinary Internal Medicine. 2017;**31**(6):1700-1707

[29] Hameed A, Hussain M, Akhtar S. Lactation Responses toward Milk Indigenous Enzymes. London, UK: Livestock Science, InTech, Selim Sekkin, IntechOpen; 2017

[30] Matos C, Ribeiro M, Guerra A. Breastfeeding: Antioxidative properties

of breast milk. Journal of Applied Biomedicine. 2015;**13**:169-180

[31] Mishra A, Chaudhary SK, Raje S, Bisht P. Effect of niacin supplementation on milk yield and composition during heat stress in dairy cows: A review. International Journal of Current Microbiology and Applied Sciences. 2018;**6**:1719-1724

[32] Pfrimer K, Ferriolli E, Takeuchi PL, Salles MS, Saran-Netto A, Zanetti MA, et al. Effects of the consumption of milk biofortified with selenium, vitamin E, and different fatty acid profile on immune response in the elderly. Molecular Nutrition & Food Research. 2018;**62**:1700307

[33] Khan IT, Nadeem M, Imran M, Ullah R, Ajmal M, Jaspal MH. Antioxidant properties of milk and dairy products: A comprehensive review of the current knowledge. Lipids in Health and Disease. 2019;**18**:1-13

[34] Lobo V, Patil A, Phatak A, Chandra N. Free radicals, antioxidants and functional foods: Impact on human health. Pharmacognosy Reviews. 2010;**4**:118

[35] Stobiecka M, Król J, Brodziak A. Antioxidant activity of milk and dairy products. Animals. 2022;**12**:245

[36] Wu X, Wu H, Liu M, Liu Z, Xu H, Lai F. Analysis of binding interaction between (−)-epigallocatechin (EGC) and β-lactoglobulin by multi-spectroscopic method. Spectrochimica Acta Part A: Molecular and Biomolecular Spectroscopy. 2011;**82**:164-168

[37] Martins A, Barros L, Carvalho AM, Santos-Buelga C, Fernandes IP, Barreiro F, et al. Phenolic extracts of *Rubus ulmifolius* Schott flowers: Characterization, microencapsulation and incorporation into yogurts as nutraceutical sources. Food & Function. 2014;**5**:1091-1100

[38] Li M, Ma Y, Ngadi MO. Binding of curcumin to β-lactoglobulin and its effect on antioxidant characteristics of curcumin. Food Chemistry. 2013;**141**:1504-1511

[39] Shpigelman A, Cohen Y, Livney YD. Thermally-induced β-lactoglobulin–EGCG nanovehicles: Loading, stability, sensory and digestive-release study. Food Hydrocolloids. 2012;**29**:57-67

[40] Mehanna NS, Hassan ZMR, El-Din HMF, Ali AAE, Amarowicz R, ElMessery TM. Effect of interaction phenolic compounds with milk proteins on cell line. Food and Nutrition Sciences. 2014;**5**:2130-2146

[41] Ozdal T, Capanoglu E, Altay F. A review on protein–phenolic interactions and associated changes. Food Research International. 2013;**51**:954-970

[42] Hermanson G. Bioconjugate Techniques. 2nd ed. Massachusetts, USA: Academic Press is an Imprint of Elsevier; 2008. pp. 77-118

[43] Abd El-Maksoud AA, Abd El-Ghany IH, El-Beltagi HS, Anankanbil S, Banerjee C, Petersen SV, et al. Adding functionality to milk-based protein: Preparation, and physico-chemical characterization of β-lactoglobulin-phenolic conjugates. Food Chemistry. 2018;**241**:281-289

[44] Abd El-Maksoud AA, Anankanbil S, Zhou Y, Abd El-Ghany IH, El-Beltagi HS, Banerjee C, et al. Grafting phenolics onto milk protein via conjugated polymerization for delivery of multiple functionalities: Synthesis and characterization. Food Chemistry. 2019;**301**:125298

[45] Ayala A, Muñoz MF, Argüelles S. Lipid peroxidation: Production, metabolism, and signaling mechanisms of malondialdehyde and 4-hydroxy-2-nonenal. Oxidative Medicine and Cellular Longevity. 2014;**2014**:360438

[46] Gad AS, Sayd AF. Antioxidant properties of rosemary and its potential uses as natural antioxidant in dairy products—A review. Food and Nutrition Sciences. 2015;**6**:179-193

[47] Król SK, Skalicka-Woźniak K, Kandefer-Szerszeń M, Stepulak A. The biological and pharmacological activity of essential oils in the treatment and prevention of infectious diseases. Postepy Higieny I Medycyny Doswiadczalnej. 2013;**67**:1000-1007

[48] Chouhan S, Sharma K, Guleria S. Antimicrobial activity of some essential oils—Present status and future perspectives. Medicines (Basel). 2017;**4**:58

[49] FAO/WHO. Guidelines for the Evaluation of Probiotics in Food. Food and Agriculture Organization of the United Nations and World Health Organization Working Group Report. Rome: Food and Agriculture Organization; 2002

[50] Elshaghabee FMF. Probiotics food supplement for NAFLD. Journal of Nutritional Health & Food Engineering. 2017;**6**:123

[51] Wang A, Yi X, Yu H, Dong B, Qiao Y. Free radical scavenging activity of *Lactobacillus fermentum* in vitro and its antioxidative effect on growing-finishing pigs. Journal of Applied Microbiology. 2009;**107**:1140-1148

[52] SM EL-D, Abd Rabo FR, Badran SM, Abd El-Fattah AM, FMF E. *In vitro* model for assessment of the health benefits of some microbial strains. International Journal of Probiotics & Prebiotics. 2010;**5**:157-163

[53] Lutgendorff F, Trulsson LM, van Minnen LP, et al. Probiotics enhance pancreatic glutathione biosynthesis and reduce oxidative stress in experimental acute pancreatitis. American Journal of Physiology. Gastrointestinal and Liver Physiology. 2008;**295**:G1111-G1121

[54] Spyropoulos BG, Misiakos EP, Fotiadis C, et al. Antioxidant properties of probiotics and their protective effects in the pathogenesis of radiation-induced enteritis and colitis. Digestive Diseases and Sciences. 2011;**56**:285-294

[55] Rossi M, Amaretti A, Raimondi S. Folate production by probiotic bacteria. Nutrients. 2011;**3**:118-134

[56] LeBlanc JG, Del Carmen S, Miyoshi A, Azevedo V, Sesma F, Langella P, et al. Use of superoxide dismutase and catalase producing lactic acid bacteria in TNBS induced Crohn's disease in mice. Journal of Biotechnology. 2011;**151**:287-293

[57] Zhang B, Zhang H, Yu Y, Zhang R, Wu Y, Yue M, et al. Effects of *Bacillus coagulans* on growth performance, antioxidant capacity, immunity function, and gut health in broilers. Poultry Science. 2021;**100**:101168

[58] Ejtahed HS, Mohtadi-Nia J, Homayouni-Rad A, Niafar M, Asghari-Jafarabadi M, Mofid V. Probiotic yogurt improves antioxidant status in type 2 diabetic patients. Nutrition. 2012;**28**:539-543

[59] Elshaghabee FMF, Rokana N, Gulhane R, Sharma C, Panwer H. *Bacillus* as potential probiotics: Status, concerns, and future perspectives. Frontiers in Microbiology. 2017;**10**:1490

[60] Qiao Y, Sun J, Ding Y, Le G, Shi Y. Alterations of the gut microbiota in high-fat diet mice is strongly linked to oxidative stress. Applied Microbiology and Biotechnology. 2013;**97**:1689-1697

[61] Jones RM, Neish AS. Redox signaling mediated by the gut microbiota. Free Radical Biology & Medicine. 2017;**105**:41-47

[62] Vanderhoof JA, Young RJ. Current and potential uses of probiotics. Annals of Allergy, Asthma & Immunology. 2004;**93**:S33-S37

[63] Kaur J, Singh BP, Chaudhary V, Elshaghabee FMF, Singh J, Singh A, et al. [Probiotics as Live Bio-Therapeutics: Prospects and Perspectives] In Advances in Probiotics for Sustainable Food and Medicine. Microorganisms for Sustainability: Springer; 2020. pp. 83-120

[64] Xin J, Zeng D, Wang H, Ni X, Yi D, Pan K, et al. Preventing non-alcoholic fatty liver disease through *Lactobacillus johnsonii* BS15 by attenuating inflammation and mitochondrial injury and improving gut environment in obese mice. Applied Microbiology and Biotechnology. 2014;**98**:6817-6829

[65] Mohamed MSM, Elshaghabee FMF, Alharbi SA, El-Hussein A. The prospective beneficial effects of red laser exposure on *Lactocaseibacillus casei* fermentation of skim milk. Biology. 2020;**9**:256

[66] Elshaghabee FMF, Abd El-Maksoud AA, Alharbi SA, Alfarraj S, Mohamed MSM. Fortification of acidophilus-bifidus-thermophilus (ABT) fermented milk with heat-treated industrial yeast enhances its selected properties. Molecules. 2021;**26**:3876

[67] Elshaghabee FMF, El-Hussein A, Mohamed MSM. Enhancement of labneh quality by laser-induced modulation of *Lactocaseibacillus casei* NRRL B-1922. Fermentation. 2022;**8**:132

[68] Lv B, Chen S, Tang C, Jin H, Du J, Huang Y. Hydrogen sulfide and vascular regulation—An update. Journal of Advanced Research. 2021;**27**:85-97

Chapter 6

Naturally Occurring Antioxidants in Seven Well-Known Fruits from the Republic of Suriname (South America): Part 1

Dennis R.A. Mans

Abstract

The dependence of humans on oxygen for their metabolism, together with their uninterrupted exposure to a wide variety of hazardous environmental chemicals, leads to the continuous formation of reactive oxygen-derived species (ROS) in the body, such as superoxide radical anion, hydrogen peroxide, peroxyl radicals, and hydroxyl radical. When in excess, ROS can damage cellular constituents such as DNA and membrane lipids causing oxidative stress, cellular injury, and, eventually, inflammatory, neoplastic, diabetic, cardiovascular, neurodegenerative, and age-related diseases. Fortunately, the body has a multitude of naturally occurring antioxidants in dietary fruits and vegetables to its disposal, including polyphenolic compounds, vitamins, and essential minerals. These antioxidants eliminate ROS by acting as reducing agents, hydrogen donors, quenchers of singlet oxygen, or chelators of metal ions that catalyze oxidation reactions, thus decreasing the risk of the abovementioned diseases. This first part of the current chapter comprehensively addresses three representative examples of fruits from the Republic of Suriname (South America) that are rich in anthocyanins, ellagitannins, and coumarins and highlights their antioxidant activity and beneficial and health-promoting effects. In part 2, four Surinamese fruits with an abundance of (pro)vitamins A, C, and E and selenium are equally extensively dealt with in light of their antioxidant activities.

Keywords: reactive oxygen species, antioxidants, fruits, Suriname, anthocyanins, ellagitannins, coumarins

1. Introduction

There is ample evidence that life on our planet has developed under anaerobic conditions [1, 2]. Most organisms that evolved from these primordial predecessors have dealt with the increasing atmospheric levels of oxygen by adapting to oxygen and its derivatives and creating antioxidant defense systems to protect themselves against the toxic effects of these compounds [3, 4]. The most notable toxic byproducts of metabolic reactions involving oxygen are reactive oxygen-derived species (ROS) such as superoxide radical anion, hydrogen peroxide, peroxyl radicals, and hydroxyl, as well as nonradical species such as hydrogen peroxide, peroxynitrite, hypochlorous acid, and ozone [5–7]. Reactive nitrogen species (RNS), such as nitric oxide, peroxynitrite, and nitrogen dioxide radical, as well as reactive chlorine species (RCS), such as hypochlorous acid, are also classified as ROS [5–7]. ROS are able to readily react with and cause damage to biomolecules including proteins, lipids, and nucleic acids, leading to cell and tissue injury [8–10]. The high reactivity of ROS derives from the presence of a single unpaired electron in their outer orbit formed as a result of incomplete reduction of the oxygen metabolites [8–10].

ROS are mainly generated in cellular organelles where oxygen consumption is high, such as mitochondria, peroxisomes, and endoplasmic reticulum [11–13]. In addition to these endogenous sources, ROS are produced from exogenous sources such as car exhaust, cigarette smoke, and industrial contaminants; peroxides, aldehydes, oxidized fatty acids, and transition metals in foods; a large variety of xenobiotics including toxins, pesticides, and herbicides; as well as various medical drugs such as narcotics, anesthetizing gases, and antineoplastic agents [5, 14, 15]. For example, γ-radiation interacts with water molecules to form water radical cations and free electrons, which react with other water molecules to form highly active hydroxyl radicals, superoxides, and organic radicals as well as organic hydroperoxides and hydrogen peroxide [16]. And the antitumor antibiotic doxorubicin generates a semiquinone derivative that can autoxidize in the presence of oxygen, producing superoxide anions following electron donation by oxidases such as mitochondrial nicotinamide adenine dinucleotide phosphate (NADPH) and nitric oxide synthases [17]. In all the cases, the ROS-induced oxidative stress results in massive damage to cellular macromolecules such as DNA, critical proteins, and membrane lipids, eventually causing, among others, neoplastic, neurodegenerative, cardiovascular, age-related, cerebrovascular, diabetic, and inflammatory diseases [18–24].

However, as mentioned above, aerobic organisms have developed mechanisms to adapt to and cope with ROS. Major adaptation mechanisms involve the utilization of oxygen and ROS as relay elements in pathways of cell signaling and homeostasis, for various metabolic reactions, to eliminate xenobiotics from the body, and to help destroy phagocytized harmful particles. For instance, ROS, in particular hydrogen peroxide, can act as messengers in the transduction of metabolic and environmental signals, which affect diverse intracellular pathways, culminating in the activation of transcription factors and other proteins, controlling their biological activities [9]. A well-investigated example is redox signaling involving the oxidation of cysteine residues of proteins by hydrogen peroxide, converting a thiolate anion in cysteine (Cys-S-) into the sulfenic form (Cys-SOH), causing the protein to undergo allosteric changes that alter its function [25]. Furthermore, the formation of adenosine triphosphate (ATP) during oxidative phosphorylation in the mitochondria is accompanied by the production of electrons in the electron transport chain for the reduction of molecular oxygen into superoxides that are subsequently transformed into the much less reactive hydrogen peroxide by superoxide dismutase [26]. In addition, the addition of oxygen atoms to xenobiotics by cytochrome P450 enzymes increases their water solubility, facilitating their removal from the body [27]. And phagocytized bacteria, bits of necrotic tissue, and foreign particles are intracellularly destroyed by macrophages and neutrophils by the so-called respiratory burst (or oxidative burst), involving the rapid release of superoxides and hydrogen peroxide following the supply of electrons by NADPH [28].

Critical mechanisms of aerobic organisms to cope with ROS involve the use of endogenous and exogenous defense systems that counter their detrimental effects. The endogenous defenses comprise enzymatic antioxidant systems such as superoxide dismutase, catalase, and glutathione peroxidase [29] and nonenzymatic mechanisms such as bilirubin and albumin [30]. The exogenous defenses complement the endogenous mechanisms and consist of antioxidants in fruits and vegetables provided through the diet [31] and include, among others, various phenolic compounds, vitamins, essential minerals, small peptides, and fatty acids [32, 33]. Like the exogenous mechanisms, the endogenous defenses prevent the formation of ROS through various mechanisms [29–31, 33, 34]. A multitude of studies have validated the critical role of exogenous dietary antioxidants in our well-being (see, for instance, [31, 32]). This has resulted in the recommendation of diets high in fruits and vegetables that are rich in these compounds to decrease the risk of developing the abovementioned degenerative diseases [35–37]. The first part of this chapter provides some information about the role of naturally occurring antioxidants as exogenous antioxidant defenses, gives some background on the Republic of Suriname, and then comprehensively addresses three representative examples of well-known Surinamese fruits that are rich in the polyphenolic compounds, such as anthocyanins, ellagitannins, and coumarins, highlighting the involvement of these naturally occurring antioxidants in the beneficial and health-promoting effects of the fruits. The second part of the chapter continues with a comprehensive overview of four additional popular Surinamese plants with an abundance of (pro)vitamins A, C, or E, or selenium and equally extensively addresses the contribution of these antioxidants to the favorable effects of the fruits on human health.

2. Exogenous antioxidant defenses: naturally occurring antioxidants

As mentioned in the previous section, whether oxidative stress and cellular damage occurs is determined by the net result of the production of ROS and their elimination by antioxidant defenses. Indeed, oxidative stress is a consequence of "a disturbance in the pro-oxidant to antioxidant balance in favor of the former, leading to potential damage" [15]. Both the endogenous and the exogenous antioxidant defenses prevent ROS from overwhelming the intracellular environment by interrupting their propagation, scavenging them, removing their intermediates in redox reactions, inhibiting oxidation reactions that generate them, and repairing oxidized molecules [29–31, 33, 34, 38]. Exogenous antioxidants are substances in the diet—particularly in fruits and vegetables—that are able to retard or prevent the oxidation of oxidizable substrates in the body at concentrations that are relatively low when compared to the substrates [32, 33]. As also mentioned before, these dietary compounds include, among others, a variety of phenolic compounds, vitamins, and essential minerals, as well as small peptides such as glutathione, and fatty acids [32, 33]. The health-promoting and preventive effects of these substances against diseases associated with oxidative stress have been well-established [18–22].

Dietary phenolic compounds acting as antioxidants mainly include phenolic acids, flavonoids, and tannins [39]. Owing to their redox properties, these compounds are able to act as antioxidants and adsorb and neutralize free radicals, quench singlet and triplet oxygen, or decompose peroxides [40, 41]. These processes are accomplished by hydrogen atom transfer, transfer of a single electron, sequential proton loss electron transfer, or chelation of transition metals [40, 41]. In addition, phenolic compounds act synergistically with other antioxidants such as (pro)vitamins A, C, and E [42] and are presumably also involved in the regulation of intracellular glutathione levels [43].

Antioxidant vitamins such as (pro)vitamins A react with peroxyl, hydroxyl, and superoxide radicals; vitamin C is able to quench ROS by donating electrons to them; and vitamins E inhibit ROS generation, preventing lipid peroxidation of cellular membranes [44, 45]. The essential minerals, such as copper, zinc, manganese, and selenium, are indirectly involved in the body's antioxidant defenses by enhancing the activities of antioxidant enzymes. Copper, zinc, and manganese are cofactors of superoxide dismutase [46], and selenium is a cofactor of glutathione transferase and other selenoproteins [47]. It has notable antioxidant activity [48] and may be beneficial in chronic conditions such as cancer [49], heart disease [50], and cognitive disorders [51]. The common dietary small peptide glutathione is able to directly scavenge ROS [52]. And polyunsaturated fatty acids in, for instance, fish oil are able to eliminate ROS and inhibit cellular processes that generate ROS, decreasing the risk of cardiovascular diseases by reducing triacylglycerol production in the plasma [53].

3. Background on Suriname

The Republic of Suriname is situated in the north-eastern part of South America at the Atlantic Ocean, just north of the Amazon delta in Brazil, and between French Guiana and Guyana (**Figure 1**). Although located in South America, Suriname is culturally considered a Caribbean rather than a Latin American country and is a member of the Caribbean Community [54]. The climate is tropical with abundant rainfall, a uniform temperature of on average 27°C, and a relatively high humidity of 81% in the capital city of Paramaribo [55]. There are four seasons, namely the long rainy season (April–July), the long dry season (August–November), the short rainy season (December–January), and the short dry season (February–March) [55].

The country's land area of roughly 165,000 km^2 can be distinguished into northern urban-coastal and rural-coastal areas as well as a southern area [55]. The urban-coastal area includes Paramaribo and the district of Wanica, and harbors approximately 80% of the population of over 600,000 [55, 56]. The rural-coastal and rural-interior areas are referred to as the hinterland, are home to the remaining 20% of Suriname's inhabitants, and encompass more than three-quarters of the country's land surface [55, 56]. These parts of the country largely consist of sparsely inhabited savanna and dense, pristine, and highly biodiverse tropical rain forest [55], making Suriname comparatively one of the most forested countries in the world [55, 57].

The urban area is characterized by a "western" lifestyle, modern health-care facilities, and an economy that is mainly based on commerce, services, and industry [58]. The hinterland societies have a more traditional way of living, lack comprehensive public health services, and have agriculture, forestry, crude oil drilling, gold mining, as well as ecotourism as major economic activities [58]. These activities have been growing in scale and economic importance in recent years and are, together with agriculture and fisheries, the country's most important means of support, contributing substantially to the gross domestic income in 2020 of USD 2.88 billion and an average per capita income of about USD 4900 [59]. This positions Suriname on the World Bank's list of upper-middle income economies [59].

Suriname's population is among the most varied in the world, comprising the Indigenous Amerindians, the original inhabitants; descendants from enslaved Africans imported between the seventeenth and the nineteenth century (called Maroons and Creoles); descendants from contract workers from China, India (called

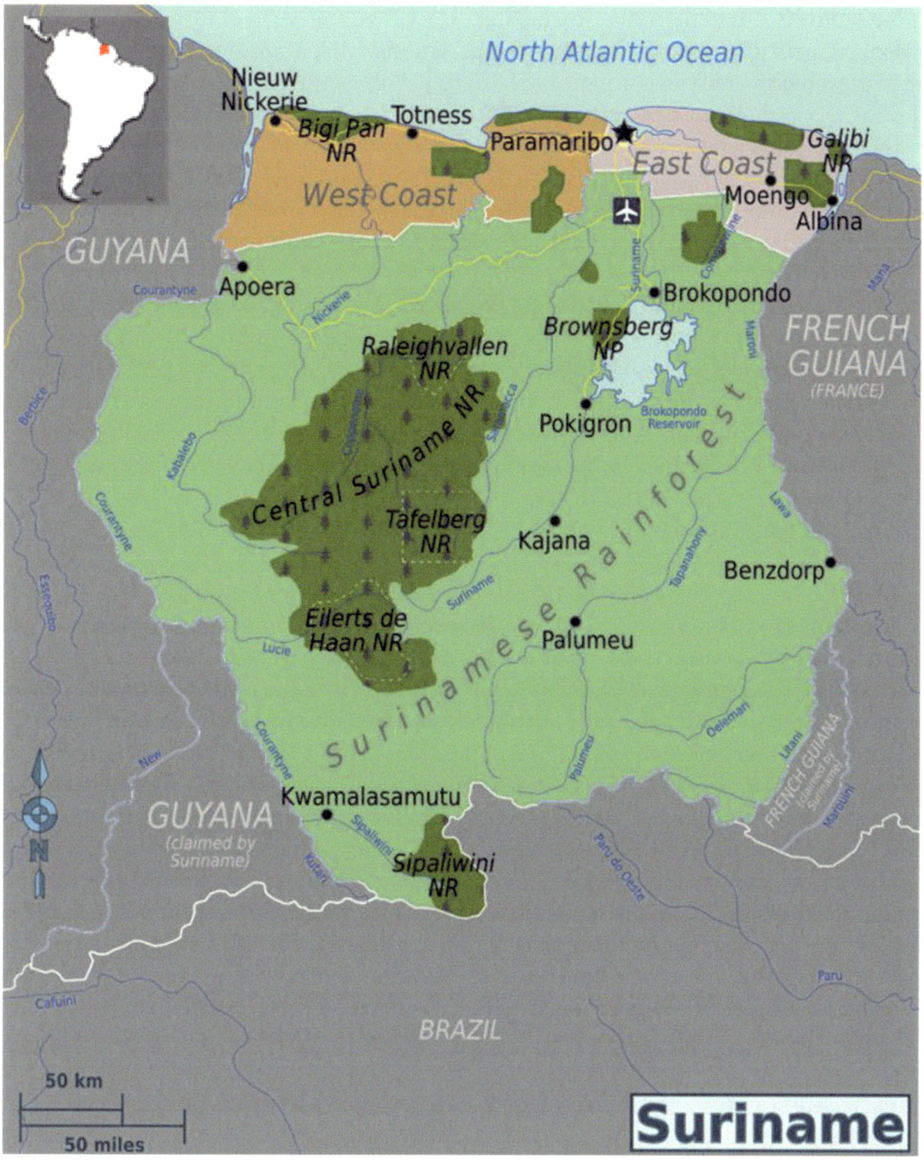

Figure 1.
Map of the Republic of Suriname (from: https://images.app.goo.gl/GrjsLhm6NEaZiDeE7). Insert: Position of Suriname in South America (from: https://images.app.goo.gl/VcvhN76aaKhkegELA).

Hindustanis), and the island of Java, Indonesia (called Javanese) attracted between the second half of the nineteenth century and the first half of the twentieth century; descendants from settlers from a number of European and Middle Eastern countries; and, more recently, immigrants from various Latin American and Caribbean countries including Brazil, Guyana, French Guiana, Haiti, and Cuba [54, 56]. Each of these groups has largely adhered to its original language, religion, and culture, including its ethnopharmacological tradition(s) [60]. This has resulted in a large array of traditional forms of medicine in the country, including those derived from traditional Indigenous, African, Chinese, Indian, Indonesian, and European origin [60].

Suriname is situated on the Guiana Shield, a 1.7-billion-year-old Precambrian geological formation in north-eastern South America that is among the regions of the highest biodiversity in the world [57, 61, 62]. This geographical location, together with the tropical climatic conditions and the variety of habitats, has substantially contributed to the country's rich fauna and flora that includes many endemic species [61, 62]. There are approximately 192 species of mammals including monkeys such as the howler monkey, predators such as the jaguar and the puma, bloodsucking vampires, anteaters, sloths, armadillos, as well as the unique South American tapir and sea cow. The bird world is very rich and includes 715 species such as the harpy eagle, the scarlet ibis, the black vulture, as well as several species of toucans and parrots. The 102 species of amphibians and the 175 species of reptiles include amphibian salamanders, the unique Surinamese toad, and poison dart frogs; caimans, iguanas, boa constrictors, anacondas, venomous bush masters, and rattlesnakes; and various terrestrial tortoises as well as aquatic and semiaquatic freshwater and sea turtles. There are 360 species of marine fish and 318 freshwater species including 61 endemic freshwater fish such as the carp salmon, the viviparous tooth carp, piranhas, electric eels, stingrays, four-eyed fish, cichlids, and many species of catfish. Lower animals are represented by giant centipedes, tarantulas, land snails that grow to over 13 cm long, and an innumerable insect world, including the intriguing lantern bearer and a variety of butterflies.

Suriname's flora roughly comprises 5100 species [63], including many species of palms, spurges, peas and beans, madders, citruses, cactuses, orchids, grasses, and bromeliads. Characteristic of Suriname's 386-km-long coastline is the presence of pristine mangrove forests, which help purify the brackish water, give protection against the sea, and provide shelter and food for many animals. The national flower of the country is the palulu *Heliconia bihai* (L.) L. (Heliconiaceae), and the national tree is the royal palm *Roystonea regia* (Kunth) O.F.Cook (Arecaceae). Popular fruit species are avocado, banana, some types of berry and cherry, a variety of citrus fruits, mango, several types of palm fruits and nuts, papaya, passion fruit, pineapple, pomegranate, tomato, and watermelon. Among the most cultivated and consumed produce items are leafy vegetables such as tannia and spinach, a number of cabbage types; various edible nightshades; legume vegetables such as black-eyed pea, lima bean, string bean, and yard-long bean; and fruiting vegetables such as bitter melon, eggplant, habanero pepper, and okra [62, 64, 65].

4. Naturally occurring antioxidants in a few well-known Surinamese fruits

Several of the plant species mentioned in the preceding paragraph are renowned for their high nutritious content and are regarded as nutraceuticals, functional food ingredients, or adaptogens [35, 66–68] and/or used as traditional medicines [69–78]. In some cases, these qualifications are attributable to an exceptionally high content of phytochemicals with antioxidant activity, including phenolic compounds such as flavonoids, lignans, and coumarins; vitamins such as (pro)vitamins A, C, and E; and trace elements such as selenium. Hereunder, each of these classes of antioxidant phytochemicals is addressed in detail, and one Surinamese fruit species representative of each class is comprehensively dealt with. All the fruits are abundantly cultivated and traded in Suriname [64] and consumed as foods and/or nutritional supplements [64] and/or used as traditional cosmeceuticals [79] and/or medicines [69–78]. The plants addressed in both parts of this chapter as well as their relevant characteristics are given in **Table 1**.

Main antioxidants	Plant family	Plant species (common vernacular; Surinamese vernacular)	Main traditional uses	Main commercialized products
Phenolic compounds—anthocyanins	Arecaceae	*Euterpe oleracea* Mart. (açai; podosiri)	Anemia; hypotension; wounds; as an external contraceptive	Health-promoting supplements and nutraceuticals
Phenolic compounds—ellagitannins	Lythraceae	*Punica granatum* L. (pomegranate; granaatappel)	Sore throat; respiratory afflictions; wounds and hemorrhages; gastrointestinal disorders; menstrual problems	Ellagitannin-enriched dietary supplements
Phenolic compounds—coumarins	Fabaceae	*Dipteryx odorata* (Aubl.) Willd (tonka bean; tonkaboon)	Hair conditions; colds and fever; respiratory disorders; gastro-intestinal disorders; menstrual problems; as an aphrodisiac	Hair care
Vitamins—vitamin A	Arecaceae	*Astrocaryum vulgare* Mart. (tucuma; awara)	Colicky babies; respiratory diseases; gastrointestinal disorders; rheumatism; pains; skin and hair problems; wounds; fractured bones; sexual underperformance and infertility	Skin and hair care
Vitamins—vitamin C	Malpighiaceae	*Malpighia glabra* L. (acerola; West-Indische kers)	Respiratory diseases; maladies of the oral cavity; cardiovascular ailments; wounds; gastrointestinal disorders; depression; cancer	Vitamin C-enriched dietary supplements and other health products
Vitamins—vitamin E	Malvaceae	*Hibiscus sabdariffa* L. (roselle; syuru)	Microbial infections; respiratory diseases; kidney problems; gastrointestinal disorders; hypertension	Skin and hair care; wound healing
Antioxidant minerals—selenium	Lecythidaceae	*Bertholletia excelsa* Humb. & Bonpl. (Brazil nut; paranoto)	Gastrointestinal disorders; burns	Skin and hair care

Table 1.
Main antioxidant compounds, traditional uses, and commercialized products of seven Surinamese types of fruits.

4.1 Antioxidant phenolic compounds

Phenolic compounds are secondary metabolites of plants that contain at least one functional phenol group [34]. These compounds are abundantly present in, among others, berries, grapes, apples, tomatoes, and apricots; artichokes, chicory, red onions, and spinach; as well as a wide diversity of beverages, food additives, and health-promoting products prepared from these fruits and vegetables [80, 81]. So far, more than 8000 phenolic compounds have been identified in natural sources, and they can be classified into flavonoids including anthocyanins, as well as tannins, coumarins, lignans, stilbenes, and phenolic acids [82]. Some of these compounds help protect plants against predators by acting as toxicants and pesticides against herbivores, nematodes, phytophagous insects, and fungal and bacterial pathogens [83, 84]. Others emanate an appealing scent and/or advertise an eye-catching pigmentation, which attracts pollinators, animals that disperse fruits, symbiotic microbes, and predators of the herbivores that act as bodyguards of the plants [85]. Still others are involved in allelopathic interactions, that is, they are released as volatiles in the air or as root exudates and affect the growth, survival, development, and reproduction of neighboring plants in the soil [86] or in water [87]. And some phenolic compounds, particularly flavonoids and isoflavonoids, are presumably involved in endomycorrhizae formation, that is, the establishment of mutually symbiotic relationship between fungi and plant roots where the roots provide carbohydrates for the fungi and the fungi transfer nutrients and water to the plant roots [88].

A high dietary intake of phenolic compounds by consuming sufficient fruits and vegetables has been related to a decreased rate of chronic diseases [89–91]. This has, for an important part, been associated with the redox properties of these compounds, which enable them to act as antioxidants, adsorbing and neutralizing free radicals, quenching singlet and triplet oxygen, and decomposing peroxides [40, 41]. These processes are accomplished by hydrogen atom transfer, transfer of a single electron, sequential proton loss electron transfer, or chelation of transition metals [40, 41]. Phenolic compounds are also able to act synergistically with the antioxidant (pro)vitamins A, C, and E [42] and are presumably also involved in the regulation of intracellular glutathione levels [43].

4.1.1 Antioxidant phenolic compounds: anthocyanins: Euterpe oleracea Mart. (Arecaceae)

Anthocyanins are water-soluble phenolic pigments belonging to the subgroup of flavonoids, and they are responsible for the red, violet, purple, and blue colors of fruits and vegetables [92]. These compounds are considered the most important group of phenolic compounds in foods [92] and are found, among others, in flower, fruit, and tuber of red and purple grapes, apples, strawberry, raspberry, blackberry, cranberry, acerola, purple potatoes, cush-cush yam, eggplant, and red cabbage [93, 94]. Anthocyanins help defend plants against attacks by microorganisms and phytopathogens; attract insects, birds, and small mammals for pollination and seed dispersal; and protect plants from the detrimental effects of ultraviolet radiation, high light intensity, drought, low temperatures, water stress, high salinity, and wounding [95, 96].

Important anthocyanins in the plant kingdom are cyanidin-3-rutinoside and cyanidin-3-glucoside [97, 98], along with pelargonidin-3-glucoside, peonidin-3-glucoside, cyanidin-3-sambubioside, and peonidin-3-rutinoside [99, 100]. These phytochemicals basically consist of an anthocyanidin (the aglycon) composed of a flavylium cation (2-phenyl-1-benzopyrilium) linked to one or more sugars such as glucose, xylose, galactose, arabinose, rhamnose, or rutinose through hydroxyl and/or methoxy groups [97–100]. Anthocyanidins exist in a variety of chemical forms depending on the conditions of the medium, which result in differently colored or colorless compounds [97–100]. For instance, at pH values less than 3, they are reddish; in the pH range of 4–5, they become colorless; and at pH values greater than 6, they have a purple, blue, bluish-green or blue/lilac coloration [97–100].

Biochemically, the flavylium moiety has an electron deficiency, which makes anthocyanins highly reactive toward ROS, rendering them powerful natural antioxidants [101, 102]. As a result, anthocyanins have the capacity to potently and readily neutralize ROS by transferring a single electron or by removing the hydrogen atom from their phenolic groups [102]. Indeed, anthocyanins obtained from various sources, including plasma from individuals who had consumed anthocyanin-rich diets, elicited substantial antioxidant effects in various *in vitro* assays (see, for instance, [103–105]). And in accordance with the apparent antioxidant and anti-inflammatory properties of anthocyanin-rich diets, the presence of these compounds in fruits and vegetables has been reported to elicit beneficial effects on human health (see, for instance, [92, 102, 106–108]).

However, there are some doubts as to whether the results from studies showing antioxidant activity of the plasma of individuals who had consumed anthocyanins must be taken as evidence of a beneficial physiological effect of these compounds in humans [105]. It is also not sure whether the plasma concentrations of anthocyanin concentrations were sufficiently high to counteract ROS *in vivo* [105]. Moreover, the instability of anthocyanins depending on the pH [97–100] as well as on temperature, light, oxygen, the presence of co-pigments, metallic ions, ascorbic acid, sugar, as well as glycosidases, peroxidases, and phenolases in the medium [109–112], also cast some uncertainty on the health-promoting effects of the abovementioned fruits and vegetables. Despite these and other reservations, the antioxidant activities of anthocyanins seem undisputable.

The açai palm *E. oleracea* Mart. (Arecaceae) is a tall, slender, multistemmed evergreen palm tree that can reach a height of 25 m, carries pinnate leaves with a length of up to 3 m, and bears 500–900 small, round, black-purple fruits of about 2.5 cm in diameter in branched, drooping panicles (**Figure 2**). The plant is indigenous to the northern, tropical parts of South America including Suriname, where it is mainly found along river edges, near swamps, and in seasonal floodplains. *E. oleracea* is also grown as an ornamental, but more often for its fruit that is commonly known as açaí berry and in Suriname as podosiri. *E. oleracea* fruit is made up of a hard endocarp that

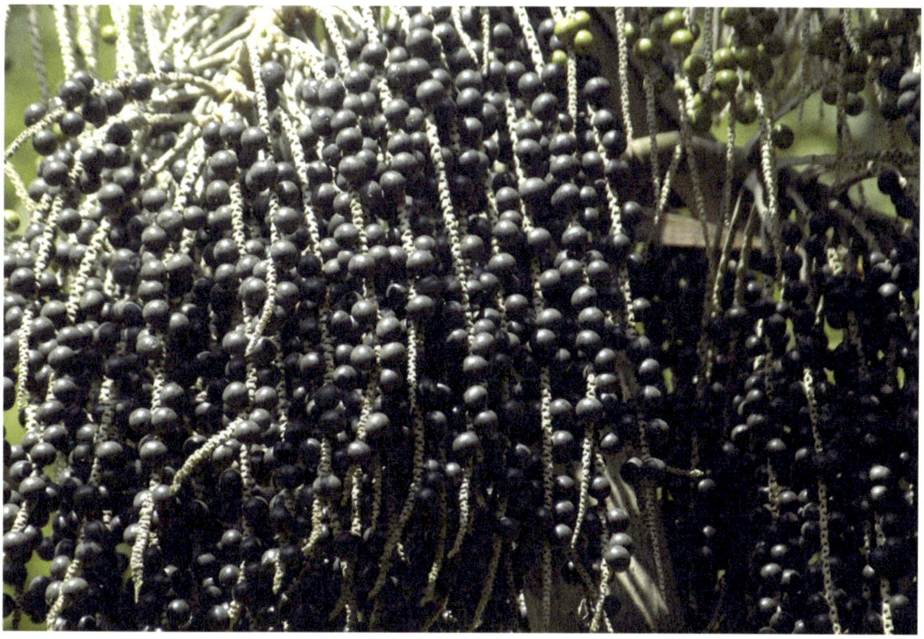

Figure 2.
Bunch of fruits of the açai Euterpe oleracea *Mart. (Arecaceae) (from: https://images.app.goo.gl/22sjzvsep94caDv2A).*

contains a single large seed of 7–10 mm in diameter, a fibrous, purple-colored, pulpy mesocarp of about 1 mm thick, and a deeply purple-colored exocarp or skin.

The pulp prepared from the mesocarp and the exocarp from *E. oleracea* fruit has a high nutritional density, containing, among others, appreciable amounts of carbohydrates, proteins, vitamin C, calcium, iron, mono- and polyunsaturated fatty acids, as well as phenolic compounds including five different types of anthocyanins with cyanidin 3-glycoside and cyanidin 3-rutinoside being the most predominant anthocyanins [99, 113]. For this reason, it has been a staple food for the Amazon indigenous peoples for centuries, either raw, prepared as a beverage, or cooked, in the latter case often together with cassava and fish [99, 114]. More recently, a multitude of commercialized *E. oleracea* fruit pulp products has entered the market, including health-promoting supplements and nutraceuticals formulated as beverages, frozen pulp, powders, tablets, and capsules, as well as ready-prepared healthy food items such as jams, ice creams and other frozen treats, as well as mousses, cakes, porridges, and bonbons [99, 101, 115].

Preparations from the fruit and other parts of *E. oleracea* are also abundantly used in various traditional medical practices in different parts of the world including Suriname. A few indications are anemia, hypotension, various types of wounds including open cuts, scorpion stings, and shot wounds; and as an external contraceptive [77, 78, 116–120]. Pharmacological studies with particularly the fruit juice have shown a wide range of activities, including antidiarrheal, anti-inflammatory, antinociceptive, antiangiogenic, antimicrobial, antileishmanial, skin regenerating and antiageing, cosmeceutical, neuroprotective, anticancer, and antioxidant effects [79, 119–122]. Particularly, the antioxidant properties of *E. oleracea* fruit preparations have been well investigated, showing an abundance of phenolic compounds with antioxidant activity [123–127], supporting some of their traditional and nutraceutical uses [79, 119–127].

Indeed, the phenolic compounds and anthocyanins in *E. oleracea* fruit pulp have been shown to very efficiently scavenge superoxide and peroxyl radicals [102]. And *E. oleracea* fruit pulp seemed to elicit a greater antioxidant power than other anthocyanin-rich fruits such as blueberries and black berries [128]. The results from clinical studies also supported the antioxidant benefits of *E. oleracea* fruit juice and related products. For instance, total anthocyanin levels in volunteers who had consumed *E. oleracea* fruit pulp and clarified fruit juice led to substantially increased plasma antioxidant capacity [129] as well as an increased catalase activity, total antioxidant capacity, and reduced ROS production in total serum of healthy women [130]. These observations support, at least partly, some of the pharmacological activities and cosmeceutical applications of *E. oleracea* fruit preparations [79, 119–122].

As indicated above, the commercial success of *E. oleracea* fruit pulp products [115] has particularly been attributed to its high content of anthocyanins—mainly cyanidin-3-glucoside [128]—with superior antioxidant activity [99, 101]. However, as also mentioned before, the chemical instability of anthocyanins may well affect their antioxidant properties [97–100, 109–112]. For this reason, the possibility exists that other, more stable phenolic compounds, vitamins, and/or fatty acids [99, 113] in *E. oleracea* fruit pulp may substantially contribute to its antioxidant activity [131].

4.1.2 Antioxidant phenolic compounds—Tannins: Punica granatum L. (Lythraceae)

Tannins are a class of astringent, water-soluble phenolic compounds that form strong complexes with macromolecules and precipitate proteins and various other organic compounds including amino acids and alkaloids [132, 133]. They occur abundantly in particularly bark, leaves, buds, unripe fruits, and seeds of many plants and play important roles in the protection of plants from predation by making them unpalatable, dissuading animals from predation [132, 133]. These compounds are responsible for the astringency, color, and some of the flavor in black and green teas [132]. The name of this group is derived from their centuries-old use for tanning animal hides in the leather processing industry [134]. Tannins are also used for dyeing fabric and making ink, as well as in the clarification of wine and beer [134]. Owing to their styptic and astringent properties, tannins have medicinally been used to treat tonsillitis, pharyngitis, hemorrhoids, and skin eruptions [135], and internally to control diarrhea, against intestinal bleeding, and to bind to and eliminate metallic, alkaloidal, and glycosidic poisons [135].

Tannins can chemically be distinguished in two major groups, namely hydrolyzable tannins and condensed tannins [136]. Hydrolyzable tannins break down in water, yielding various water-soluble products, and are subdivided in gallotannins and ellagitannins [136]. The gallotannins release gallic acid and glucose by hydrolysis at low ambient pH and can be encountered in, among others, the pods of the tara *Tara spinosa* (Feuillée ex Molina) Britton & Rose (Fabaceae) [137] and the gallnuts of the Aleppo oak *Quercus infectoria* Oliv. (Fagaceae) [138]. The ellagitannins are made up of ellagic acid glycosides, and are ingredients of the wood of several species of oak in the family Fagaceae such as that of the common oak *Quercus robur* L and the white oak *Quercus alba* L. [139], as well as the gallnuts of the myrobalan *Terminalia chebula* Retz. (Combretaceae) [140].

Condensed tannins are the larger group of tannins, form reddish-colored, water-insoluble phenolic precipitates called tanner's reds or phlobaphenes, and are less astringent when compared to hydrolysable tannins [136]. They are polymers of monomeric flavonoids, are also called proanthocyanidins because they yield anthocyanidins when depolymerized under oxidative conditions, and include, among others, the procyanidins, propelargonidins, prodelphinidins, profisetinidins, proteracacinidins, proguibourtinidins or prorobinetidins [136]. Some of these compounds are naturally present in the skin and seed of the red grape *Vitis vinifera* L. (Vitaceae) and are, therefore, present in red wines [141]. Other important sources of condensed tannins are the extracts from various genera and species of mangrove [142] and acacia [143].

With more than 1000 natural ellagitannins identified to date, this subgroup constitutes the largest among the hydrolyzable tannins [144, 145]. Examples of these compounds are punicalagin, sanguiin H6, lambertianin C, pedunculagin, vescalagin, castalagin, casuarictin, and potentillin [146] in, among others, walnuts and almonds in the genera *Juglans* (Juglandaceae) and *Prunus* (Rosaceae), respectively; oak-aged wines; berries in the genera *Rubus* and Fragaria (Rosaceae); and the pomegranate *P. granatum* L. (Lythraceae) [147, 148]. Like other tannins [135], ellagitannins, along with some of its metabolites, have been reported to exhibit various beneficial effects on human health including anti-inflammatory, anticancer, prebiotic, cardioprotective, as well as antioxidant properties [149, 150]. After ingestion, ellagitannins are hydrolytically fractionated in the stomach and the duodenum, yielding ellagic acids [132, 133, 151], which are partially metabolized to urolithins by gut microbiota [149, 151]. Both the ellagic acids and the urolithins elicited *in vitro* antioxidant activity [152, 153] and might be responsible for (some of) the pharmacological activities of ellagitannins [154]. These findings are consistent with the assumption that the potential health benefits of ellagitannins could not solely be attributed to these compounds themselves [155].

The pomegranate *P. granatum* L. (Lythraceae) is a long-lived, deciduous shrub or small tree with multiple spiny branches that grows between 5 and 10 m tall. The plant originates from the Mediterranean region and has been introduced into the New

World in the late sixteenth century by Spanish colonizers. It is now widely cultivated for its edible fruit in various countries in the Americas as well as in parts of the Mediterranean Basin, north and tropical Africa, Iran, Armenia, the Middle East and Caucasus region, the Indian subcontinent, and the drier parts of Southeast Asia. The rounded fruit measures 5–12 cm in diameter, develops from bright red flowers, and is made up of a red-purpled colored husk consisting of an outer, hard exocarp, and an inner, white, spongy mesocarp that forms chambers that contain 200–1400 seeds inside pulpy, succulent sarcotestas (**Figure 3**). The juice obtained from the sarcotesta is sweet-sour-tasting and is used in baking, cooking, juice blends, meal garnishes, smoothies, and alcoholic beverages such as cocktails and wines.

P. granatum is much appreciated in many parts of the world including Suriname, where the fresh fruit is recommended for the promotion of general health and as a remedy for bleeding gums, lung afflictions, and tuberculosis [70, 156], while preparations from various parts of the fruit are used against small wounds in the oral cavity; hemorrhage; sore throat; shortness of breath; ulcers, diarrhea, and dysentery; menstrual pain, and tapeworm infection [69, 70, 75, 78, 156–158]. These uses are partially supported by the many pharmacological activities of this plant including antidiabetic, antitumor, anti-inflammatory, antimicrobial, antiparasitic, antiviral, antifibrotic, and other effects [156, 159, 160]. And several of these activities have been associated with the antioxidant activities of the many bioactive compounds in the plant including the ellagitannins [156].

Notably, *P. granatum* sarcotesta juice has a relatively high content of ellagitannins [161–164], in addition to anthocyanins which give the juice its red color [164, 165]. In fact, ellagitannins, particularly punicalagin isomers, are presumably the major phenolics in pomegranate fruit and juice [163]. These compounds probably account for more than 90% of the antioxidant activity of the juice, exceeding that of other red-purple fruits,

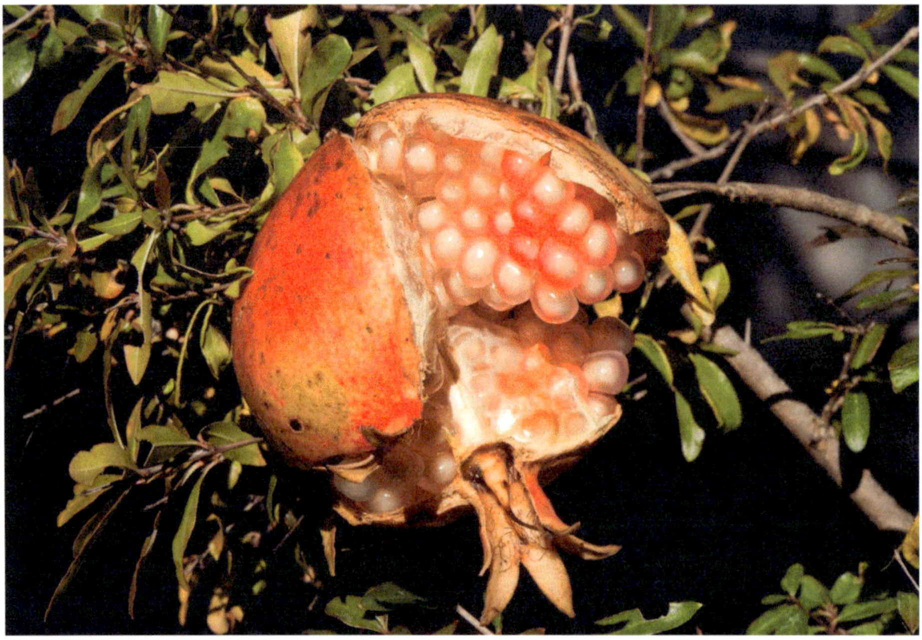

Figure 3.
Open fruit of the pomegranate Punica granatum *L. (Lythraceae) showing seeds inside sarcotestas (from: https://images.app.goo.gl/zyYerutR5BTYZ87f8).*

red wine, and green tea [161, 162]. Indeed, ellagitannins from various sources including *P. granatum* fruit as well as their metabolites such as urolithin, elicited substantial antioxidant effects in several *in vitro* assays [166] and *in vivo* models [167]. Of note, the plasma of individuals given a *P. granatum* ellagitannin-enriched polyphenolic dietary supplement also elicited meaningful *in vitro* antioxidant activity [168]. These observations support the use of *P. granatum* fruit preparations as health-promoting substances.

4.1.3 Antioxidant phenolic compounds: coumarins: Dipteryx odorata (Aubl.) Willd (Fabaceae)

Coumarins, including the type compound coumarin, also known as 2H-chromen-2-one, 2H-1-benzopyran-2-one, 1,2-benzopyrone, and o-hydroxycinnamic acid lactone, are phenolic compounds that were first isolated from the seed of the tonka bean *D. odorata* Willd. (Fabaceae) [169]. Subsequently, these compounds appeared to be present in many other plants including species of cinnamon, strawberries, black currants, apricots, and cherries [170]. They have a bitter taste that helps protect the plants from herbivory by acting as appetite suppressants [171]. To date, about 800 naturally occurring coumarins have been identified in about 600 genera of 100 families of plants [172]. Coumarins can be distinguished into simple coumarins (e.g., coumarin, as well as umbelliferone, also known as 7-hydroxycoumarin, in Apiaceae members such as carrot and coriander), furanocoumarines (e.g., psoralen in the seed of the Indian medicinal plant *Psoralea corylifolia* L. (Fabaceae), pyranocoumarins (e.g., the natural vasodilator visnadin in the bishop's weed *Visnaga daucoides* Gaertn. (Apiaceae), and pyrone-substituted coumarins (e.g., the 4-hydroxycoumarin dicoumarol, a naturally occurring anticoagulant that depletes vitamin K stores similarly to warfarin) [172]. Warfarin is a synthetic anticoagulant produced on the basis of dicoumarol's structure [173].

Coumarin itself is of relatively low toxicity to humans when consumed in moderation [174]. However, at large (infused) doses, it may cause liver damage, hemorrhages, and paralysis of the heart [174]. It is, therefore, controlled as a food additive by many governments [175] and has even been banned in the USA [176]. Warfarin, acenocoumarol, and phenprocoumon are commonly prescribed to patients suffering from atrial fibrillation, deep venous thrombosis, or pulmonary embolism, or to individuals with artificial heart valves, in order to prevent the formation of blood clots and reduce the risk of embolism [177, 178]. Warfarin is also widely used as a rat poison [179]. Other well-known industrial applications of coumarins are their use as agrochemicals, materials for food processing, optical brighteners, and dispersed fluorescent and laser dyes (see, for instance, [40, 179]).

Besides anticoagulant activity, coumarins have been found to elicit a host of other pharmacological activities including antitumor, photochemotherapeutic, anti-HIV, antimicrobial, anti-inflammatory, triglyceride-lowering, central nervous system-stimulating, and menopausal distress-preventing effects [180–182]. These beneficial health effects are believed to be mainly related to their antioxidant activities, providing protection against oxidative stress by scavenging ROS such as superoxide, hypochlorous acid, and hydroxyl radicals [183]. Indeed, numerous studies with natural and synthetic coumarins using a variety of assays have shown strong *in vitro* antioxidant effects (see, for instance, [184–186]). At least one of the mechanisms involved in the antioxidant activity of coumarins is the donation of hydrogen to ROS in its reduction to nonreactive species, removing the odd electron responsible for radical reactivity [187, 188].

The tonka bean *D. odorata* (Aubl.) Willd., called "tonkaboon" in Suriname, is a large semideciduous evergreen tree with a small, rounded crown that can reach a height of 30 m. The plant is native to Central America and the northern parts of South America. It is sometimes cultivated but is mostly harvested from the wild for its seed that becomes black and wrinkled with a smooth, brown interior after steeping for 24 hours in alcohol and drying (**Figure 4**). As mentioned above, the seed is rich in phenolic compounds including coumarin and several of its derivatives [169]. These compounds have a strong sweet and spicy fragrance that is reminiscent of new mown hay, vanilla, and almond [189]. For this reason, they are abundantly used as key fragrances of fougère perfumes, as a substitute for vanilla, and as flavoring agents for desserts and stews as well as tobacco and whisky [175]—in addition to the applications mentioned above—despite the safety concerns [174]. Besides coumarins, *D. odorata* seed contains various other bioactive phenolic compounds, particularly isoflavones, mostly in the endocarp [190] but also in some of its other parts [191, 192].

Preparations from *D. odorata* seed have many traditional uses, among others, to fortify the scalp and improve hair growth; as a remedy for colds, fever, coughing, asthma, and tuberculosis; for treating stomach pain and diarrhea; against dysentery and schistosomiasis; as an emmenagogue, and as an aphrodisiac [117, 193, 194]. In Suriname, *D. odorata* seed is mainly used as an ingredient of products to treat hair loss, dandruff, and an itching scalp; against colds; and to command luck [78, 195].

Some of these traditional uses are in accordance with the results from the above-mentioned pharmacological studies with coumarin analogues—from the seed as well as other parts of the plant—showing a wide range of pharmacological activities [180–182]. This suggests that at least some of the traditional uses of *D. odorata* seed preparations are also attributable to antioxidant activities. Indeed, the coumarin-rich oil from *D. odorata* seed displayed meaningful antioxidant activity in several *in vitro* free radical scavenging assays but also had a substantial total phenolic content [196].

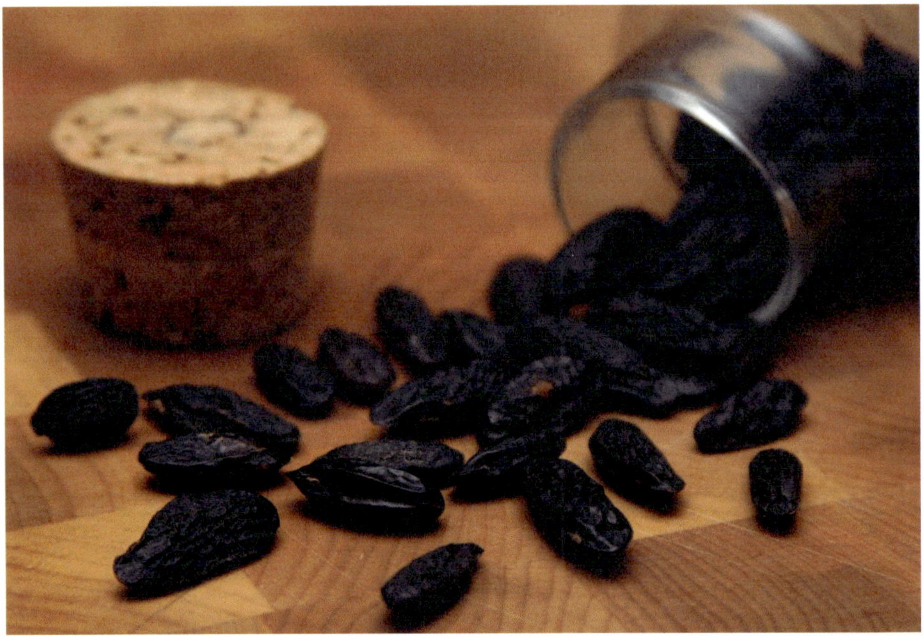

Figure 4.
Dried fruits of the Tonka bean Dipteryx odorata *(Aubl.) Willd (Fabaceae) (from: https://images.app.goo.gl/Jw7f48V1kARX9vgE9).*

And raw, roasted, and boiled *D. odorata* seeds had a considerable coumarin, total phenolic, and total flavonoid contents and displayed meaningful free radical scavenging activity, superoxide dismutase activity, as well as ferric reducing antioxidant power [197]. However, both coumarins and flavonoids in *D. odorata* seed preparations elicited antioxidant activities [180, 184, 185] and can be classified as phenylpropanoid-derived natural products. This makes it difficult to determine whether and to which extent the traditional and pharmacological activities of *D. odorata* seed preparations can only be associated with antioxidant activities due to coumarins.

5. Concluding remarks

Naturally occurring antioxidants in fruits and vegetables provided through the diet represent vital components of the exogenous defense mechanisms of the body to manage oxidative stress caused by ROS, minimizing the chances of developing, among others, inflammatory disorders, cancer, diabetes mellitus, cardiovascular diseases, and cognitive ailments. Important classes of such naturally occurring antioxidants are anthocyanins, ellagitannins, coumarins, (pro)vitamins A, C, and E, as well as selenium. In this chapter, seven well-known Surinamese fruits, each of which known to contain one of these compounds at appreciably high concentrations, have elaborately been dealt with. The fruits were those from the açai palm *E. oleracea*, the pomegranate *P. granatum*, the tonka bean *D. odorata*, the tucumã *Astrocaryum vulgare*, the acerola *Malpighia glabra*, the roselle *Hibiscus sabdariffa*, and the Brazil nut *Bertholletia excelsa*. These fruits are widely consumed in Suriname and various other countries throughout the world, either raw or incorporated into dishes, or prepared into traditional medicines, food additives, nutraceuticals, or cosmeceuticals. Numerous pharmacological studies with a wide range of assays have provided support that these beneficial health effects are associated with the powerful antioxidant activities of one or more of the phytochemical classes mentioned above.

However, many studies have also suggested that the antioxidant activities of the fruits must probably be attributed to the combined effects of several classes of biologically active compounds rather than to one specific phytochemical. For instance, the antioxidant activities of *E. oleracea* fruit pulp products [99, 101] are presumably not only due to their high content of mainly the anthocyanin cyanidin-3-glucoside, but also due to other phenolic compounds, vitamins, and/or fatty acids [99, 113, 128, 131]. Similarly, as mentioned in part 2 of this chapter, the antioxidant activity of the mesocarp of the tucumã or awara *Astrocaryum vulgare* Mart. (Arecaceae) *A. vulgare* [198, 199] may be partly ascribed to phytosterols and vitamin E derivatives in addition to its high content of carotenoids [198, 199]. And those of preparations from the seed of the Brazil nut or paranoto *Bertholletia excelsa* Humb. & Bonpl. (Lecythidaceae) [200–202] might be due to the combined actions of selenium with phenolic compounds, tocopherols, and unsaturated fatty acids [203–206].

These considerations indicate the need to more precisely identify the pharmacologically active phytochemicals, particularly those with antioxidant activity, in raw natural products, traditional medicines, and commercial plant-based products with purported health beneficial properties. This is the more important in the case of substances containing chemically instable ingredients such as anthocyanins [97–100, 109–112], and those that may generate pro-oxidant radical species such as carotenoids [207, 208], or display pro-oxidant properties at, for instance, relatively low concentration such as vitamin C [209].

Author details

Dennis R.A. Mans
Faculty of Medical Sciences, Department of Pharmacology, Anton de Kom University of Suriname, Paramaribo, Suriname

*Address all correspondence to: dennismans16@gmail.com;
dennis_mans@yahoo.com

References

[1] Canfield DE, Rosing MT, Bjerrum C. Early anaerobic metabolisms. Philosophical Transactions of the Royal Society B: Biological Sciences. 2006;**361**:1819-1834. discussion 1835-1836. DOI: 10.1098/rstb.2006.1906

[2] Martin WF, Sousa FL. Early microbial evolution: The age of anaerobes. Cold Spring Harbor Perspectives in Biology. 2015;**8**:a018127. DOI: 10.1101/cshperspect.a018127

[3] Birben E, Sahiner UM, Sackesen C, Erzurum S, Kalayci O. Oxidative stress and antioxidant defense. World Allergy Organization Journal. 2012;**5**:9-19. DOI: 10.1097/WOX.0b013e3182439613

[4] Noori S. An overview of oxidative stress and antioxidant defensive system. Open Access Scientific Reports. 2012;**1**:413. DOI: 10.4172/scientificreports

[5] Kumar V, Abdussalam A. A review on reactive oxygen and nitrogen species. Era's Journal of Medical Research. 2017;**4**:1-5

[6] Checa J, Aran JM. Reactive oxygen species: Drivers of physiological and pathological processes. Journal of Inflammation Research. 2020;**13**:1057-1073. DOI: 10.2147/JIR.S275595

[7] Juan CA, Pérez de la Lastra JM, Plou FJ, Pérez-Lebeña E. The chemistry of reactive oxygen species (ROS) revisited: Outlining their role in biological macromolecules (DNA, lipids and proteins) and induced pathologies. International Journal of Molecular Sciences. 2021;**22**:4642. DOI: 10.3390/ijms22094642

[8] Pham-Huy LA, He H, Pham-Huy C. Free radicals, antioxidants in disease and health. International Journal of Biomedical Sciences. 2008;**4**:89-96

[9] Schieber M, Chandel NS. ROS function in redox signaling and oxidative stress. Current Biology. 2014;**24**:R453-R462. DOI: 10.1016/j.cub.2014.03.034

[10] Bardaweel SK, Gul M, Alzweiri M, Ishaqat A, Salamat HA, Bashatwah RM. Reactive oxygen species: The dual role in physiological and pathological conditions of the human body. Eurasian Journal of Medicine. 2018;**50**:193-201

[11] Turrens JF. Mitochondrial formation of reactive oxygen species. Journal of Physiology. 2003;**552**(Pt 2):335-344. DOI: 10.1113/jphysiol.2003.049478

[12] Fransen M, Nordgren M, Wang B, Apanasets O. Role of peroxisomes in ROS/RNS-metabolism: Implications for human disease. Biochimica et Biophysica Acta. 2012;**1822**:1363-1373. DOI: 10.1016/j.bbadis.2011.12.001

[13] Zeeshan HM, Lee GH, Kim HR, Chae HJ. Endoplasmic reticulum stress and associated ROS. International Journal of Molecular Sciences. 2016;**17**:327. DOI: 10.3390/ijms17030327

[14] Li R, Jia Z, Trush MA. Defining ROS in biology and medicine. Reactive Oxygen Species (Apex). 2016;**1**:9-21. DOI: 10.20455/ros.2016.803

[15] Sies H, Jones DP. Reactive oxygen species (ROS) as pleiotropic physiological signalling agents. Nature Reviews: Molecular Cell Biology. 2020;**21**:363-383. DOI: 10.1038/s41580-020-0230-3

[16] Spitz DR, Azzam EI, Li JJ, Gius D. Metabolic oxidation/reduction reactions

and cellular responses to ionizing radiation: A unifying concept in stress response biology. Cancer Metastasis Reviews. 2004;**23**:311-322. DOI: 10.1023/B:CANC.0000031769.14728.bc

[17] Kong CY, Guo Z, Song P, Zhang X, Yuan YP, Teng T, et al. Underlying the mechanisms of doxorubicin-induced acute cardiotoxicity: Oxidative stress and cell death. International Journal of Biological Sciences. 2022;**18**:760-770. DOI: 10.7150/ijbs.65258

[18] Klaunig JE, Kamendulis LM. The role of oxidative stress in carcinogenesis. Annual Review of Pharmacology and Toxicology. 2004;**44**:239-267. DOI: 10.1146/annurev.pharmtox.44.101802.121851

[19] Markesbery WR, Lovell MA. DNA oxidation in Alzheimer's disease. Antioxidants and Redox Signaling. 2006;**8**:2039-2045. DOI: 10.1089/ars.2006.8.2039

[20] Elahi MM, Kong YX, Matata BM. Oxidative stress as a mediator of cardiovascular disease. Oxidative Medicine and Cellular Longevity. 2009;**2**:259-269. DOI: 10.4161/oxim.2.5.9441

[21] Cui H, Kong Y, Zhang H. Oxidative stress, mitochondrial dysfunction, and aging. Journal of Signal Transduction. 2012;**2012**:646354. DOI: 10.1155/2012/646354

[22] Shirley R, Ord EN, Work LM. Oxidative stress and the use of antioxidants in stroke. Antioxidants (Basel). 2014;**3**:472-501. DOI: 10.3390/antiox3030472

[23] Asmat U, Abad K, Ismail K. Diabetes mellitus and oxidative stress—A concise review. Saudi Pharmaceutical Journal. 2016;**24**:547-553. DOI: 10.1016/j.jsps.2015.03.013

[24] Soomro S. Oxidative stress and inflammation. Open Journal of Immunology. 2019;**9**:1-20. DOI: 10.4236/oji.2019.91001

[25] Rhee SG. Cell signaling. H_2O_2, a necessary evil for cell signaling. Science. 2006;**312**:1882-1883. DOI: 10.1126/science.1130481

[26] Zhao RZ, Jiang S, Zhang L, Yu ZB. Mitochondrial electron transport chain, ROS generation and uncoupling (review). International Journal of Molecular Medicine. 2019;**44**:3-15. DOI: 10.3892/ijmm.2019.4188

[27] Banerjee S, Ghosh J, Sil PC. Drug metabolism and oxidative stress: Cellular mechanism and new therapeutic insights. Biochemistry and Analytical Biochemistry. 2016;**5**:255. DOI: 10.4172/2161-1009.1000255

[28] Thomas DC. The phagocyte respiratory burst: Historical perspectives and recent advances. Immunology Letters. 2017;**192**:88-96. DOI: 10.1016/j.imlet.2017.08.016

[29] Ighodaro OM, Akinloye OA. First line defence antioxidants-superoxide dismutase (SOD), catalase (CAT) and glutathione peroxidase (GPX): Their fundamental role in the entire antioxidant defence grid. Alexandria Journal of Medicine. 2018;**54**:287-293. DOI: 10.1016/j.ajme.2017.09.001

[30] Mirończuk-Chodakowska I, Witkowska AM, Zujko ME. Endogenous non-enzymatic antioxidants in the human body. Advances in Medical Sciences. 2018;**63**:68-78. DOI: 10.1016/j.advms.2017.05.005

[31] Lobo V, Patil A, Phatak A, Chandra N. Free radicals, antioxidants and functional foods: Impact on human health. Pharmacognosy

Reviews. 2010;**4**:118-126. DOI: 10.4103/0973-7847.70902

[32] Balsano C, Alisi A. Antioxidant effects of natural bioactive compounds. Current Pharmaceutical Design. 2009;**15**:3063-3073. DOI: 10.2174/138161209789058084

[33] Briggs MA. From foods to chemotherapeutics: The antioxidant potential of dietary phytochemicals. PRO. 2022;**10**:1222. DOI: 10.3390/pr10061222

[34] Miguel-Chávez R. Phenolic antioxidant capacity: A review of the state of the art. In: Soto-Hernandez M, Palma-Tenango M, Garcia-Mateos M, editors. Phenolic Compounds: Biological Activity. London: IntechOpen; 2017. pp. 59-74. DOI: 10.5772/66897

[35] Caleja C, Ribeiro A, Barreiro MF, Ferreira ICFR. Phenolic compounds as nutraceuticals or functional food ingredients. Current Pharmaceutical Design. 2017;**23**:2787-2806. DOI: 10.2174/1381612822666161227153906

[36] Aune D, Keum N, Giovannucci E, Fadnes LT, Boffetta P, Greenwood DC, et al. Dietary intake and blood concentrations of antioxidants and the risk of cardiovascular disease, total cancer, and all-cause mortality: A systematic review and dose-response meta-analysis of prospective studies. American Journal of Clinical Nutrition. 2018;**108**:1069-1091. DOI: 10.1093/ajcn/nqy097

[37] Jayedi A, Rashidy-Pour A, Parohan M, Zargar MS, Shab-Bidar S. Dietary antioxidants, circulating antioxidant concentrations, total antioxidant capacity, and risk of all-cause mortality: A systematic review and dose-response meta-analysis of prospective observational studies. Advances in Nutrition. 2018;**9**:701-716. DOI: 10.1093/advances/nmy040

[38] Gutteridge JMC, Halliwell B. Antioxidants in Nutrition, Health and Disease. Oxford: Oxford University Press; 1994

[39] Spencer JP, Abd El Mohsen MM, Minihane AM, Mathers JC. Biomarkers of the intake of dietary polyphenols: Strengths, limitations and application in nutrition research. British Journal of Nutrition. 2008;**99**:12-22. DOI: 10.1017/S0007114507798938

[40] Pereira DM, Valentão P, Pereira JA, Andrade PB. Phenolics: From chemistry to biology. Molecules. 2009;**14**:2202-2211. DOI: 10.3390/molecules14062202

[41] Zeb A. Concept, mechanism, and applications of phenolic antioxidants in foods. Journal of Food Biochemistry. 2020;**44**:e13394. DOI: 10.1111/jfbc.13394

[42] Croft KD. The chemistry and biological effects of flavonoids and phenolic acids. Annals of the New York Academy of Sciences. 1998;**854**:435-442. DOI: 10.1111/j.1749-6632.1998.tb09922.x

[43] Myhrstad MC, Carlsen H, Nordström O, Blomhoff R, Moskaug JØ. Flavonoids increase the intracellular glutathione level by transactivation of the gamma-glutamylcysteine synthetase catalytical subunit promoter. Free Radical Biology and Medicine. 2002;**32**:386-393. DOI: 10.1016/s0891-5849(01)00812-7

[44] Sinbad OO, Folorunsho AA, Olabisi OL, Ayoola OA, Temitope RJ. Vitamins as antioxidants. Journal of Food Science and Nutrition Research. 2019;**2**:214-235. DOI: 10.26502/jfsnr.2642-11000021

[45] Khadim RM, Al-Fartusie FS. Antioxidant vitamins and their effect

on immune system. Journal of Physics Conference Series. 2021;**1853**:012065. DOI: 10.1088/1742-6596/1853/1/012065

[46] Reddi AR, Jensen LT, Naranuntarat A, Rosenfeld L, Leung E, Shah R, et al. The overlapping roles of manganese and Cu/Zn SOD in oxidative stress protection. Free Radical Biology and Medicine. 2009;**46**:154-162. DOI: 10.1016/j.freeradbiomed.2008.09.032

[47] Hariharan S, Dharmaraj S. Selenium and selenoproteins: Its role in regulation of inflammation. Inflammopharmacology. 2020;**28**:667-695. DOI: 10.1007/s10787-020-00690-x

[48] Schnabel R, Lubos E, Messow CM, Sinning CR, Zeller T, Wild PS, et al. Selenium supplementation improves antioxidant capacity *in vitro* and *in vivo* in patients with coronary artery disease. The SElenium therapy in coronary artery disease patients (SETCAP) study. American Heart Journal. 2008;**156**(1201):e1-e11. DOI: 10.1016/j.ahj.2008.09.004

[49] Cai X, Wang C, Yu W, Fan W, Wang S, Shen N, et al. Selenium exposure and cancer risk: An updated meta-analysis and meta-regression. Scientific Reports. 2016;**6**:19213. DOI: 10.1038/srep19213

[50] Ju W, Li X, Li Z, Wu GR, Fu XF, Yang XM, et al. The effect of selenium supplementation on coronary heart disease: A systematic review and metaanalysis of randomized controlled trials. Journal of Trace Elements in Medicine and Biology. 2017;**44**:8-16. DOI: 10.1016/j.jtemb.2017.04.009

[51] Santos JR, Gois AM, Mendonça DM, Freire MA. Nutritional status, oxidative stress and dementia: The role of selenium in Alzheimer's disease. Frontiers in Aging Neuroscience. 2014;**6**:206. DOI: 10.3389/fnagi.2014.00206

[52] Minich DM, Brown BI. A review of dietary (phyto)nutrients for glutathione support. Nutrients. 2019;**11**:2073. DOI: 10.3390/nu11092073

[53] Saini RK, Prasad P, Sreedhar RV, Akhilender Naidu K, Shang X, Keum YS. Omega-3 polyunsaturated fatty acids (PUFAs): Emerging plant and microbial sources, oxidative stability, bioavailability, and health benefits—A review. Antioxidants (Basel). 2021;**10**:1627. DOI: 10.3390/antiox10101627

[54] Bakker E, Dalhuisen L, Donk R, Hassankhan M, Steegh F. Geschiedenis van Suriname: Van Stam tot Staat (History of Suriname: From Tribe to State). Zutphen: Walburg Pers; 1998

[55] Algemeen Bureau voor de Statistiek/Conservation International Suriname. In: Suriname in cijfers 286-2012/04 (General Bureau of Statistics/Conservation International Suriname. Suriname in Numbers 286-2012/04). Milieustatistieken (Environment Statistics). Paramaribo: Algemeen Bureau voor de Statistiek; 2012

[56] Algemeen Bureau voor de Statistiek/Censuskantoor. Suriname in Cijfers 2013/05. Resultaten Achtste (8ste) Volks- en Woningtelling in Suriname (Volume 1) (General Bureau of Statistics/Census Office. Suriname in Numbers 2013/05. Results of the Eight General Census of Suriname). Demografische en Sociale Karakteristieken en Migratie (Demographic and Social Characteristics and Migration). Paramaribo: Algemeen Bureau voor de Statistiek; 2013

[57] Hammond DS. Forest conservation and management in the Guiana shield. In: Hammond DS, editor. Tropical Rainforests of the

Guiana Shield. Wallingford: CABI Publishing; 2005. pp. 481-520. DOI: 10.1079/9780851995366.0481

[58] Algemeen Bureau voor de Statistiek. Suriname in Cijfers 303-2014-04 (General Bureau of Statistics. Suriname in Numbers 303-2014-04). Basis Indicatoren (Basic Indicators). Paramaribo: Algemeen Bureau voor de Statistiek; 2014

[59] The World Bank Group. Data - Suriname. Washington, DC: World Bank Group; 2021

[60] Mans DRA, Ganga D, Kartopawiro J. Meeting of the minds: Traditional herbal medicine in multiethnic Suriname. In: El-Shemy H, editor. Aromatic and Medicinal Plants - Back to Nature. Rijeka: InTech; 2017. pp. 111-132. DOI: 10.5772/66509

[61] Forget P-M, Hammond DS. Rainforest vertebrates and food plant diversity in the Guiana shield. In: Hammond DS, editor. Tropical Rainforests of the Guiana Shield. Wallingford: CABI Publishing; 2005. pp. 233-294. DOI: 10.1079/9780851995366.0481

[62] Algemeen Bureau voor de Statistiek (General Bureau of Statistics). Milieustatistieken (Environment statistics). Paramaribo: Algemeen Bureau voor de Statistiek; 2016

[63] Berry PE, Weitzman AL. Checklist of the Plants of the Guiana Shield (Venezuela: Amazonas, Bolivar, Delta Amacuro; Guyana, Suriname, French Guiana). In: Funk VA, Hollowell TH, Berry PE, Kelloff CL, Alexander SN, Eds. Checklist of the Plants of the Guiana Shield (Venezuela: Amazonas, Bolivar, Delta Amacuro; Guyana, Surinam, French Guiana). Washington, DC: United States National Herbarium, Smithsonian Institution; 2007

[64] Ministry of Agriculture, Animal Husbandry and Fisheries. Beplante Arealen, Productie en Export van Groenten (Cultivated Areas, Production, and export of Vegetables). Unpublished manuscript; 2015

[65] Abdoel Wahid F, Wickliffe J, Wilson M, Van Sauers A, Bond N, Hawkins W, et al. Presence of pesticide residues on produce cultivated in Suriname. Environmental Monitoring and Assessment. 2017;**189**:303. DOI: 10.1007/s10661-017-6009-0

[66] Panossian A. Understanding adaptogenic activity: Specificity of the pharmacological action of adaptogens and other phytochemicals. Annals of the New York Academy of Sciences. 2017;**1401**:49-64. DOI: 10.1111/nyas.13399

[67] Tungmunnithum D, Thongboonyou A, Pholboon A, Yangsabai A. Flavonoids and other phenolic compounds from medicinal plants for pharmaceutical and medical aspects: An overview. Medicines (Basel). 2018;**5**:93. DOI: 10.3390/medicines5030093

[68] Mans DRA, Friperson P, Pawirodihardjo J, Djotaroeno M. Antioxidant activity of Surinamese medicinal plants with adaptogenic properties and correlation with total phenolic contents. Journal of Antioxidant Activity. 2020;**2**:11-28. DOI: 10.14302/issn.2471-2140.jaa-20-3478

[69] Stephen HJM. Geneeskruiden Van Suriname: Hun Toepassing in de Volksgeneeskunde en in de Magie (Herbal Medicines from Suriname: Their Applications in Folk Medicine and Wizardry). Amsterdam: De Driehoek; 1979

[70] May AF, Dresi SO. Surinaams Kruidenboek (Surinamese Folk Medicine. A Collection of Surinamese

Medicinal Herbs). Paramaribo: De Walburg Pers; 1982

[71] Titjari. Famiri-Encyclopedia foe da Natoera Dresi-Fasi. Gezinskruidenboek van de Natuurgeneeswijzen. Natuurgeneeswijzen uit het Zonnige Suriname (Encyclopedia of Plant-Based Forms of Treatment. Folk Medicines from Sunny Suriname). Amsterdam: Sangrafoe; 1985

[72] Heyde H. Surinaamse Medicijnplanten (Surinamese Medicinal Plants). 2nd ed. Paramaribo: Westfort; 1987

[73] Tjong AG. Het Gebruik van Medicinale Planten Door de Javanen in Suriname (the Use of Medicinal Plants by the Javanese in Suriname). Paramaribo: Instituut voor de Opleiding van Leraren; 1989

[74] Slagveer JL. Surinaams Groot Kruidenboek: Sranan Oso Dresie (A Surinamese Herbal: Surinamese Traditional Medicines). Paramaribo: De West; 1990

[75] Sedoc NO. Afrosurinaamse Natuurgeneeswijzen: Bevattende meer dan Tweehonderd Meest Gebruikelijke Geneeskrachtige Kruiden (Afro-Surinamese Natural Remedies: Over Two hundred Commonly Used Medicinal Herbs). Paramaribo: Vaco Press; 1992

[76] Raghoenandan UPD. Een Ethnobotanisch Onderzoek onder de Hindustanen in Suriname (An Ethnobotanical Survey among Hindustanis in Suriname). Paramaribo: Anton de Kom Universiteit van Suriname; 1994

[77] DeFilipps RA, Maina SL, Crepin J. Medicinal Plants of the Guianas (Guyana, Surinam, French Guiana). Washington, DC: Smithsonian Institution; 2004

[78] Van Andel TR, Ruysschaert S. Medicinale en Rituele Planten van Suriname (Medicinal and Ritual Plants of Suriname). Amsterdam: KIT Publishers; 2011

[79] Mans DRA, Grant A. "A thing of beauty is a joy forever". Plants and plant-based preparations for facial care in Suriname. Clinical and Medical Investigations. 2017;**2**:1-16. DOI: 10.15761/CMI.1000143

[80] Lima GPP, Vianello F, Corrêa CR, da Silva Campos RA, Borguini MG. Polyphenols in fruits and vegetables and its effect on human health. Food and Nutrition Sciences. 2014;**5**:1065-1082. DOI: 10.4236/fns.2014.511117

[81] Nardini M. Phenolic compounds in food: Characterization and health benefits. Molecules. 2022;**27**:783. DOI: 10.3390/molecules27030783

[82] Christophe H. Plant polyphenols, more than just simple natural antioxidants: Oxidative stress, aging and age-related diseases. Medicine. 2020;7:26. DOI: 10.3390/medicines7050026

[83] Klepacka J, Gujska E, Michalak J. Phenolic compounds as cultivar- and variety-distinguishing factors in some plant products. Plant Foods for Human Nutrition. 2011;**66**:64-69. DOI: 10.1007/s11130-010-0205-1

[84] Timperio AM, D'Alessandro A, Fagioni M, Magro P, Zolla L. Production of the phytoalexins trans-resveratrol and delta-viniferin in two economy-relevant grape cultivars upon infection with Botrytis cinerea in field conditions. Plant Physiology and Biochemistry. 2012;**50**:65-71. DOI: 10.1016/j.plaphy.2011.07.008

[85] Bhattacharya A, Sood P, Citovsky V. The roles of plant phenolics

in defence and communication during *Agrobacterium* and *Rhizobium* infection. Molecular Plant Pathology. 2010;**11**:705-719. DOI: 10.1111/j.1364-3703.2010.00625.x

[86] Blum U, Shafer SR, Lehman ME. Evidence for inhibitory allelopathic interactions involving phenolic acids in field soils: Concepts vs. an experimental model. Critical Reviews in Plant Sciences. 1999;**18**:673-693. DOI: 10.1080/07352689991309441

[87] Nakai S. *Myriophyllum spicatum*-released allelopathic polyphenols inhibiting growth of blue-green algae Microcystis aeruginosa. Water Research. 2000;**34**:3026-3032. DOI: 10.1016/S0043-1354(00)00039-7

[88] Morandi D. Occurrence of phytoalexins and phenolic compounds in endomycorrhizal interactions, and their potential role in biological control. Plant and Soil. 1996;**185**:241-305. DOI: 10.1007/BF02257529

[89] Roleira FM, Tavares-da-Silva EJ, Varela CL, Costa SC, Silva T, Garrido J, et al. Plant derived and dietary phenolic antioxidants: Anticancer properties. Food Chemistry. 2015;**183**:235-258. DOI: 10.1016/j.foodchem.2015.03.039

[90] Lin D, Xiao M, Zhao J, Li Z, Xing B, Li X, et al. An overview of plant phenolic compounds and their importance in human nutrition and management of type 2 diabetes. Molecules. 2016;**21**:1374. DOI: 10.3390/molecules21101374

[91] Lutz M, Fuentes E, Ávila F, Alarcón M, Palomo I. Roles of phenolic compounds in the reduction of risk factors of cardiovascular diseases. Molecules. 2019;**24**:366. DOI: 10.3390/molecules24020366

[92] Khoo HE, Azlan A, Tang ST, Lim SM. Anthocyanidins and anthocyanins: Colored pigments as food, pharmaceutical ingredients, and the potential health benefits. Food and Nutrition Research. 2017;**61**:1361779. DOI: 10.1080/16546628.2017.1361779

[93] Horbowicz M, Kosson R, Grzesiuk A, Dębski H. Anthocyanins of fruits and vegetables—Their occurrence, analysis and role in human nutrition. Journal of Fruit and Ornamental Plant Research. 2008;**68**:5-22. DOI: 10.2478/v10032-008-0001-8

[94] Ramos P, Herrera R, Moya-León MA. Anthocyanins: Food sources and benefits to consumer's health. In: Warner LM, editor. Handbook of Anthocyanins. New York: Nova Science Publishers; 2014. pp. 373-394

[95] Takahama U. Oxidation of vacuolar and apoplastic phenolic substrates by peroxidase: Physiological significance of the oxidation reactions. Phyto B:PHYT.0000047805.08470.e3

[96] Pervaiz T, Songtao J, Faghihi F, Haider MS, Fang J. Naturally occurring anthocyanin, structure, functions and biosynthetic pathway in fruit plants. Journal of Plant Biochemistry and Physiology. 2017;**5**:2. DOI: 10.4172/2329-9029.1000187

[97] Gallori S, Bilia AR, Bergonzi MC, Barbosa WLR, Vincieri FF. Polyphenolic constituents of fruit pulp of *Euterpe oleracea* Mart. (Açai palm). Chromatographia. 2004;**59**:739-743. DOI: 10.1365/s10337-004-0305-x

[98] Bichara CMG, Rogez H. Açai (*Euterpe oleracea* Martius). In: Yahia EM, editor. Postharvest Biology and Technology of Tropical and Subtropical Fruits. Volume 2. Cambridge: Woodhead Publishing; 2011. pp. 1-27. DOI: 10.1533/9780857092762.1

[99] Schauss A, Wu X, Prior R, Ou B, Patel D, Huang D, et al. Phytochemical and nutrient composition of the freeze-dried Amazonian palm berry, *Euterpe oleraceae* Mart. (Açai). Journal of Agricultural and Food Chemistry. 2006;**54**:8598-8603. DOI: 10.1021/jf060976g

[100] Rosso VV, Hillebrand S, Montilla EC, Bobbio FO, Winterhalter P, Mercadante AZ. Determination of anthocyanins from acerola (*Malpighia emarginata* DC) and açai (*Euterpe oleracea* Mart.) by HPLC-PDA-MS/MS. Journal of Food Composition and Analysis. 2008;**21**:291-299. DOI: 10.1016/j.jfca.2008.01.001

[101] Schauss AG, Wu X, Prior RL, Ou B, Huang D, Owens J, et al. Antioxidant capacity and other bioactivities of the freeze-dried Amazonian palm berry, *Euterpe oleraceae* Mart. (açaí). Journal of Agricultural and Food Chemistry. 2006;**54**:8604-8610. DOI: 10.1021/jf0609779

[102] De Pascual-Teresa S, Sanchez-Ballesta MT. Anthocyanins: From plant to health. Phytochemistry Reviews. 2008;**7**:281-299. DOI: 10.1007/s11101-007-9074-0

[103] Miguel MG. Anthocyanins: Antioxidant and/or anti-inflammatory activities. Journal of Applied Pharmaceutical Science. 2011;**1**:7-15

[104] Bueno JM, Sáez-Plaza P, Ramos-Escudero F, Jiménez AM, Fett R, Asuero AG. Analysis and antioxidant capacity of anthocyanin pigments. Part II: Chemical structure, color, and intake of anthocyanins. Critical Reviews in Analytical Chemistry. 2012;**42**:126-151. DOI: 10.1080/10408347.2011.632314

[105] Tena N, Martín J, Asuero AG. State of the art of anthocyanins: Antioxidant activity, sources, bioavailability, and therapeutic effect in human health. Antioxidants (Basel). 2020;**9**:451. DOI: 10.3390/antiox9050451

[106] Lucioli S. Anthocyanins: Mechanism of action and therapeutic efficacy. In: Capasso A, editor. Medicinal Plants as Antioxidant Agents: Understanding their Mechanism of Action and Therapeutic Efficacy. Kerala: Research Signpost; 2012. pp. 27-57

[107] Khoo HE, Lim SM, Azlan A. Evidence-based therapeutic effects of anthocyanins from foods. Pakistan Journal of Nutrition. 2019;**18**:1-11. DOI: 10.3923/pjn.2019.1.11

[108] Nistor M, Pop R, Daescu A, Pintea A, Socaciu C, Rugina D. Anthocyanins as key phytochemicals acting for the prevention of metabolic diseases: An overview. Molecules. 2022;**27**:4254. DOI: 10.3390/molecules27134254

[109] Laleh GH, Frydoonfar H, Heidary R, Jameei R, Zare S. The effect of light, temperature, pH and species on stability of anthocyanin pigments in four *Berberis* species. Pakistan Journal of Nutrition. 2006;**5**:90-92. DOI: 10.3923/pjn.2006.90.92

[110] West ME, Mauer LJ. Color and chemical stability of a variety of anthocyanins and ascorbic acid in solution and powder forms. Journal of Agricultural and Food Chemistry. 2013;**61**:4169-4179. DOI: 10.1021/jf400608b

[111] Contreras-Lopez E, Castañeda-Ovando A, González-Olivares LG, Añorve-Morga J, Jaimez-Ordaz J. Effect of light on stability of anthocyanins in ethanolic extracts of *Rubus fruticosus*. Food and Nutrition Sciences. 2014;**5**:488-494. DOI: 10.4236/fns.2014.56058

[112] Enaru B, Drețcanu G, Pop TD, Stănilă A, Diaconeasa Z. Anthocyanins:

Factors affecting their stability and degradation. Antioxidants (Basel). 2021;**10**:1967. DOI: 10.3390/antiox10121967

[113] Panche AN, Diwan AD, Chandra SR. Flavonoids: An overview. Journal of Nutritional Science. 2016;**5**:e47. DOI: 10.1017/jns.2016.41

[114] Brondízio ES, Safar CA, Siqueira AD. The urban market of açaí fruit (*Euterpe oleracea* Mart.) and rural land use change: Ethnographic insights into the role of price and land tenure constraining agricultural choices in the Amazon estuary. Urban Ecosystem. 2002;**6**:67-97. DOI: 10.1023/A:1025966613562

[115] Sabbe S, Verbeke W, Van Damme P. Analysing the market environment for açaí (*Euterpe oleracea* Mart.) juices in Europe. Fruits. 2009;**64**:273-284. DOI: 10.1051/fruits/2009022

[116] Plotkin MJ, Balick MJ. Medicinal uses of south American palms. Journal of Ethnopharmacology. 1984;**10**:157-179. DOI: 10.1016/0378-8741(84)90001-1

[117] Bourdy G, DeWalt SJ, de Michel LRC, Roca A, Deharo E, Muñoz V, et al. Medicinal plants uses of the Tacana, an Amazonian Bolivian ethnic group. Journal of Ethnopharmacology. 2000;**70**:87-109. DOI: 10.1016/s0378-8741(99)00158-0

[118] Sosnowska J, Balslev H. American palms used for medicine, in the ethnobotanical and pharmacological publications. Revista Peruana de Biología. 2008;**15**:143-146

[119] Portinho JA, Zimmermann LM, Bruck MR. Beneficial effects of açai. International Journal of Nutrology. 2012;**5**:15-20

[120] Da Silva MACN, do Desterro MSBN, de Carvalho JE. Traditional uses, phytochemistry, pharmacology and anticancer activity of açaí (*Euterpe oleracea* Mart): A narrative review. Current Traditional Medicine. 2021;7:e070520181766. DOI: 10.2174/2215083806999200508081308

[121] De Oliveira NKS, Almeida MRS, Pontes FMM, Barcelos MP, de Paula da Silva CHT, Rosa JMC, et al. Antioxidant effect of flavonoids present in *Euterpe oleracea* Martius and neurodegenerative diseases: A literature review Central Nervous System Agents in Medicinal Chemistry. 2019;19:75-99. DOI: 10.2174/1871524919666190502105855

[122] De Almeida Magalhães TSS, de Oliveira Macedo PC, Converti A, Neves de Lima ÁA. The use of *Euterpe oleracea* Mart. as a new perspective for disease treatment and prevention. Biomolecules. 2020;**10**:813. DOI: 10.3390/biom10060813

[123] Pacheco-Palencia LA, Mertens-Talcott S, Talcott ST. Chemical composition, antioxidant properties, and thermal stability of a phytochemical enriched oil from açai (*Euterpe oleracea* Mart.). Journal of Agricultural and Food Chemistry. 2008;**56**:4631-4636. DOI: 10.1021/jf800161u

[124] Kang J, Li Z, Wu T, Jensen GS, Schauss AG, Wu X. Anti-oxidant capacities of flavonoid compounds isolated from açai pulp (*Euterpe oleracea* Mart). Food Chemistry. 2010;**122**:610-617. DOI: 10.1016/j.foodchem.2010.03.020

[125] Thummayot S, Tocharus C, Pinkaew D, Viwatpinyo K, Sringarm K, Tocharus J. Neuroprotective effect of purple rice extract and its constituent against amyloid beta-induced neuronal cell death in SK-N-SH cells. Neurotoxicology. 2014;**45**:149-158. DOI: 10.1016/j.neuro.2014.10.010

[126] Yamaguchi KK, Pereira LF, Lamarão CV, Lima ES, da Veiga-Junior VF. Amazon açai: Chemistry and biological activities: A review. Food Chemistry. 2015;**179**:137-151. DOI: 10.1016/j.foodchem.2015.01.055

[127] Garzón GA, Narváez-Cuenca CE, Vincken JP, Gruppen H. Polyphenolic composition and antioxidant activity of açai (*Euterpe oleracea* Mart.) from Colombia. Food Chemistry. 2017;**217**:364-372. DOI: 10.1016/j.foodchem.2016.08.107

[128] Cesar LT, de Freitas CM, Maia GA, de Figueiredo RW, de Miranda MR, de Sousa PH, et al. Effects of clarification on physicochemical characteristics, antioxidant capacity and quality attributes of açaí (*Euterpe oleracea* Mart.) juice. Journal of Food Science and Technology. 2014;**51**:3293-2300. DOI: 10.1007/s13197-012-0809-6

[129] Mertens-Talcott SU, Rios J, Jilma-Stohlawetz P, Pacheco-Palencia LA, Meibohm B, Talcott ST, et al. Pharmacokinetics of anthocyanins and antioxidant effects after the consumption of anthocyanin-rich açai juice and pulp (*Euterpe oleracea* Mart.) in human healthy volunteers. Journal of Agricultural and Food Chemistry. 2008;**56**:7796-7802. DOI: 10.1021/jf8007037

[130] Barbosa PO, Pala D, Silva CT, de Souza MO, do Amaral JF, Vieira RA, et al. Açai (*Euterpe oleracea* Mart.) pulp dietary intake improves cellular antioxidant enzymes and biomarkers of serum in healthy women. Nutrition. 2016;**32**:674-680. DOI: 10.1016/j.nut.2015.12.030

[131] Pina F, Oliveira J, de Freitas V. Anthocyanins and derivatives are more than flavylium cations. Tetrahedron. 2015;**71**:3107-3114. DOI: 10.1016/j.tet.2014.09.051

[132] Khanbabaee K, van Ree T. Tannins: Classification and definition. Natural Product Reports. 2001;**18**:641-649. DOI: 10.1039/b101061l

[133] Tong Z, He W, Fan X, Guo A. Biological function of plant tannin and its application in animal health. Frontiers in Veterinary Science. 2022;**8**:803657. DOI: 10.3389/fvets.2021.803657

[134] Dasa AK, Islamb MN, Farukb MO, Ashaduzzamanb M, Dunganic R. Review on tannins: Extraction processes, applications and possibilities. South African Journal of Botany. 2020;**135**:58-70

[135] Koleckar V, Kubikova K, Rehakova Z, Kuca K, Jun D, Jahodar L, et al. Condensed and hydrolysable tannins as antioxidants influencing the health. Mini-Reviews in Medicinal Chemistry. 2008;**8**:436-447. DOI: 10.2174/138955708784223486

[136] Bule M, Khan F, Nisar MF, Kamal NK. Tannins (hydrolysable tannins, condensed tannins, phlorotannins, flavono-ellagitannins). In: Silva AS, Nabavi SF, Saeedi M, Nabavi SM, editors. Recent Advances in Natural Products Analysis. Amsterdam: Elsevier; 2020. pp. 132-146. DOI: 10.1016/C2018-0-00121-8

[137] Castell JC, Sorolla S, Jorba M, Aribau J, Bacardit A, Ollé L. Tara (*Caesalpinia spinosa*): The sustainable source of tannins for innovative tanning processes. Journal of the American Leather Chemists Association. 2012;**108**:221-230

[138] Ahmad W, Zeenat F, Hasan A, Abdullah A, Nargis A, Mazu TT. *Quercus infectoria* Oliv.—An overview. Indian Journal of Unani Medicine. 2011;**4**:17-22

[139] Mämmelä P, Savolainen H, Lindroos L, Kangas J, Vartiainen T.

Analysis of oak tannins by liquid chromatography-electrospray ionisation mass spectrometry. Journal of Chromatography A. 2000;**891**:75-83. DOI: 10.1016/S0021-9673(00)00624-5

[140] Lee DY, Kim HW, Yang H, Sung SH. Hydrolyzable tannins from the fruits of *Terminalia chebula* Retz and their α-glucosidase inhibitory activities. Phytochemistry. 2017;**137**:109-116. DOI: 10.1016/j.phytochem.2017.02.006

[141] Monagas M, Gómez-Cordovés C, Bartolomé B, Laureano O, Ricardo da Silva JM. Monomeric, oligomeric, and polymeric flavan-3-ol composition of wines and grapes from *Vitis vinifera* L. cv. Graciano, Tempranillo, and Cabernet Sauvignon. Journal of Agricultural and Food Chemistry. 2003;**51**:6475-6481. DOI: 10.1021/jf030325+

[142] Zhang LL, Lin YM, Zhou HC, Wei SD, Chen JH. Condensed tannins from mangrove species *Kandelia candel* and *Rhizophora mangle* and their antioxidant activity. Molecules. 2010;**15**:420-431. DOI: 10.3390/molecules15010420

[143] Bharudin MA, Zakaria S, Chia CH. Condensed tannins from *Acacia mangium* bark: Characterization by spot tests and FTIR. AIP Conference Proceedings. 2013;**1571**:153. DOI: 10.1063/1.4858646

[144] Yamada H, Wakamori S, Hirokane T, Ikeuchi K, Matsumoto S. Structural revisions in natural ellagitannins. Molecules. 2018;**23**:1901. DOI: 10.3390/molecules23081901

[145] Yoshida T, Amakura Y, Yoshimura M. Structural features and biological properties of ellagitannins in some plant families of the order Myrtales. International Journal of Molecular Sciences. 2010;**11**:79-106. DOI: 10.3390/ijms11010079

[146] Smeriglio A, Barreca D, Bellocco E, Trombetta D. Proanthocyanidins and hydrolysable tannins: Occurrence, dietary intake and pharmacological effects. British Journal of Pharmacology. 2017;**174**:1244-1262. DOI: 10.1111/bph.13630

[147] Lipińska L, Klewicka E, Sójka M. The structure, occurrence and biological activity of ellagitannins: A general review. Acta Scientiarum Polonorum, Technologia Alimentaria. 2014;**13**:289-299. DOI: 10.17306/j.afs.2014.3.7

[148] Lorenzo JM, Munekata PE, Putnik P, Kovačević DB, Muchenje V, Barba FJ. Sources, chemistry, and biological potential of ellagitannins and ellagic acid derivatives. Studies in Natural Products Chemistry. 2019;**60**:189-221. DOI: 10.1016/B978-0-444-64181-6.00006-1

[149] Landete JM. Ellagitannins, ellagic acid and their derived metabolites: A review about source, metabolism, functions and health. Food Research International. 2011;**44**:1150-1160. DOI: 10.1016/j.foodres.2011.04.027

[150] Cortés-Martín A, Selma MV, Espín JC, García-Villalba R. The human metabolism of nuts proanthocyanidins does not reveal urinary metabolites consistent with distinctive gut microbiota metabotypes. Molecular Nutrition and Food Research. 2019;**63**:e1800819. DOI: 10.1002/mnfr.201800819

[151] Aguilar-Zarate P, Wong-Paz JE, Buenrostro-Figueroa JJ, Ascacio JA, Contreras-Esquivel JC, Aguilar CN. Ellagitannins: Bioavailability, purification and biotechnological degradation. Mini-Reviews in Medicinal Chemistry. 2018;**18**:1244-1252. DOI: 10.2174/1389557517666170208144742

[152] Ito H. Metabolites of the ellagitannin geraniin and their antioxidant activities. Planta Medica. 2011;**77**:1110-1115. DOI: 10.1055/s-0030-1270749

[153] Sharifi-Rad J, Quispe C, Castillo CMS, Caroca R, Lazo-Vélez MA, Antonyak H, et al. Ellagic acid: A review on its natural sources, chemical stability, and therapeutic potential. Oxidative Medicine and Cellular Longevity. 2022;**2022**:3848084. DOI: 10.1155/2022/3848084

[154] Liberal J, Carmo A, Gomes C, Cruz MT, Batista MT. Urolithins impair cell proliferation, arrest the cell cycle and induce apoptosis in UMUC3 bladder cancer cells. Investigational New Drugs. 2017;**35**:671-681. DOI: 10.1007/s10637-017-0483-7

[155] Villalba KJO, Barka FV, Pasos CV, Rodríguez PE. Food ellagitannins: Structure, metabolomic fate, and biological properties. In: Aires A, editor. Tannins—Structural Properties, Biological Properties and Current Knowledge. London: IntechOpen; 2019. pp. 26-46. DOI: 10.5772/intechopen.86420

[156] Maphetu N, Unuofin JO, Masuku NP, Olisah C, Lebelo SL. Medicinal uses, pharmacological activities, phytochemistry, and the molecular mechanisms of *Punica granatum* L. (pomegranate) plant extracts: A review. Biomedicine and Pharmacotherapy. 2022;**153**:113256. DOI: 10.1016/j.biopha.2022.113256

[157] Viuda-Martos M, Fernandez-Lopez J, Perez-Alvarez JA. Pomegranate and its many functional components as related to human health: A review. Comprehensive Reviews in Food Science and Food Safety. 2010;**9**:635-654

[158] Bhowmik D, Gopinath H, Kumar BP, Duraivel S, Aravind G, Kumar KPS. Medicinal uses of *Punica granatum* and its health benefits. Journal of Pharmacognosy and Phytochemistry. 2013;**1**:28-35

[159] Jasuja ND, Saxena R, Chandra S, Sharma R. Pharmacological characterization and beneficial uses of *Punica granatum*. Asian Journal of Plant Sciences. 2012;**11**:251-267. DOI: 10.3923/ajps.2012.251.267

[160] Rahimi HR, Arastoo M, Ostad SN. A comprehensive review of *Punica granatum* (pomegranate) properties in toxicological, pharmacological, cellular and molecular biology researches. Iranian Journal of Pharmaceutical Research. 2012;**11**:e125841. DOI: 10.22037/ijpr.2012.1148

[161] Gil MI, Tomás-Barberán FA, Hess-Pierce B, Holcroft DM, Kader AA. Antioxidant activity of pomegranate juice and its relationship with phenolic composition and processing. Journal of Agricultural and Food Chemistry. 2000;**48**:4581-4589. DOI: 10.1021/jf000404a

[162] Rosenblatt M, Aviram M. Antioxidative properties of pomegranate. In: Seeram NP, Schulman RN, Heber D, editors. Pomegranates: Ancient Roots Modern Medicine; Medicinal and Aromatic Plant Series. Boca Raton: CRC Press/Taylor and Francis; 2006. pp. 310-343

[163] Heber D. Pomegranate ellagitannins. In: Benzie IFF, Wachtel-Galor S, editors. Herbal Medicine: Biomolecular and Clinical Aspects. 2nd ed. Boca Raton: CRC Press/Taylor & Francis; 2011. Chapter 10

[164] Gómez Caravaca AM, Verardo V, Toselli M, Segura Carretero A, Fernández Gutiérrez A, Caboni MF. Determination of the major phenolic compounds in pomegranate juices by HPLC–DAD–ESI-MS. Journal of Agricultural and Food Chemistry. 2013;**61**:5328-5337. DOI: 10.1021/jf400684n

[165] Hernández F, Melgarejo P, Tomás-Barberán FA, Artés F. Evolution of juice anthocyanins during ripening

of new selected pomegranate (*Punica granatum*) clones. European Food Research and Technology. 1999;**210**:39-42. DOI: 10.1007/s002170050529

[166] Kähkönen M, Kylli P, Ollilainen V, Salminen JP, Heinonen M. Antioxidant activity of isolated ellagitannins from red raspberries and cloudberries. Journal of Agricultural and Food Chemistry. 2012;**60**:1167-1174. DOI: 10.1021/jf203431g

[167] Ishimoto H, Shibata M, Myojin Y, Ito H, Sugimoto Y, Tai A, et al. *In vivo* anti-inflammatory and antioxidant properties of ellagitannin metabolite urolithin A. Bioorganic and Medicinal Chemistry Letters. 2011;**21**:5901-5904. DOI: 10.1016/j.bmcl.2011.07.086

[168] Heber D, Seeram NP, Wyatt H, Henning SM, Zhang Y, Ogden LG, et al. Safety and antioxidant activity of a pomegranate ellagitannin-enriched polyphenol dietary supplement in overweight individuals with increased waist size. Journal of Agricultural and Food Chemistry. 2007;**55**:10050-10054. DOI: 10.1021/jf071689v

[169] Annunziata F, Pinna C, Dallavalle S, Tamborini L, Pinto A. An overview of coumarin as a versatile and readily accessible scaffold with broad-ranging biological activities. International Journal of Molecular Sciences. 2020;**21**:4618. DOI: 10.3390/ijms21134618

[170] Sproll C, Ruge W, Andlauer C, Godelmann R, Lachenmeier DW. HPLC analysis and safety assessment of coumarin in foods. Food Chemistry. 2008;**109**:462-469. DOI: 10.1016/j.foodchem.2007.12.068

[171] Menezes JCJMDS, Diederich MF. Natural dimers of coumarin, chalcones, and resveratrol and the link between structure and pharmacology. European Journal of Medicinal Chemistry. 2019;**182**:111637. DOI: 10.1016/j.ejmech.2019.111637

[172] Murray RD. The naturally occurring coumarins. Fortschritte der Chemie Organischer Naturstoffe. 2002;**83**:1-619. DOI: 10.1007/978-3-7091-6172-2_1

[173] Kresge N, Simoni RD, Hill RL. Hemorrhagic sweet clover disease, dicumarol, and warfarin: The work of Karl Paul link. Journal of Biological Chemistry. 2005;**280**:e5

[174] Loprinzi CL, Sloan J, Kugler J. Coumarin-induced hepatotoxicity. Journal of Clinical Oncology. 1997;**15**:3167-3168. DOI: 10.1200/JCO.1997.15.9.3167

[175] Lončar M, Jakovljević M, Šubarić D, Pavlić M, Buzjak Služek V, Cindrić I, et al. Coumarins in food and methods of their determination. Food. 2020;**9**:645. DOI: 10.3390/foods9050645

[176] Abraham K, Wöhrlin F, Lindtner O, Heinemeyer G, Lampen A. Toxicology and risk assessment of coumarin: Focus on human data. Molecular Nutrition and Food Research. 2010;**54**:228-239. DOI: 10.1002/mnfr.200900281

[177] Kuruvilla M, Gurk-Turner C. A review of warfarin dosing and monitoring. Proceedings/Baylor University Medical Center. 2001;**14**:305-396. DOI: 10.1080/08998280.2001.11927781

[178] Ramachandran S, Pitchai S. Story of warfarin: From rat poison to lifesaving drug. Indian Journal of Vascular and Endovascular Surgery. 2018;**5**:174-175

[179] Hussain MI, Qamar Abbas S, Reigosa MJ. Activities and novel applications of secondary metabolite coumarins. Planta Daninha.

2018;**36**:e018174040. DOI: 10.1590/S0100-8358201836010001

[180] Venugopala KN, Rashmi V, Odhav B. Review on natural coumarin lead compounds for their pharmacological activity. BioMed Research International. 2013;**2013**:963248. DOI: 10.1155/2013/963248

[181] Srikrishna D, Godugu C, Dubey PK. A review on pharmacological properties of coumarins. Mini-Reviews in Medicinal Chemistry. 2018;**18**:113-141. DOI: 10.2174/1389557516666160801094919

[182] Gouda MA, Salem MA, Helal MH. A review on synthesis and pharmacological activity of coumarins and their analogs. Current Bioactive Compounds. 2020;**16**:818-836. DOI: 10.2174/1573407215666190405154406

[183] Paya M, Halliwell B, Hoult JR. Interactions of a series of coumarins with reactive oxygen species. Scavenging of superoxide, hypochlorous acid and hydroxyl radicals. Biochemical Pharmacology. 1992;**44**:205-214. DOI: 10.1016/0006-2952(92)90002-Z

[184] Fylaktakidou KC, Hadjipavlou-Litina DJ, Litinas KE, Nicolaides DN. Natural and synthetic coumarin derivatives with anti-inflammatory/antioxidant activities. Current Pharmaceutical Design. 2004;**10**:3813-3833. DOI: 10.2174/1381612043382710

[185] Bubols GB, da Rocha VD, Medina-Remon A, von Poser G, Lamuela-Raventos RM, Eifler-Lima VL, et al. The antioxidant activity of coumarins and flavonoids. Mini-Reviews in Medicinal Chemistry. 2013;**13**:318-334. DOI: 10.2174/1389557511313030002

[186] Al-Majedy Y, Al-Amiery A, Kadhum AA, Mohamad AB. Antioxidant activity of coumarins. Systematic Reviews in Pharmacy. 2017;**8**:24-30

[187] Al-Majedy YK, Al-Duhaidahawi DL, Al-Azawi KF, Al-Amiery AA, Kadhum AAH, Mohamad AB. Coumarins as potential antioxidant agents complemented with suggested mechanisms and approved by molecular modeling studies. Molecules. 2016;**21**:135. DOI: 10.3390/molecules21020135

[188] Tataringa G, Zbancioc AM. Coumarin derivatives with antimicrobial and antioxidant activities. In: Rao V, Mans D, Rao L, editors. Phytochemicals in Human Health. Rijeka: IntechOpen; 2019. pp. 139-158. DOI: 10.5772/intechopen.88096

[189] Sarker SD, Nahar L. Progress in the chemistry of naturally occurring coumarins. In: Kinghorn A, Falk H, Gibbons S, Kobayashi J, editors. Progress in the Chemistry of Organic Natural Products. Cham: Springer; 2017. pp. 241-304. DOI: 10.1007/978-3-319-59542-9_3

[190] Da Cunha CP, Godoy RLO, Braz FR. Isolation of flavonoids from *Dipteryx odorata* by high-performance liquid chromatography. Revista Virtual de Química. 2016;**8**:43-56. DOI: 10.5935/1984-6835.20160004

[191] Socorro MP, Pinto AC, Kaiser CR. New isoflavonoid from *Dipteryx odorata*. Zeitschrift für Naturforschung. 2003;**58B**:1206-1209

[192] Januário AH, Lourenço MV, Domézio LA, Pietro RCLR, Castilho MS, Tomazela DM, et al. Isolation and structure determination of bioactive isoflavones from callus culture of *Dipteryx odorata*. Chemical and Pharmaceutical Bulletin. 2005;**53**:740-742. DOI: 10.1248/cpb.53.740

[193] De Oliveira PC, de Oliveira Queiroz de Sou BC. Traditional knowledge of

forest medicinal plants of Munduruku indigenous people - Ipaupixuna European Journal of Medicinal Plants. 2020;31:20-35. DOI: 10.9734/ejmp/2020/v31i1330309

[194] Heghes SC, Vostinaru O, Mogosan C, Miere D, Iuga CA, Filip L. Safety profile of nutraceuticals rich in coumarins: An update. Frontiers in Pharmacology. 2022;**13**:803338. DOI: 10.3389/fphar.2022.803338

[195] Van Andel T, Behari-Ramdas J, Havinga R, Groenendijk S. The medicinal plant trade in Suriname. Ethnobotany Research and Applications. 2007;**5**:351-372

[196] Fetzer DEL. Extraction of *Dipteryx odorata* (Aubl.) Willd. Coumarin-Rich Seed Oil Using High-Pressure Trending Technology. Curitiba: Universidade Federal do Paraná; 2021

[197] Kim D-S, Iida F. Nutritional composition of Tonka bean (*Dipteryx odorata*) and its application as an elder-friendly food with gelling agent. Gels. 2022;**8**:704. DOI: 10.3390/gels8110704

[198] Bony E, Boudard F, Brat P, Dussossoy E, Portet K, Poucheret P, et al. Awara (*Astrocaryum vulgare* M.) pulp oil: Chemical characterization, and anti-inflammatory properties in a mice model of endotoxic shock and a rat model of pulmonary inflammation. Fitoterapia. 2012;**83**:33-43. DOI: 10.1016/j.fitote.2011.09.007

[199] Bony E, Boudard T, Dussossoy E, Portet K, Brat P, Giaimis J, et al. Chemical composition and anti-inflammatory properties of the unsaponifiable fraction from Awara (*Astrocaryum vulgare* M.) pulp oil in activated J774 macrophages and in a mice model of endotoxic shock. Plant Foods for Human Nutrition. 2012;**67**:384-392. DOI: 10.1007/s11130-012-0323-z

[200] Da Silva A, Silveira BKS, de Freitas BVM, Hermsdorff HHM, Bressan J. Effects of regular Brazil nut (*Bertholletia excelsa* H.B.K.) consumption on health: A systematic review of clinical trials. Food. 2022;**11**:2925. DOI: 10.3390/foods11182925

[201] Cardoso BR, Duarte GBS, Reis BZ, Cozzolino SMF. Brazil nuts: Nutritional composition, health benefits and safety aspects. Food Research International. 2017;**100**:9-18. DOI: 10.1016/j.foodres.2017.08.036

[202] Eslami O, Shidfar F, Dehnad A. Inverse association of long-term nut consumption with weight gain and risk of overweight/obesity: A systematic review. Nutrition Research. 2019;**68**:1-8. DOI: 10.1016/j.nutres.2019.04.001

[203] National Institutes of Health. Office of Dietary Supplements. Fact Sheet for Health Professionals: Selenium; 2021

[204] Chunhieng T, Pétritis K, Elfakir C, Brochier J, Goli T, Montet D. Study of selenium distribution in the protein fractions of the Brazil nut, *Bertholletia excelsa*. Journal of Agricultural and Food Chemistry. 2004;**52**:4318-4322. DOI: 10.1021/jf049643e

[205] Chunhieng T, Hafidi A, Pioch D, Brochier J, Montet D. Detailed study of Brazil nut (*Bertholletia excelsa*) oil microcompounds: Phospholipids, tocopherols and sterols. Journal of the Brazilian Chemical Society. 2008;**19**:1374-1380. DOI: 10.1590/S0103-50532008000700021

[206] John JA, Shahidi F. Phenolic compounds and antioxidant activity of Brazil nut (*Bertholletia excels*a). Journal of Functional Foods. 2010;**2**:196-209. DOI: 10.1016/j.jff.2010.04.00

[207] El-Agamey A, Lowe GM, McGarvey DJ, Mortensen A, Philip DM, Truscott TG, et al. Carotenoid radical chemistry and antioxidant/pro-oxidant

properties. Archives of Biochemistry and Biophysics. 2004;**430**:37-48. DOI: 10.1016/j.abb.2004.03.007

[208] Burke M, Edge R, Land EJ, McGarvey DJ, Truscott TG. One-electron reduction potentials of dietary carotenoid radical cations in aqueous micellar environments. FEBS Letters. 2001;**500**:132-136. DOI: 10.1016/S0014-5793(01)02601-1

[209] Kaźmierczak-Barańska J, Boguszewska K, Adamus-Grabicka A, Karwowski BT. Two faces of viamin C—Anti-oxidative and pro-oxidative agent. Nutrients. 2020;**12**:1501. DOI: 10.3390/nu12051501

Chapter 7

Naturally Occurring Antioxidants in Seven Well-Known Fruits from the Republic of Suriname (South America): Part 2

Dennis R.A. Mans

Abstract

The dependence of humans on oxygen for their metabolism, together with their uninterrupted exposure to a wide variety of hazardous environmental chemicals, leads to the continuous formation of reactive oxygen-derived species (ROS) in the body such as superoxide radical anion, hydrogen peroxide, peroxyl radicals, and hydroxyl radical. When in excess, ROS can damage cellular constituents such as DNA and membrane lipids causing oxidative stress, cellular injury, and eventually, inflammatory, neoplastic, diabetic, cardiovascular, neurodegenerative, and age-related diseases. Fortunately, the body has a multitude of naturally occurring antioxidants in dietary fruits and vegetables to its disposal, including polyphenolic compounds, vitamins, and essential minerals. These antioxidants eliminate ROS by acting as reducing agents, hydrogen donors, quenchers of singlet oxygen, or chelators of metal ions that catalyze oxidation reactions, thus decreasing the risk of the above-mentioned diseases. Part 1 of this chapter has comprehensively addressed three representative examples of fruits from the Republic of Suriname (South America) that are rich in the polyphenolics anthocyanins, ellagitannins, and coumarins and has highlighted their antioxidant activity and beneficial and health-promoting effects. This second part deals with four Surinamese fruits with an abundance of (pro)vitamins A, C, and E and selenium in light of their antioxidant activities.

Keywords: antioxidants, fruits, Suriname, (pro)vitamin A, vitamin C, vitamin E, selenium

1. Introduction

There is ample evidence that life on our planet has developed under anaerobic conditions [1, 2]. Most organisms that evolved from these primordial predecessors have dealt with the increasing atmospheric levels of oxygen by adapting to oxygen and its derivatives and creating antioxidant defense systems to protect themselves against the toxic effects of these compounds [3, 4]. The most notable toxic byproducts of metabolic reactions involving oxygen are reactive oxygen-derived species (ROS) such as superoxide radical anion, hydrogen peroxide, peroxyl radicals, and hydroxyl radical, as well as non-radical species such as hydrogen peroxide, peroxynitrite, hypochlorous acid, and ozone [5–7]. Reactive nitrogen species (RNS) such as nitric oxide, peroxynitrite, and nitrogen dioxide radical, as well as reactive chlorine species (RCS) such as hypochlorous acid, are also classified as ROS [5–7]. ROS are able to readily react with and cause damage to biomolecules including proteins, lipids, and nucleic acids, leading to cell and tissue injury [8–10]. The high reactivity of ROS derives from the presence of a single unpaired electron in their outer orbit formed as a result of incomplete reduction of the oxygen metabolites [8–10].

ROS are mainly generated in cellular organelles where oxygen consumption is high, such as mitochondria, peroxisomes, and endoplasmic reticulum [11–13]. In addition to these endogenous sources, ROS are produced from exogenous sources such as car exhaust, cigarette smoke, and industrial contaminants; peroxides, aldehydes, oxidized fatty acids, and transition metals in foods; a large variety of xenobiotics including toxins, pesticides, and herbicides; as well as various medical drugs such as narcotics, anesthetizing gases, and antineoplastic agents [5, 14, 15]. For example, γ-radiation interacts with water molecules to form water radical cations and free electrons which react with other water molecules to form highly active hydroxyl radical, superoxides, and organic radicals as well as organic hydroperoxides and hydrogen peroxide [16]. And the antitumor antibiotic doxorubicin generates a semiquinone derivative that can autoxidize in the presence of oxygen, producing superoxide anions following electron donation by oxidases such as mitochondrial NADPH and nitric oxide synthases [17]. In all cases, the ROS-induced oxidative stress results in massive damage to cellular macromolecules such as DNA, critical proteins, and membrane lipids, eventually causing, among others, neoplastic, neurodegenerative, cardiovascular, age-related, cerebrovascular, diabetic, and inflammatory diseases [18–24].

However, as mentioned above, aerobic organisms have developed mechanisms to adapt to and cope with ROS. Major adaptation mechanisms involve the utilization of oxygen and ROS as relay elements in pathways of cell signaling and homeostasis, for various metabolic reactions, to eliminate xenobiotics from the body, and to help destroy phagocytized harmful particles. For instance, ROS, in particular hydrogen peroxide, can act as messengers in the transduction of metabolic and environmental signals which affect diverse intracellular pathways, culminating in the activation of transcription factors and other proteins, controlling their biological activities [9]. A well-investigated example is redox signaling involving the oxidation of cysteine residues of proteins by hydrogen peroxide, converting a thiolate anion in cysteine (Cys-S-) into the sulfenic form (Cys-SOH), causing the protein to undergo allosteric changes that alter its function [25]. Furthermore, the formation of ATP during oxidative phosphorylation in the mitochondria is accompanied by the production of electrons in the electron transport chain for the reduction of molecular oxygen into superoxides which are subsequently transformed into the much less reactive hydrogen peroxide by superoxide dismutase [26]. As well, the addition of oxygen atoms to xenobiotics by cytochrome P450 enzymes increases their water solubility, facilitating their removal from the body [27]. And phagocytized bacteria, bits of necrotic tissue, and foreign particles are intracellularly destroyed by macrophages and neutrophils by the so-called respiratory burst (or oxidative burst), involving the rapid release of superoxides and hydrogen peroxide following the supply of electrons by NADPH [28].

Critical mechanisms of aerobic organisms to cope with ROS involve the use of endogenous and exogenous defense systems that counter their detrimental effects. The endogenous defenses comprise enzymatic antioxidant systems such as superoxide dismutase, catalase, and glutathione peroxidase [29] and nonenzymatic mechanisms such as bilirubin and albumin [30]. The exogenous defenses complement the endogenous mechanisms and consist of antioxidants in fruits and vegetables provided through the diet [31] and include, among others, various phenolic compounds, vitamins, essential minerals, small peptides, and fatty acids [32, 33]. Like the exogenous mechanisms, the endogenous defenses prevent the formation of ROS through various mechanmsm [29–31, 33, 34]. A multitude of studies have validated the critical role of exogenous dietary antioxidants in our well-being (see, for instance, references [31, 32]). This has resulted in the recommendation of diets high in fruits and vegetables that are rich in these compounds to decrease the risk of developing the above-mentioned degenerative diseases [35–37]. The first part of this chapter provided some background information about the role of naturally occurring antioxidants as exogenous antioxidant defenses, gave some background on the Republic of Suriname, then comprehensively addressed three representative examples of well-known Surinamese fruits that are rich in the polyphenolic compounds anthocyanins, ellagitannins, and coumarins, highlighting the involvement of these naturally occurring antioxidants in the beneficial and health-promoting effects of the fruits. This second part of the chapter continues with a comprehensive overview of four additional popular Surinamese plants with an abundance of (pro)vitamins A, C, or E, or selenium, and equally extensively addresses the contribution of these antioxidants to the favorable effects of the fruits on human health.

2. (Pro)vitamins A, C, and/or E, and selenium in four well-known Surinamese fruits

Like the three Surinamese fruits that have in detail been addressed in the first part of this chapter, the four fruits dealt with in this part are abundantly cultivated and traded in Suriname [38], consumed as foods and/or nutritional supplements [38], and/or used as traditional cosmeceuticals [39] and/or medicines [40–49]. The plants addressed in both parts of this chapter as well as their relevant characteristics are given in **Table 1**.

2.1 Antioxidant vitamins

Vitamins are essential organic compounds that must be obtained from the diet and are required in minute amounts for: supporting normal growth, development, and reproduction; fortifying the immune system and fighting infections; proper wound healing; strengthening bones, ligaments, muscles, teeth, and nails; regulating hormones; and processing of energy in cells [50]. Insufficient intake of vitamins may cause deficiency diseases such as xerophthalmia, scurvy, beri-beri, and pellagra (particularly in developing countries [50]), but resupplying these nutrients can help ease the symptoms of these conditions [50].

Vitamins can be divided into fat-soluble compounds (vitamins A, D, E, and K) [50, 51] and water-soluble compounds such as vitamins of the B complex (vitamins B_1, B_2, B_3, B_5, B_6, B_9, B_{12}, and biotin) as well as vitamin C [50, 52]. The fat-soluble vitamins dissolve in fat before they are absorbed in the bloodstream to carry out their functions [50, 51]. Excesses of these vitamins are stored in the liver and fatty

Main antioxidants	Plant family	Plant species (common vernacular; Surinamese vernacular)	Main traditional uses	Main commercialized products
Phenolic compounds—anthocyanins	Arecaceae	*Euterpe oleracea* Mart. (açai; podosiri)	Anemia; hypotension; wounds; as an external contraceptive	Health-promoting supplements and nutraceuticals
Phenolic compounds—ellagitannins	Lythraceae	*Punica granatum* L. (pomegranate; granaatappel)	Sore throat; respiratory afflictions; wounds and hemorrhages; gastrointestinal disorders; menstrual problems	Ellagitannin-enriched dietary supplements
Phenolic compounds—coumarins	Fabaceae	*Dipteryx odorata* (Aubl.) Willd (tonka bean; tonkaboon)	Hair conditions; colds and fever; respiratory disorders; gastrointestinal disorders; menstrual problems; as an aphrodisiac	Hair care
Vitamins—vitamin A	Arecaceae	*Astrocaryum vulgare* Mart. (tucuma; awara)	Colicky babies; respiratory diseases; gastrointestinal disorders; rheumatism; pains; skin and hair problems; wounds; fractured bones; sexual underperformance and infertility	Skin and hair care
Vitamins—vitamin C	Malpighiaceae	*Malpighia glabra* L. (acerola; West-Indische kers)	Respiratory diseases; maladies of the oral cavity; cardiovascular ailments; wounds; gastrointestinal disorders; depression; cancer	Vitamin C-enriched dietary supplements and other health products
Vitamins—vitamin E	Malvaceae	*Hibiscus sabdariffa* L. (roselle; syuru)	Microbial infections; respiratory diseases; kidney problems; gastrointestinal disorders; hypertension	Skin and hair care; wound healing
Antioxidant minerals—selenium	Lecythidaceae	*Bertholletia excelsa* Humb. & Bonpl. (Brazil nut; paranoto)	Gastrointestinal disorders; burns	Skin and hair care

Table 1.
Main antioxidant compounds, traditional uses, and commercialized products of seven Surinamese types of fruits.

tissues; for this reason, they are not needed in the daily diet [50, 51]. Notably, excessive intake of fat-soluble vitamins may lead to toxicity and potential health problems [50, 51]. Water-soluble vitamins dissolve in water and are not stored in the body and must therefore be acquired via the daily diet [50, 52]. Unlike the fat-soluble vitamins, excessive intake of water-soluble vitamins is readily eliminated in the urine and does not cause health problems [50, 52].

Apart from the functions mentioned in the preceding paragraph, vitamins function as antioxidants [53, 54]. The best studied antioxidant vitamins are (pro)vitamin A, vitamin C, and vitamin E; other vitamins such as vitamin K, vitamin D, vitamin B_2, vitamin B_3, and vitamin B_6 have not adequately been evaluated for their antioxidant potential [54]. Vitamin C is able to quench ROS by donating electrons to them; vitamin D inhibits ROS generation, preventing lipid peroxidation of cellular membranes; and vitamin A reacts with peroxyl, hydroxyl, and superoxide radicals [53, 54].

2.1.1 Antioxidant vitamins: Vitamin A: Astrocaryum vulgare Mart. (Arecaceae)

Vitamin A is the collective name of a group of fat-soluble organic compounds which are essential for humans (and other vertebrates) and comprise vitamin A alcohols (retinols), vitamin A aldehydes (retinals), retinyl acids (retinoic acids), and retinyl esters [55, 56]. All-*trans*-retinol is the primary homeostatically regulated vitamin A species in the body, all-*trans*-retinal and 11-*cis*-retinal are vitamin A derivatives involved in photoperception, and retinyl esters like retinyl palmitate are the storage form of vitamin A in mainly the liver [55, 56]. Preformed vitamins A are provided by consuming animal products such as meat, fish, poultry, and dairy foods, either as retinol or bound to a fatty acid to become a retinyl ester [57]. The body can also synthesize the preformed vitamins A from provitamin A carotenoids including carotenes such as α- and β-carotene and the xanthophyll β-cryptoxanthin [58]. This mainly occurs in the mucosa of the terminal small intestine using the enzyme β-carotene 15-15′-oxygenase [58]. Conversely, non-provitamin A carotenoids such as the carotene lycopene and the xanthophylls lutein and zeaxanthin cannot be converted into retinol and other preformed vitamins A [55, 56]. Carotenoids are bright yellow-, red-, or orange-colored and are found in, among others, mango, grapefruit, watermelon, papaya, tomato, tangerine, and guava, as well as carrot and yellow corn [57]. The recommended dietary allowance for men and women is 900 and 700 μg retinol activity equivalents, respectively, per day [59].

Vitamins A are involved, among others, in cell growth and fetal development; male and female reproductive health; the condition of surface tissues such as skin, intestines, lungs, bladder, and inner ear; the growth and distribution of T cells and in this way, immune function; and the health of cornea and conjunctiva as well as the capacity of both low-light vision and color vision [55, 56]. These functions and most of vitamins A's biological effects are carried out following its binding to and activation of the nuclear retinoic acid receptors RARα, RARβ, and RARγ [60]. Chronic shortages of vitamins A and/or carotenoids in the diet result in vitamin A deficiency that typically manifests as night blindness and dry skin, and if prolonged and severe, can even lead to total and irreversible blindness [56].

Vitamins A may also help protect the body from oxidative stress. This is supported by the results from *in vitro* studies indicating that retinoic acid inhibited the activity of thioredoxin-interacting protein [61], an enyme known to bind to and inhibit the activity of ubiquitous cytosolic and mitochondrial antioxidant oxidase-reductase enzymes called thioredoxins [62]. Furthermore, retinoic acid upregulated the expression of antioxidant-related genes [63] and increased superoxide dismutase and glutathione transferase activities while decreasing those of malondialdehyde and ROS [64].

Experimental data on the antioxidant properties of carotenoids—both carotenes and xanthophylls—are more compelling [65, 66], showing that these compounds efficiently quenched singlet molecular oxygen and potently scavenged other ROS such as peroxyl radicals [67–71]. Not surprisingly, diets high in carotenoids have been associated with a lower risk of, among others, heart disease, lung cancer, and diabetes mellitus [72–74]. However, it should be taken into account that the elimination of ROS by carotenoids may be accompanied by the formation of several potentially harmful pro-oxidant carotenoid radical derivatives [75]. For instance, carotenoid radical cations may oxidize the tyrosine and cysteine moieties of cellular proteins, damaging their structure and impairing their function [76].

A well-known source of vitamin A in Suriname is the fruit of the tucuma or awara *Astrocaryum vulgare* Mart. (Arecaceae). *A. vulgare* is a multi-stemmed, spiny, evergreen, feather palm that can be found in the forested parts, savannas, and lowlands of the country but is also cultivated for its edible fruit that is produced in clusters on the tree. *A. vulgare* grows in a small bunch of unbranched stems of 10–20 cm in diameter which can reach a height of 4–10 m and are covered with black spines of about 2 cm long. The fruit is globose to ovoid, 35–45 mm long and 25–35 mm wide, and consists of a fleshy orange-red, fatty mesocarp (pulp) that covers a single large seed (**Figure 1**). The mesocarp is slightly sweet and has a flavor reminiscent of apricots and is very nutritious, containing a relatively high concentration of carotenoids with a very high concentration of β-carotene (about 52 mg per 100 g), in addition to appreciable amounts of vitamin E, vitamin B_2 (riboflavin), as well as carbohydrates, proteins, and saturated fatty acids (such as oleic acid and palmitic acid), and polyunsaturated fatty acids (such as omega-3, omega-6, and omega-9 fatty acids) [77, 78].

A. vulgare fruit is eaten raw, prepared into juices, and used as an indispensable ingredient of the very popular French Guianan dish "*bouillon d'awara*" that is traditionally eaten during Easter. Cold-pressing of the mesocarp gives tucuma oil, and cold-pressing of the hard, white endosperm from the rigid, black seed gives tucuma butter that has an unusually high concentration of the fatty acid lauric acid in addition to myristic acid and oleic acid [79, 80]. Both tucuma oil and tucuma butter are edible and suitable for cooking and also for preparing nourishing and moisturizing beauty products, anti-aging creams, soaps, body lotions, and products for damaged hair [80, 81]. And the immature endosperm gives a juice called *vino de tucuma* that is used for preparing tasty beverages and culinary delicacies.

Preparations from the mesocarp of *A. vulgare* fruit are traditionally used to replenish vitamin A deficiency in individuals suffering from xerophthalmia, to calm colicky babies, and to treat coughs and as a breath freshener [78, 82]. The seed oil is used as a laxative, for treating rheumatism, pain, earache, as a topical diaphoretic to stimulate perspiration in patients with fever, and as an ingredient of treatments of furuncles [78, 82]. In Suriname's traditional medicine, preparations from several parts of the fruit are used for skin care, to repair damaged hair, against coughing, as an ingredient of dressings for open wounds and fractured bones, against fleas and lice, for treating impotence, and to prevent miscarriage and increase fertility [43, 49].

Some of these uses may be related to the antioxidant activities of the constituents of *A. vulgare* mesocarp including β-carotene. This could be derived from the anti-inflammatory properties of the pulp oil in both acute and chronic *in vivo* models of inflammation which could be localized to an unsaponifiable fraction [83, 84] that displayed antioxidant effects in cultured J774 macrophages activated by lipopolysaccharide plus interferon-γ, as well as an animal model of endotoxic shock resulting from the systemic release of inflammatory mediators [83, 84]. However, this fraction contained not only carotenoids but also phytosterols as well as vitamin E derivatives [83–85] which have been shown to be partly responsible for the biological properties

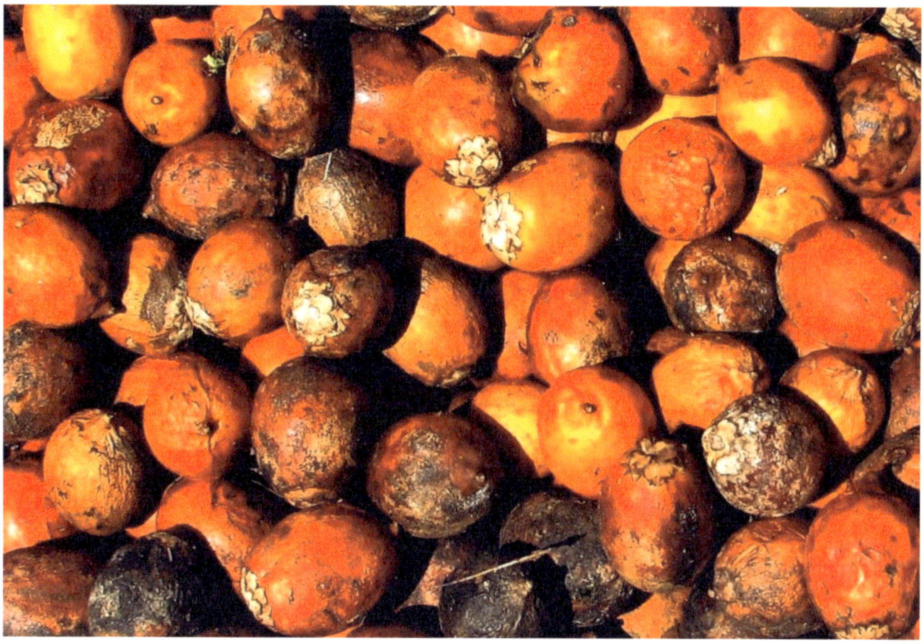

Figure 1.
Fruits of the tucumã Astrocaryum vulgare Mart. (Arecaceae) (from: https://images.app.goo.gl/ohwh8G8BwHZBiUk8A).

of vegetable oils [86]. This suggests that the beneficial effects and traditional uses of *A. vulgare* should be credited to its contents of other antioxidant compounds in addition to provitamins A and/or vitamins A.

2.1.2 Antioxidant vitamins: vitamin C: Malpighia glabra L. (Malpighiaceae)

Ascorbic acid, more precisely, L-ascorbic acid, also known as vitamin C, is a water-soluble vitamin that is essential for: the formation and repair of collagen required for, among others, skin, tendons, ligaments, and blood vessels; the healing of wounds and the formation of scar tissue; the repair and maintenance of cartilage, bones, and teeth; carnitine and catecholamine metabolism; the maintenance of a healthy immune system; and the resorption of dietary iron into the body [87, 88]. As a result, vitamin C deficiency leads to impaired collagen synthesis, scurvy, impaired healing of wounds and fractured bones, bleeding gums, achy joints, tiredness, an increased susceptibility to viral infections, skin issues, an increased risk of soft tissue infections with potentially lethal complications, and a decline of general health [87, 88].

Humans as well as primates and a few other animals such as guinea pigs lack the ability to synthesize vitamin C due to the absence of L-gulono-1,4-lactone oxidase, the enzyme that catalyzes the conversion of L-gulonolactone into vitamin C [89]. For this reason, humans depend on the regular intake of vitamin C through the diet in sufficient amounts to prevent the above-mentioned diseases [90]. This is readily achieved by consuming fruits that contain relatively high levels of vitamin C such as strawberries, citrus fruits, watermelon, berries, pineapple, kiwi fruits, mangoes, and tomatoes as well as cherries [91, 92].

Many of the health-promoting effects of vitamin C have been attributed—directly or indirectly—to its notable antioxidant activity. This held true for, for instance, its strong anti-inflammatory and antihistaminic activity and its ability to inhibit several types of inflammatory mediators such as tumor necrosis factor-α [93]; its inhibitory effects on signaling for lipopolysaccharide formation and ROS production during infection [94]; its anti-aging effect due to the stimulation of collagen formation and the protection of particularly elastin from ROS-mediated damage [95]; and its cytotoxicity (in mega-doses) against cancer [96, 97], and perhaps also against diabetes mellitus, cardiovascular ailments, metabolic syndrome, and ocular diseases [98–101]. All these beneficial effects have been associated with vitamin C's capacity to generate cytotoxic ascorbyl radicals which do not harm normal cells [102], its antibacterial effects due to its ability to neutralize bacterial endotoxins [102] and impede bacterial replication [103]; and its immune-stimulatory properties by promoting the phagocytic properties of neutrophils and macrophages, the production and titer of antibodies, and the activity of lymphocytes [104].

Vitamin C elicits its antioxidant effects by acting as a reducing agent, donating an electron to potentially harmful ROS such as hydroxyl radical, hydrogen peroxide, and singlet oxygen, and scavenging these species and preventing them from inflicting oxidative damage to lipids and other macromolecules [105, 106]. At the same time, vitamin C is oxidized to a relatively stable, unreactive ascorbyl-free radical (semi-dehydrovitamin C) with a lifetime of 10–15 s [107, 108]. In a subsequent electron-donating reaction, semi-dehydroascorbic acid is transformed into a dehydroascorbic acid that is also relatively stable and lasts for a few minutes [87, 107, 108]. These properties of the vitamin C metabolites render them harmless to surrounding cells [87, 107, 108]. Apart from eliminating ROS, vitamin C protects cells from oxidative stress-induced damage by vitamin E-dependent neutralization of lipid hydroperoxyl radicals in a one-electron reduction reaction via the vitamin E redox cycle, regenerating the antioxidant form of vitamin E (α-tocopherol) by reducing tocopheroxyl radicals [109, 110]. However, there are reports mentioning that vitamin C can also act as a pro-oxidant at relatively low doses [111].

The acerola, also known as Barbados cherry and West Indian cherry (or West-Indische kers in Suriname), with the scientific names *M. glabra* L., *Malpighia punicifolia* L., and *Malpighia emarginata* DC. (Malpighiaceae), is a small tree with spreading, somewhat drooping branches on a short trunk that usually grows to a height of 2–3 m. It is indigenous to the area ranging from Central America and Mexico to the Caribbean and the northern parts of South America including Suriname. *M. glabra* fruit is ovoid, bright red-colored, sweet- to somewhat acid-tasting, has a diameter of 10–35 mm (**Figure 2**), and can be eaten raw, cooked, stewed, and made into juices, sauces, jellies, jams, wines, or purees. Because the fruit rapidly deteriorates, it is immediately after harvesting processed into pulp and clarified juice which are frozen and stored for later use. The global market for these products is enormous and is estimated to reach USD 17.5 billion by 2026, with Brazil as the major producer and exporter [112].

M. glabra fruit is also traditionally used against flu, colds, sore throat, coughing, and hay fever; to prevent scurvy and treat gum infections as well as tooth decay; to avert heart disease and treat atherosclerosis and blood clots; against various types of wounds ranging from pimples to pressure sores; for remedying gastrointestinal problems; as an antidepressant; and for treating cancer [49, 113]. *M. glabra* fruit has been used to produce vitamin C concentrates, dietary supplements, and in the enrichment of other processed health products [114]. Pharmacological studies with preparations

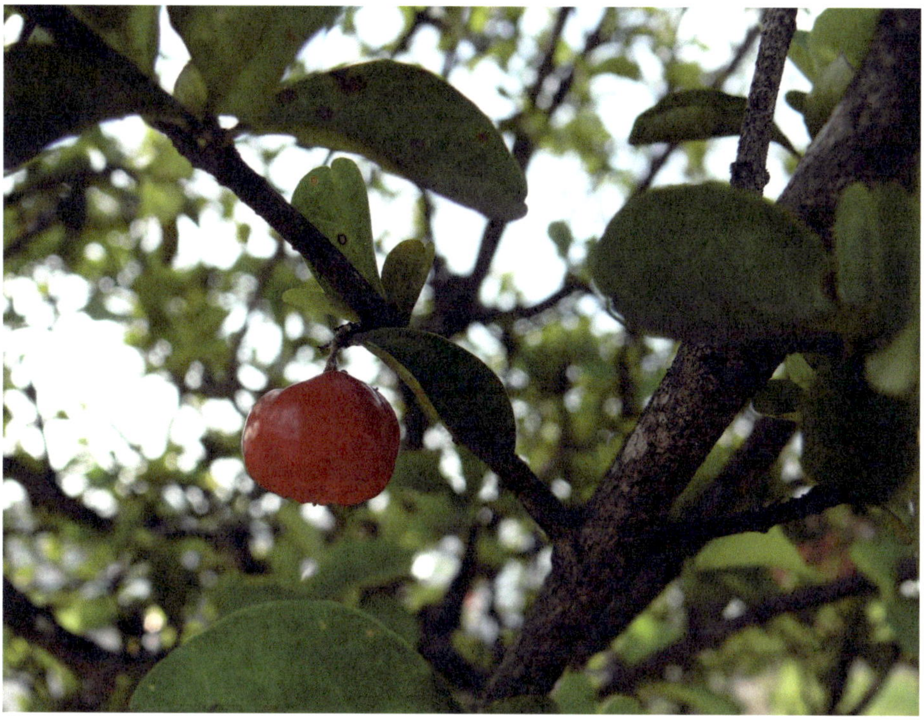

Figure 2.
Fruit of the acerola Malpighia glabra L. (Malpighiaceae) (from: https://images.app.goo.gl/SXvp1ifwFFRWLm TU7).

from *M. glabra* fruit extracts showed, among others, anti-inflammatory, antihyperglycemic, antitumor, antigenotoxic, and hepatoprotective activity [115–118].

The beneficial health effects of *M. glabra* fruit have been associated with its powerful antioxidant effects in several *in vitro* assays [119–121] which, in their turn, have been attributed to its abundant amount of vitamin C as well as phenolic compounds (including benzoic acid derivatives, phenylpropanoid derivatives, flavonoids, and anthocyanins) and carotenoids [114, 122–125]. Notably, the vitamin C content of *M. glabra* fruit is 1000–4500 mg per 100 g, which is 50–100 times that of an orange or a lemon [125]. When considering that the recommended dietary allowances of vitamin C are 75 mg/day for women and 90 mg/day for men [126], the consumption of three *M. glabra* fruits per day would satisfy the required daily vitamin C intake for an adult [127].

Several investigators also reported that *M. glabra* fruit extracts displayed a relatively high total phenolic content and *in vitro* antioxidant activity which correlated well with each other [114, 125, 128–130]. Thus, the remarkable antioxidant activity of *M. glabra* fruit is most probably not only attributable to its relatively high content of vitamin C but also to phenolic phytonutrients with antioxidant activity which may act synergistically with vitamin C [123]. Indeed, the contribution of vitamin C to the hydrophilic antioxidant activity in *M. glabra* fruit, commercial pulps, and juices ranged from 40 to 83%, while the remaining activity was due to phenolic compounds, mainly phenolic acids [123]. And the antioxidant activity of *M. glabra* fruit juices depended on the synergistic action of the constituents of different fractions, with most significant components being phenolic compounds and vitamin C [122].

2.1.3 Antioxidant vitamins: vitamin E: *Hibiscus sabdariffa* L. (Malvaceae)

In its broadest sense, vitamin E is a collective term of a group of lipid-soluble compounds called tocochromanols which are present in fat-containing foods [131]. Vitamins E can be divided into tocopherols and tocotrienols, which in their turn, can be subdivided into eight naturally occurring forms, namely the α, β, γ, and δ classes of tocopherol and tocotrienol [131, 132]. All these derivatives are synthesized by plants from the phenolic acid homogentisic acid [131]. The major form of vitamin E used by the human body is α-tocopherol [132]. The richest dietary sources of α-tocopherol are nuts and seeds such as dry roasted peanuts, almonds, and hazelnuts (2.2–6.8 mg per serving); green leafy vegetables such as spinach (0.6 mg per serving); fruits such as mango, tomato, and kiwi (0.7–1.1 mg per serving); as well as edible vegetable oils such as sunflower oil and wheat germ oil (5.6–20.3 mg per serving) [133]. The recommended dietary allowance for α-tocopherol for individuals aged 14 years and older including pregnant women is 15 mg per day [134]. Breast feeding women need slightly more of this compound, namely 19 mg or 28 IU daily [134].

α-Tocopherol is involved in various important functions in the body, including maintaining the proper organization of and repairing damage to cellular membranes [135–137]; the inhibition of platelet aggregation by promoting the release of prostacyclin from the endothelium, decreasing the adhesion of blood cell components to the endothelium [138], stimulating phospholipase A2 and cyclooxygenase-1 activities and the subsequent release of prostacyclin [139]; and inhibiting nitric oxide synthase activation [140].

These properties of α-tocopherol are for an important part attributable to its potent activity against ROS-mediated lipid peroxidation [141]. Indeed, α-tocopherol appeared to be a powerful chain-breaking antioxidant that inhibits the production of ROS when lipids undergo oxidation and during the propagation of free radical reactions [142]. Not surprisingly, it is primarily located in cellular membranes (such as the membranes of the mitochondria and endoplasmic reticulum in heart and lungs) where it acts as the first line of defense against lipid peroxidation [141]. Due to its peroxyl radical-scavenging activity, α-tocopherol also protects the polyunsaturated fatty acids in membrane phospholipids and plasma lipoproteins [143]. As a result, α-tocopherol has been associated with the prevention of, among others, neurological disorders, cardiovascular diseases, cancer, aging, arthritis, age-related eye and skin damage, and infertility [144, 145]. Because it is able to inhibit air oxidation, it is also used to fortify and extend the lifetime of foods, oils, and industrial materials [146].

The roselle or syuru *H. sabdariffa* L. (Malvaceae) is an erect, branched, annual to perennial plant with a woody stem that grows to an average height of 2–2.5 m. It probably originates from India and the adjoining regions and has been introduced into Africa, from where enslaved Africans have brought it to the new World including Suriname [147]. *H. sabdariffa* is now cultivated in many tropical countries, mostly for its conspicuously crimson red-colored fleshy calyces (**Figure 3**), which develop from white to pale yellow flowers, each petal of which has a dark red spot at the base. The dried calyces taste like cranberry and are used to prepare a variety of teas, jams, sauces, and even beer [41, 45, 46].

The calyx contains a number of constituents with known antioxidant activity, including phenolic acids, a number of anthocyanins, β-carotene, ascorbic acid, as well as α-tocopherol and other tocopherols [148–151]. Due to this favorable

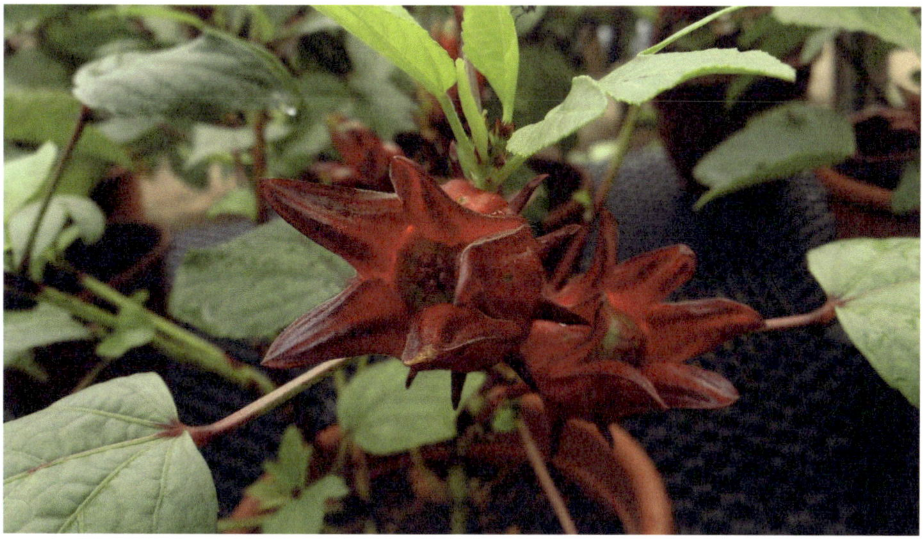

Figure 3.
Calyx of the roselle Hibiscus sabdariffa L. (Malvaceae) (from: https://images.app.goo.gl/5M5iBiBb4nHwcTFk6).

phytochemical composition, extracts from *H. sabdariffa* calyx have been included in skin care products, skin-protecting agents, anti-aging creams, and hair care products [152]. Furthermore, a polysaccharide-enriched crude extract from *H. sabdariffa* flower potently stimulated the proliferation of cultured keratinocytes [153], which may explain the addition of these preparations to *H. sabdariffa* skin care products. As well, a water in oil cream of the methanol extract of the calyces has been prepared as a potential commercial wound healing substance [154, 155]. Preparations from *H. sabdariffa* calyx are also traditionally used in various countries including Suriname, for treating a broad range of conditions such as microbial infections, cough and bronchitis, kidney problems, various gastrointestinal conditions, and hypertension [49, 151, 156, 157].

It is likely that some of these uses can be attributed to the antioxidant activity of *H. sabdariffa* calyx [158, 159]. For instance, the antioxidant activity of calyx preparations has been held responsible for their efficacy against bacterial infections [149, 151, 158, 160]. And the regular use of *H. sabdariffa* calyx preparations would decrease the oxidative stress involved in the development of atherosclerosis, lipid disorders, and hypertension [161]. Indeed, aqueous and alcoholic extracts of the (dried) calyx elicited appreciable antioxidant activities in various *in vitro* assays [158, 159, 162, 163]. However, the antioxidant activity has not only been associated with α-tocopherol [163] but also with various types of phenolic compounds such as anthocyanins [163–165] and phenolic acids such as protocatechuic acid [160]. Thus, as may hold true for *A. vulgare* and *M. glabra* fruit, the benefical effcts of *H. sabdariffa* calyx preparations also seem attributable to multiple bioactive phytochemicals rather than only one compound, in the present case, vitamin E.

2.2 Antioxidant minerals

Minerals are inorganic substances that are present in all body tissues and fluids, and although not yielding energy, are necessary for the maintenance and the progression of many physicochemical processes which are essential to life [166–168]. They can be classified into macroelements, microelements, and trace elements [166–168]. The macroelements comprise elements which are abundantly found in nature and which the body needs in relatively large amounts (in excess of 100 mg/dL), and they include hydrogen, oxygen, carbon, nitrogen, calcium, and phosphorus [166–168]. These compounds comprise together about 99% of the body mass, are present in most tissues and organs, represent the most important constituents of DNA, enzymes, cellular membranes, as well as inter- and intracellular liquids, and are essential for almost all metabolic processes [166–168]. Microelements are required in the body in relatively modest amounts (less than 100 mg/dL), only comprise 0.85% of the body mass, and include potassium, sulfur, sodium, chlorine, and magnesium [166–168]. They fulfill more or less the same functions as the macroelements but are required in smaller amounts [166–168].

Trace elements are present in the body at concentrations of much less than 0.1% and are required in parts per million [166–168]. Nevertheless, in these minute amounts, they are vital for proper growth and development and are therefore also referred to as essential minerals [166–168]. They include, among others, iron, copper, zinc, molybdenum, manganese, chromium, cobalt, cadmium, and selenium [166–168]. Iron, copper, zinc, manganese, and selenium are indirectly involved in the body's antioxidant defenses by enhancing the activities of antioxidant enzymes (see, for instance, reference [169]). And copper, zinc, and manganese are cofactors of superoxide dismutase [170]. Similarly to vitamins, essential minerals must be acquired through the diet, and deficiencies may occur because of inadequate diets [166–168].

2.2.1 Antioxidant minerals: selenium: Bertholletia excelsa Humb. and Bonpl. (Lecythidaceae)

Selenium is a trace element that is essential for many functions in humans, particularly as part of innate antioxidant defense mechanisms [166–168]. It is present in soils as inorganic selenites and selenates which are accumulated and converted by plants into the amino acids selenocysteine and selenomethionine and their methylated derivatives [171, 172]. On the basis of the amount of selenium plants accumulate inside their cells, they can be classified as hyperaccumulators, secondary accumulators, and non-accumulators [173]. These groups of plants accumulate selenium at concentrations in excess of 1000 mg, 100–1000 mg, and less than 100 mg, respectively, per kilogram dry weight [173]. The precise functions of selenium in plants is still controversial, but at low doses it seems to protect plants from a variety of abiotic stresses such as cold, drought, desiccation, and metal stress [174].

Humans do not synthesize selenocysteine and selenomethionine *de novo* but obtain them from dietary sources such as the Brazil nut *Bertholletia excelsa* Humb. & Bonpl. (Lecythidaceae), grains, wheat, and corn used for bread and cereals, as well as poultry, eggs, animal meats, sea food, and dairy products [175, 176]. These amino acids are, in their turn, constituents of selenoproteins such as glutathione peroxidases, thyroid hormone deiodinases, and thioredoxin reductases, in which selelenium acts as the catalytic center (see, for instance, references [177, 178]). Skeletal muscle is the major site of selenium storage, accounting for approximately 28–46% of the total selenium pool in the body [179]. There are more than two dozen selenoproteins, and they play vital roles in reproduction, thyroid hormone metabolism, DNA synthesis, and protection from oxidative damage and infection [180].

The recommended dietary allowance for selenium for adult men and women is 55 μg daily [181]. The amount of selenium in soil and groundwater is a major determinant of the amount of selenium in plant-based foods (as well sources of foods from animals feeding on these plants [176, 182]). As a result, selenium concentrations in plant-based foods often vary widely by geographic location [183], which may lead to either deficiencies or toxicities. Severe selenium deficiency (7–11 μg/dL) may occur in areas with soils poor in selenium and can lead to a congestive cardiac myopathy called Keshan disease after Keshan County in north-eastern China where it was first described [184]; Kashin-Beck disease, a chronic, endemic osteochondropathy with joint necrosis that has mainly been seen in some Eastern parts of Eurasia [185]; and myxedematous endemic cretinism and mental retardation caused by thyroid atrophy that is highly prevalent in Central Africa [186]. On the other hand, excess selenium (>100μg/dL) may cause selenosis, manifesting as hair loss, white blotchy nails, a garlic breath, gastrointestinal disorders, fatigue, irritability, and neurological damage [187].

The selenium taken up in the body—in the form of organic selenium (as selenocysteine and selenomethionine) and inorganic selenium (in general as selenite and selenite)—is used for the biosynthesis of selenium-containing proteins [188–190]. As mentioned above, selenoproteins are crucial to, among others, reproduction, thyroid hormone metabolism, DNA synthesis, immune function, and the protection of cells from oxidative damage, inflammation, and cancer [169, 182, 191, 192]. Particularly the critical association of glutathione peroxidases with the innate antioxidant defense mechanisms has meticulously been investigated, and the involvement of these enzymes in the protection against oxidative stress has now been well established [178, 192, 193]. These cytosolic enzymes appeared to catalyze the reduction of hydrogen peroxide to water and oxygen and that of peroxide radicals to alcohols and oxygen, inhibiting DNA damage and the development of cancer [178, 192, 193]. Notably, the beneficial health effects of selenium (as part of selenoproteins) because of its notable antioxidant activity have been supported by the results from varous clinical studies with patients suffering from coronary heart disease [194], cancer [195], and cognitive disorders [196].

The Brazil nut (or paranoto in Surinamese) *B. excelsa* is native to the northern parts of South America and is one of the largest and longest-living trees in the Amazon rainforest, reaching ages of 500 years or more. It can achieve a height of 50 m and a trunk diameter of 1–2 m and has grayish and smooth bark. It produces small, greenish-white flowers in panicles which must be pollinated by specific bee genera in order to develop into fruits. *B. excelsa* fruit is rigid and heavy, weighing as much as 2 kg (**Figure 4**), and contains 8–24 wedge-shaped edible seeds of 4–5 cm long (the so-called "Brazil nuts") which are packed like the segments of an orange and are encapsulated by a woody shell of 8–12 mm thickness.

B. excelsa fruit is rich in dietary fiber, vitamins, and dietary minerals and has been a staple diet of the natives residing in the Amazon forest since the Upper Paleolithic era, 11,000 years ago [197]. It also has a long history of traditional use. For instance, a tea prepared of the seed husks would alleviate stomach aches and other gastrointestinal complaints, the oil from the seed is applied to burns, and a decoction of the stembark would cure liver disorders [48]. Currently, the seeds are commercially harvested from the wild for inclusion into mixed nuts and confections coated with chocolate [197]. The oil extracted from the seeds contains 75% unsaturated fatty acids mainly composed of oleic and linoleic acids, as well as phytosterols, several phenolic compounds such as gallic acid and ellagic acid, tocopherols, and selenium [198–200]. It is used in creams, lotions, conditioners, and hair care products, as well

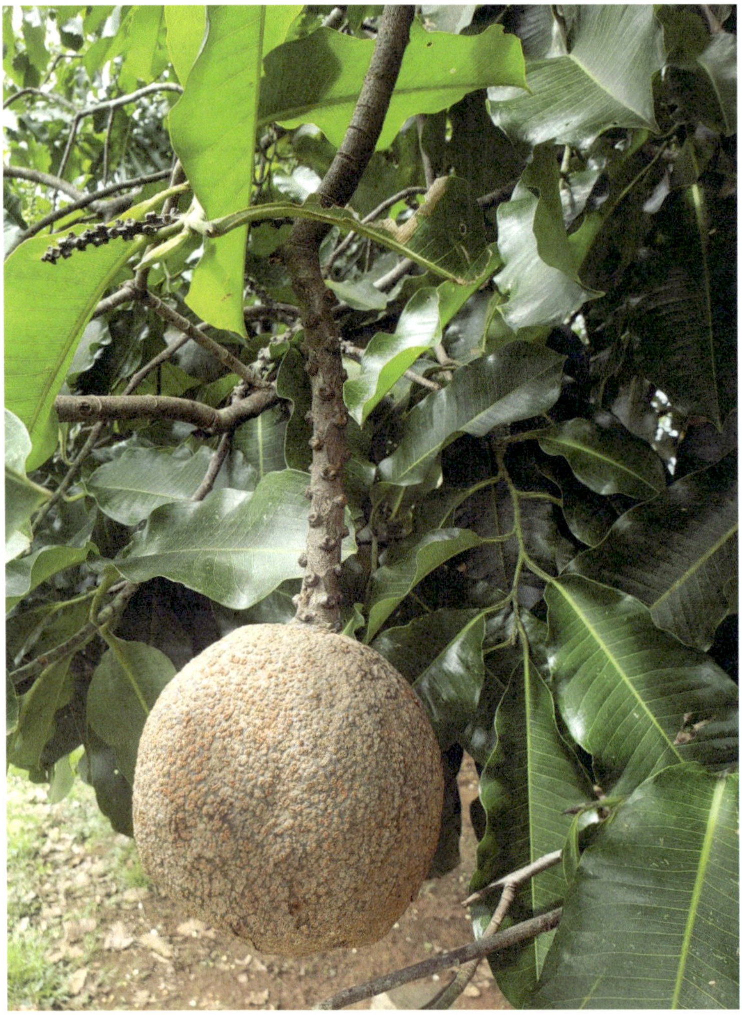

Figure 4.
Fruit of the Brazil nut Bertholletia excelsa Humb. & Bonpl. (Lecythidaceae) (from: https://images.app.goo.gl/Ju62ZypEttADRQVH8).

as formulations for alleviating dry, flaky skin, aging skin, acne, and skin inflammation. These applications may be supported by the moisturizing effects of the fatty acids [200, 201].

As a selenium hyperaccumulator [173], selenium levels of *B. excelsa* seed are remarkably high, with one nut of on average 5 g containing on average 96 μg selenium, i.e., more than the recommended dietary allowance of 55 μg daily [181]. In fact, despite considerable variations within batches of the amount of selenium [202], the Brazil nut is considered one of the richest natural sources of selenium [203]. Not surprisingly, many of the positive effects of *B. excelsa* fruit preparations have been attributed to its high selenium content and antioxiodant activity. Indeed, the consumption of *B. excelsa* fruit would improve antioxidant status in humans through increased levels of selenium and/or glutathione peroxidase activity in plasma, serum, whole blood, and/or erythrocytes [204] and would decrease the risk of overweight/obesity and various degenerative diseases such as cardiovascular, neoplastic, and cognitive disorders [205, 206]. However, several studies with the whole fruit of *B. excelsa*, parts of the fruit, and products derived from the fruit such as "Brazil nut milk," a cake fraction, and a fat fraction, showed appreciable antioxidant activity in various *in vitro* assays, as well as the presence of phenolic compounds, tocopherols, and a high level of selenium [200, 207]. Thus, when considering all the phytochemical constituents with antioxidant properties identified in *B. excelsa* seed [181, 198–200], its beneficial health effects may also be attributable to the combined effects of selenium, phenolic compounds, tocopherols, and unsaturated fatty acids.

3. Concluding remarks

Naturally occurring antioxidants in fruits and vegetables provided through the diet represent vital components of the exogenous defense mechanisms of the body to manage oxidative stress caused by ROS, minimizing the chances of developing, among others, inflammatory disorders, cancer, diabetes mellitus, cardiovascular diseases, and cognitive ailments. Important classes of such naturally occurring antioxidants are anthocyanins, ellagitannins, coumarins, (pro)vitamins A, C, and E, as well as selenium. In this chapter, seven well-known Surinamese fruits, each of which known to contain one of these compounds at appreciably high concentrations, have elaborately been dealt with. The fruits were those from the açai palm *E. oleracea*, the pomegranate *Punica granatum*, the tonka bean *D. odorata*, the tucumã *A. vulgare*, the acerola *M. glabra*, the roselle *H. sabdariffa*, and the Brazil nut *B. excelsa*, respectively. These fruits are widely consumed in Suriname and various other countries throughout the world, either raw or incorporated into dishes, or prepared into traditional medicines, food additives, nutraceuticals, or cosmeceuticals. Numerous pharmacological studies with a wide range of assays have provided support that these beneficial health effects are associated with the powerful antioxiodant activities of one or more of the phytochemical classes mentioned above.

However, many studies have also suggested that the antioxidant activities of the fruits must probably be attributed to the combined effects of several classes of biologically active compounds rather than to one specific phytochemical. For instance, the antioxidant activity of *A. vulgare* mesocarp [83, 84] may be partly ascribed to phytosterols and vitamin E derivatives in addition to its high content of carotenoids [83, 84]. And those of *B. excelsa* seed preparations [204–206] might be due to the combined actions of selenium with phenolic compounds, tocopherols, and unsaturated fatty acids [181, 198–200]. And as mentioned in part 1 of this chapter, the antioxidant activities of products from the fruit pulp of the açai or podosiri *Euterpe oleracea* Mart. (Arecaceae) [208, 209] is presumably not only due to its high content of mainly the anthocyanin cyanidin-3-glucoside, but also to other phenolic compounds, vitamins, and/or fatty acids [208, 210–212].

These considerations indicate the need to more precisely identify the pharmacologically active phytochemicals, particularly those with antioxidant activity, in raw natural products, traditional medicines, and commercial plant-based products with purported health benefical properties. This is the more important in the case of substances containing chemically instable ingredients such as anthocyanins [209, 213–218], and those that may generate pro-oxidant radical species such as carotenoids [75, 76] or display pro-oxidant properties at, for instance, relatively low concentration such as vitamin C [111].

Author details

Dennis R.A. Mans
Faculty of Medical Sciences, Department of Pharmacology, Anton de Kom University of Suriname, Paramaribo, Suriname

Address all correspondence to: dennismans16@gmail.com;
dennis_mans@yahoo.com

References

[1] Canfield DE, Rosing MT, Bjerrum C. Early anaerobic metabolisms. Philosophical Transactions of the Royal Society B: Biological Sciences. 2006;**361**:1819-1834; discussion 1835-1836. DOI: 10.1098/rstb.2006.1906

[2] Martin WF, Sousa FL. Early microbial evolution: The age of anaerobes. Cold Spring Harbor Perspectives in Biology. 2015;**8**:a018127. DOI: 10.1101/cshperspect.a018127

[3] Birben E, Sahiner UM, Sackesen C, Erzurum S, Kalayci O. Oxidative stress and antioxidant defense. World Allergy Organization Journal. 2012;**5**:9-19. DOI: 10.1097/WOX.0b013e3182439613

[4] Noori S. An overview of oxidative stress and antioxidant defensive system. Open Access Scientific Reports. 2012;**1**:413. DOI: 10.4172/scientificreports

[5] Kumar V, Abdussalam A. A review on reactive oxygen and nitrogen species. Era's Journal of Medical Research. 2017;**4**:1-5

[6] Checa J, Aran JM. Reactive oxygen species: Drivers of physiological and pathological processes. Journal of Inflammation Research. 2020;**13**:1057-1073. DOI: 10.2147/JIR.S275595

[7] Juan CA, Pérez de la Lastra JM, Plou FJ, Pérez-Lebeña E. The chemistry of reactive oxygen species (ROS) revisited: Outlining their role in biological macromolecules (DNA, lipids and proteins) and induced pathologies. International Journal of Molecular Sciences. 2021;**22**:4642. DOI: 10.3390/ijms22094642

[8] Pham-Huy LA, He H, Pham-Huy C. Free radicals, antioxidants in disease and health. International Journal of Biomedical Sciences. 2008;**4**:89-96

[9] Schieber M, Chandel NS. ROS function in redox signaling and oxidative stress. Current Biology. 2014;**24**:R453-R462. DOI: 10.1016/j.cub.2014.03.034

[10] Bardaweel SK, Gul M, Alzweiri M, Ishaqat A, Salamat HA, Bashatwah RM. Reactive oxygen species: The dual role in physiological and pathological conditions of the human body. Eurasian Journal of Medicine. 2018;**50**:193-201

[11] Turrens JF. Mitochondrial formation of reactive oxygen species. Journal of Physiology. 2003;**552**(Pt 2):335-344. DOI: 10.1113/jphysiol.2003.049478

[12] Fransen M, Nordgren M, Wang B, Apanasets O. Role of peroxisomes in ROS/RNS-metabolism: Implications for human disease. Biochimica et Biophysica Acta. 2012;**1822**:1363-1373. DOI: 10.1016/j.bbadis.2011.12.001

[13] Zeeshan HM, Lee GH, Kim HR, Chae HJ. Endoplasmic reticulum stress and associated ROS. International Journal of Molecular Sciences. 2016;**17**:327. DOI: 10.3390/ijms17030327

[14] Li R, Jia Z, Trush MA. Defining ROS in biology and medicine. Reactive Oxygen Species (Apex). 2016;**1**:9-21. DOI: 10.20455/ros.2016.803

[15] Sies H, Jones DP. Reactive oxygen species (ROS) as pleiotropic physiological signalling agents. Nature Reviews: Molecular Cell Biology. 2020;**21**:363-383. DOI: 10.1038/s41580-020-0230-3

[16] Spitz DR, Azzam EI, Li JJ, Gius D. Metabolic oxidation/reduction reactions and cellular responses to ionizing radiation: A unifying concept in stress response biology. Cancer Metastasis

Reviews. 2004;**23**:311-322. DOI: 10.1023/B:CANC.0000031769.14728.bc

[17] Kong CY, Guo Z, Song P, Zhang X, Yuan YP, Teng T, et al. Underlying the mechanisms of doxorubicin-induced acute cardiotoxicity: Oxidative stress and cell death. International Journal of Biological Sciences. 2022;**18**:760-770. DOI: 10.7150/ijbs.65258

[18] Klaunig JE, Kamendulis LM. The role of oxidative stress in carcinogenesis. Annual Review of Pharmacology and Toxicology. 2004;**44**:239-267. DOI: 10.1146/annurev.pharmtox.44.101802.121851

[19] Markesbery WR, Lovell MA. DNA oxidation in Alzheimer's disease. Antioxidants and Redox Signaling. 2006;**8**:2039-2045. DOI: 10.1089/ars.2006.8.2039

[20] Elahi MM, Kong YX, Matata BM. Oxidative stress as a mediator of cardiovascular disease. Oxidative Medicine and Cellular Longevity. 2009;**2**:259-269. DOI: 10.4161/oxim.2.5.9441

[21] Cui H, Kong Y, Zhang H. Oxidative stress, mitochondrial dysfunction, and aging. Journal of Signal Transduction. 2012;**2012**:646354. DOI: 10.1155/2012/646354

[22] Shirley R, Ord EN, Work LM. Oxidative stress and the use of antioxidants in stroke. Antioxidants (Basel). 2014;**3**:472-501. DOI: 10.3390/antiox3030472

[23] Asmat U, Abad K, Ismail K. Diabetes mellitus and oxidative stress—A concise review. Saudi Pharmaceutical Journal. 2016;**24**:547-553. DOI: 10.1016/j.jsps.2015.03.013

[24] Soomro S. Oxidative stress and inflammation. Open Journal of Immunology. 2019;**9**:1-20. DOI: 10.4236/oji.2019.91001

[25] Rhee SG. Cell signaling. H_2O_2, a necessary evil for cell signaling. Science. 2006;**312**:1882-1883. DOI: 10.1126/science.1130481

[26] Zhao RZ, Jiang S, Zhang L, Yu ZB. Mitochondrial electron transport chain, ROS generation and uncoupling (review). International Journal of Molecular Medicine. 2019;**44**:3-15. DOI: 10.3892/ijmm.2019.4188

[27] Banerjee S, Ghosh J, Sil PC. Drug metabolism and oxidative stress: Cellular mechanism and new therapeutic insights. Biochemistry and Analytical Biochemistry. 2016;**5**:255. DOI: 10.4172/2161-1009.1000255

[28] Thomas DC. The phagocyte respiratory burst: Historical perspectives and recent advances. Immunology Letters. 2017;**192**:88-96. DOI: 10.1016/j.imlet.2017.08.016

[29] Ighodaro OM, Akinloye OA. First line defence antioxidants-superoxide dismutase (SOD), catalase (CAT) and glutathione peroxidase (GPX): Their fundamental role in the entire antioxidant defence grid. Alexandria Journal of Medicine. 2018;**54**:287-293. DOI: 10.1016/j.ajme.2017.09.001

[30] Mirończuk-Chodakowska I, Witkowska AM, Zujko ME. Endogenous non-enzymatic antioxidants in the human body. Advances in Medical Sciences. 2018;**63**:68-78. DOI: 10.1016/j.advms.2017.05.005

[31] Lobo V, Patil A, Phatak A, Chandra N. Free radicals, antioxidants and functional foods: Impact on human health. Pharmacognosy Reviews.

2010;**4**:118-126. DOI: 10.4103/0973-7847.70902

[32] Balsano C, Alisi A. Antioxidant effects of natural bioactive compounds. Current Pharmaceutical Design. 2009;**15**:3063-3073. DOI: 10.2174/138161209789058084

[33] Briggs MA. From foods to chemotherapeutics: The antioxidant potential of dietary phytochemicals. PRO. 2022;**10**:1222. DOI: 10.3390/pr10061222

[34] Miguel-Chávez R. Phenolic antioxidant capacity: A review of the state of the art. In: Soto-Hernandez M, Palma-Tenango M, Garcia-Mateos M, editors. Phenolic Compounds: Biological Activity. London: IntechOpen; 2017. pp. 59-74. DOI: 10.5772/66897

[35] Caleja C, Ribeiro A, Barreiro MF, Ferreira ICFR. Phenolic compounds as nutraceuticals or functional food ingredients. Current Pharmaceutical Design. 2017;**23**:2787-2806. DOI: 10.2174/1381612822666161227153906

[36] Aune D, Keum N, Giovannucci E, Fadnes LT, Boffetta P, Greenwood DC, et al. Dietary intake and blood concentrations of antioxidants and the risk of cardiovascular disease, total cancer, and all-cause mortality: A systematic review and dose-response meta-analysis of prospective studies. American Journal of Clinical Nutrition. 2018;**108**:1069-1091. DOI: 10.1093/ajcn/nqy097

[37] Jayedi A, Rashidy-Pour A, Parohan M, Zargar MS, Shab-Bidar S. Dietary antioxidants, circulating antioxidant concentrations, total antioxidant capacity, and risk of all-cause mortality: A systematic review and dose-response meta-analysis of prospective observational studies. Advances in Nutrition. 2018;**9**:701-716. DOI: 10.1093/advances/nmy040

[38] Ministry of Agriculture, Animal Husbandry and Fisheries. Beplante Arealen, Productie en Export van Groenten (Cultivated Areas, Production, and export of Vegetables). Unpublished manuscript; 2015

[39] Mans DRA, Grant A. "A thing of beauty is a joy forever". Plants and plant-based preparations for facial care in Suriname. Clinical and Medical Investigations. 2017;**2**:1-16. DOI: 10.15761/CMI.1000143

[40] Stephen HJM. Geneeskruiden Van Suriname: Hun Toepassing in de Volksgeneeskunde en in de Magie (Herbal Medicines from Suriname: Their Applications in Folk Medicine and Wizardry). Amsterdam: De Driehoek; 1979

[41] May AF. Sranan Oso Dresi. Surinaams Kruidenboek (Surinamese Folk Medicine. A Collection of Surinamese Medicinal Herbs). Paramaribo: De Walburg Pers; 1982

[42] Titjari. Famiri-Encyclopedia foe da Natoera Dresi-Fasi. Gezinskruidenboek van de Natuurgeneeswijzen. Natuurgeneeswijzen uit het Zonnige Suriname (Encyclopedia of Plant-Based Forms of Treatment. Folk Medicines from Sunny Suriname). Amsterdam: Sangrafoe; 1985

[43] Heyde H. Surinaamse Medicijnplanten (Surinamese Medicinal Plants). 2nd ed. Paramaribo: Westfort; 1987

[44] Tjong AG. Het Gebruik van Medicinale Planten Door de Javanen in Suriname (The Use of Medicinal Plants by the Javanese in Suriname).

Paramaribo: Instituut voor de Opleiding van Leraren; 1989

[45] Slagveer JL. Surinaams Groot Kruidenboek: Sranan Oso Dresie (A Surinamese Herbal: Surinamese Traditional Medicines). Paramaribo: De West; 1990

[46] Sedoc NO. Afrosurinaamse Natuurgeneeswijzen: Bevattende meer dan Tweehonderd Meest Gebruikelijke Geneeskrachtige Kruiden (Afro-Surinamese Natural Remedies: Over Two hundred Commonly Used Medicinal Herbs). Paramaribo: Vaco Press; 1992

[47] Raghoenandan UPD. Een Ethnobotanisch Onderzoek onder de Hindustanen in Suriname (An Ethnobotanical Survey among Hindustanis in Suriname). Paramaribo: Anton de Kom Universiteit van Suriname; 1994

[48] DeFilipps RA, Maina SL, Crepin J. Medicinal Plants of the Guianas (Guyana, Surinam, French Guiana). Washington, DC: Smithsonian Institution; 2004

[49] Van Andel TR, Ruysschaert S. Medicinale en Rituele Planten van Suriname (Medicinal and Ritual Plants of Suriname). Amsterdam: KIT Publishers; 2011

[50] Akram M, Munir N, Daniyal M, Egbuna C, Găman M-A, Onyekere PF, et al. Vitamins and minerals: Types, sources and their functions. In: Egbuna C, Dable Tupas G, editors. Functional Foods and Nutraceuticals. Cham: Springer; 2020. pp. 149-172. DOI: 10.1007/978-3-030-42319-3_9

[51] Ravisankar P, Reddy AA, Nagalakshmi B, Koushik OS, Kumar BV, Anvith PS. The comprehensive review on fat soluble vitamins. IOSR Journal of Pharmacy. 2015;**5**:12-28

[52] Said HM. Water-soluble vitamins. World Review of Nutrition and Dietetics. 2015;**111**:30-37. DOI: 10.1159/000362294

[53] Abba Y, Hassim HA, Hamzah H, Noordin MM. Antioxidant vitamins, oxidant injuries and diseases. Pertanika Journal of Scholarly Research Reviews. 2015;**1**:58-66

[54] Sinbad OO, Folorunsho AA, Olabisi OL, Ayoola OA, Temitope RJ. Vitamins as antioxidants. Journal of Food Science and Nutrition Research. 2019;**2**:214-235. DOI: 10.26502/jfsnr.2642-11000021

[55] Edem DO. Vitamin A: A review. Asian Journal of Clinical Nutrition. 2009;**1**:65-82

[56] Carazo A, Macáková K, Matoušová K, Krčmová LK, Protti M, Mladěnka P. Vitamin A update: Forms, sources, kinetics, detection, function, deficiency, therapeutic use and toxicity. Nutrients. 2021;**13**:1703. DOI: 10.3390/nu13051703

[57] Maiani G, Castón MJ, Catasta G, Toti E, Cambrodón IG, Bysted A, et al. Carotenoids: Actual knowledge on food sources, intakes, stability and bioavailability and their protective role in humans. Molecular Nutrition and Food Research. 2009;**53**:S194-S218. DOI: 10.1002/mnfr.200800053

[58] Dela Seña C, Riedl KM, Narayanasamy S, Curley RW Jr, Schwartz SJ, Harrison EH. The human enzyme that converts dietary provitamin A carotenoids to vitamin A is a dioxygenase. Journal of Biological Chemistry. 2014;**289**:13661-12666. DOI: 10.1074/jbc.M114.557710

[59] Institute of Medicine (US) Panel on Micronutrients. Dietary Reference Intakes for Vitamin A, Vitamin K,

Arsenic, Boron, Chromium, Copper, Iodine, Iron, Manganese, Molybdenum, Nickel, Silicon, Vanadium, and Zinc. Washington (DC): National Academies Press (US); 2001

[60] Balmer JE, Blomhoff R. Gene expression regulation by retinoic acid. Journal of Lipid Research. 2002;**43**:1773-1808. DOI: 10.1194/jlr.r100015-jlr200

[61] Shimizu H, Tsubota T, Kanki K, Shiota G. All-trans retinoic acid ameliorates hepatic stellate cell activation via suppression of thioredoxin interacting protein expression. Journal of Cellular Physiology. 2018;**233**:607-616. DOI: 10.1002/jcp.25921

[62] Shah A, Xia L, Goldberg H, Lee KW, Quaggin SE, Fantus IG. Thioredoxin-interacting protein mediates high glucose-induced reactive oxygen species generation by mitochondria and the NADPH oxidase, Nox4, in mesangial cells. Journal of Biological Chemistry. 2013;**288**:6835-6848. DOI: 10.1074/jbc.M112.419101

[63] Gad A, Abu Hamed S, Khalifa M, Amin A, El-Sayed A, Swiefy SA, et al. Retinoic acid improves maturation rate and upregulates the expression of antioxidant-related genes in in vitro matured buffalo (*Bubalus bubalis*) oocytes. International Journal of Veterinary Science and Medicine. 2018;**6**:279-285. DOI: 10.1016/j.ijvsm.2018.09.003

[64] Malivindi R, Rago V, De Rose D, Gervasi MC, Cione E, Russo G, et al. Influence of all-trans retinoic acid on sperm metabolism and oxidative stress: Its involvement in the physiopathology of varicocele-associated male infertility. Journal of Cellular Physiology. 2018;**233**:9526-9537. DOI: 10.1002/jcp.26872

[65] Fiedor J, Burda K. Potential role of carotenoids as antioxidants in human health and disease. Nutrients. 2014;**6**:466-388. DOI: 10.3390/nu6020466

[66] Young AJ, Lowe GL. Carotenoids—Antioxidant properties. Antioxidants (Basel). 2018;**7**:28. DOI: 10.3390/antiox7020028

[67] Fiedor J, Fiedor L, Haessner R, Scheer H. Cyclic endoperoxides of beta-carotene, potential pro-oxidants, as products of chemical quenching of singlet oxygen. Biochimica et Biophysica Acta. 2005;**1709**:1-4. DOI: 10.1016/j.bbabio.2005.05.008

[68] Rózanowska M, Cantrell A, Edge R, Land EJ, Sarna T, Truscott TG. Pulse radiolysis study of the interaction of retinoids with peroxyl radicals. Free Radical Biology and Medicine. 2005;**39**:1399-1405. DOI: 10.1016/j.freeradbiomed.2005.07.018

[69] Galano A, Vargas R, Martinez A. Carotenoids can act as antioxidants by oxidizing the superoxide radical anion. Physical Chemistry Chemical Physics. 2010;**12**:193-200. DOI: 10.1039/b917636e

[70] Fiedor J, Sulikowska A, Orzechowska A, Fiedor L, Burda K. Antioxidant effects of carotenoids in a model pigment-protein complex. Acta Biochimica Polonica. 2012;**59**:61-64. DOI: https://doi.org/10.18388/abp.2012_2172

[71] Edge R, Truscott TG. Singlet oxygen and free radical reactions of retinoids and carotenoids—A review. Antioxidants (Basel). 2018;**7**:5. DOI: 10.3390/antiox7010005

[72] Gammone MA, Riccioni G, D'Orazio N. Carotenoids: Potential allies of cardiovascular health? Food and

Nutrition Research. 2015;**59**:26762. DOI: 10.3402/fnr.v59.26762

[73] Shareck M, Rousseau MC, Koushik A, Siemiatycki J, Parent ME. Inverse association between dietary intake of selected carotenoids and vitamin C and risk of lung cancer. Frontiers in Oncology. 2017;**7**:23. DOI: 10.3389/fonc.2017.00023

[74] She C, Shang F, Zhou K, Liu N. Serum carotenoids and risks of diabetes and diabetic retinopathy in a Chinese population sample. Current Molecular Medicine. 2017;**17**:287-297. DOI: 10.2174/1566524017666171106112131

[75] El-Agamey A, Lowe GM, McGarvey DJ, Mortensen A, Philip DM, Truscott TG, et al. Carotenoid radical chemistry and antioxidant/pro-oxidant properties. Archives of Biochemistry and Biophysics. 2004;**430**:37-48. DOI: 10.1016/j.abb.2004.03.007

[76] Burke M, Edge R, Land EJ, McGarvey DJ, Truscott TG. One-electron reduction potentials of dietary carotenoid radical cations in aqueous micellar environments. FEBS Letters. 2001;**500**:132-136. DOI: 10.1016/S0014-5793(01)02601-1

[77] Bony E, Dussossoy E, Michel A, Brat P, Boudard F, Giaimis J, et al. Chemical composition and anti-inflammatory activities of an unsaponifiable fraction of pulp oil from Awara (*Astrocaryum vulgare* M.). Acta Horticulturae. 2014;**1040**:43-48. DOI: 10.17660/ActaHortic.2014.1040.4

[78] Guex CG, Cassanego GB, Dornelles RC, Casoti R, Engelmann AM, Somacal S, et al. Tucumã (*Astrocaryum aculeatum*) extract: Phytochemical characterization, acute and subacute oral toxicity studies in Wistar rats. Drug and Chemical Toxicology. 2022;**45**:810-821. DOI: 10.1080/01480545.2020.1777151

[79] Silva M, Grimaldi L, Godoi K, Lüdtke F, Silva T, Grimaldi R, et al. Physicochemical and thermal behavior of tucumã oil and butter. INFORM International News on Fats, Oils, and Related Materials. 2021;**32**:24-27. DOI: 10.21748/inform.03.2021.24

[80] Teixeira GL, Ibañez E, Block JM. Emerging lipids from Arecaceae palm fruits in Brazil. Molecules. 2022;**27**:4188. DOI: 10.3390/molecules27134188

[81] Dourado D, Barreto C, Fernandes RS, Blanco IMR, Oliveira D, Pereira N, et al. Development and evaluation of emulsifying systems of the material grease from Brazilian flora. Journal of Pharmacy and Pharmacognosy Research. 2015;**3**:130-140

[82] Kahn F. The genus *Astrocaryum* (Arecaceae). Revista Peruana de Biología. 2008;**15**:31-48

[83] Bony E, Boudard F, Brat P, Dussossoy E, Portet K, Poucheret P, et al. Awara (*Astrocaryum vulgare* M.) pulp oil: Chemical characterization, and anti-inflammatory properties in a mice model of endotoxic shock and a rat model of pulmonary inflammation. Fitoterapia. 2012;**83**:33-43. DOI: 10.1016/j.fitote.2011.09.007

[84] Bony E, Boudard T, Dussossoy E, Portet K, Brat P, Giaimis J, et al. Chemical composition and anti-inflammatory properties of the unsaponifiable fraction from Awara (*Astrocaryum vulgare* M.) pulp oil in activated J774 macrophages and in a mice model of endotoxic shock. Plant Foods for Human Nutrition. 2012;**67**:384-392. DOI: 10.1007/s11130-012-0323-z

[85] Ryan E, Galvin K, O'Connor TP, Maguire AR, O'Brien NM. Phytosterol,

squalene, tocopherol content and fatty acid profile of selected seeds, grains, and legumes. Plant Foods for Human Nutrition. 2007;**62**:85-91. DOI: 10.1007/s11130-007-0046-8

[86] Bester D, Esterhuyse AJ, Truter EJ, van Rooyen J. Cardiovascular effects of edible oils: A comparison between four popular edible oils. Nutrition Research Reviews. 2010;**23**:334-348. DOI: 10.1017/S0954422410000223

[87] Yussif NM, Vitamin C. In: JG LB, editor. Vitamin C—An Update on Current Uses and Functions. London: IntechOpen; 2018. Chapter 2. DOI: 10.5772/intechopen.81783

[88] Doseděl M, Jirkovský E, Macáková K, Krčmová LK, Javorská L, Pourová J, et al. Vitamin C—Sources, physiological role, kinetics, deficiency, use, toxicity, and determination. Nutrients. 2021;**13**:615. DOI: 10.3390/nu13020615

[89] Nishikimi M, Fukuyaman R, Minoshiman I, Shimizux N, Yag K. Cloning and chromosomal mapping of the human non-functional gene for l-gulono-y-lactone oxidase, the enzyme for l-ascorbic acid biosynthesis missing in man. Journal of Biological Chemistry. 1994;**269**:13685-13688

[90] Garriguet D. The effect of supplement use on vitamin C intake. Statistics Canada. 2010;**21**:1-7

[91] Akhtar HMN, Rahman SMM, Muslim T. Comparative study of the content of vitamin C in fresh fruits and different types of food prepared from them. Dhaka University Journal of Science. 2010;**58**:55-57

[92] Fenech M, Amaya I, Valpuesta V, Botella MA. Vitamin C content in fruits: Biosynthesis and regulation. Frontiers in Plant Science. 2019;**9**:2006. DOI: 10.3389/fpls.2018.02006

[93] Gęgotek A, Skrzydlewska E. Antioxidative and anti-inflammatory activity of ascorbic acid. Antioxidants (Basel). 2022;**11**:1993. DOI: 10.3390/antiox11101993

[94] Chen Y, Luo G, Yuan J, Wang Y, Yang X, Wang X, et al. Vitamin C mitigates oxidative stress and tumor necrosis factor-alpha in severe community-acquired pneumonia and LPS-induced macrophages. Mediators of Inflammation. 2014;**2014**:426740. DOI: 10.1155/2014/426740

[95] Riordan NH, Riordan HD, Casciari JJ. Clinical and experimental experiences with intravenous vitamin C. Journal of Orthomolecular Medicine. 2000;**15**:201-213

[96] Sakagami H, Satoh K, Hakeda Y, Kumegawa M. Apoptosis-inducing activity of vitamin C and vitamin K. Cellular and Molecular Biology (Noisy-le-Grand, France). 2000;**46**:129-143

[97] Grad JM, Bahlis NJ, Reis I, Oshiro MM, Dalton WS, Boise LH. Ascorbic acid enhances arsenic trioxide-induced cytotoxicity in multiple myeloma cells. Blood. 2001;**98**:805-813. DOI: 10.1182/blood.v98.3.805

[98] Devanandan P, Chowdary PR, Muthukumar VA. Association of vitamin C status in diabetes mellitus: Prevalence and predictors of vitamin C deficiency. Future Journal of Pharmaceutical Sciences. 2020;**6**:30. DOI: 10.1186/s43094-020-00040-2

[99] Morelli MB, Gambardella J, Castellanos V, Trimarco V, Santulli G. Vitamin C and cardiovascular disease: An update. Antioxidants (Basel). 2020;**9**:1227. DOI: 10.3390/antiox9121227

[100] Wong SK, Chin K-Y, Ima-Nirwana S. Vitamin C: A review on its role in the

management of metabolic syndrome. International Journal of Medical Sciences. 2020;**17**:1625-1638. DOI: 10.7150/ijms.47103

[101] Fogagnolo P, De Cilla' S, Alkabes M, Sabella P, Rossetti L. A review of topical and systemic vitamin supplementation in ocular surface diseases. Nutrients. 2021;**13**:1998. DOI: 10.3390/nu13061998

[102] Cadenas S, Cadenas AM. Fighting the stranger—Antioxidant protection against endotoxin toxicity. Toxicology. 2002;**180**:45-63. DOI: 10.1016/s0300-483x(02)00381-5

[103] Voigt K, Kontush A, Stuerenburg HJ, Muench-Harrach D, Hansen HC, Kunze K. Decreased plasma and cerebrospinal fluid ascorbate levels in patients with septic encephalopathy. Free Radical Research. 2002;**36**:735-739. DOI: 10.1080/10715760290032557

[104] Tewary A, Patra BC. Use of vitamin C as an immunostimulant. Effect on growth, nutritional quality, and immune response of Labeo rohita (Ham.). Fish Physiology and Biochemistry. 2008;**34**:251-259. DOI: 10.1007/s10695-007-9184-z

[105] Arrigoni O, De Tullio MC. Ascorbic acid: Much more than just an antioxidant. Biochimica et Biophysica Acta. 2002;**1569**:1-9. DOI: 10.1016/s0304-4165(01)00235-5

[106] Hacışevki A. An overview of ascorbic acid biochemistry. Journal of Faculty of Pharmacy. 2009;**38**:233-255

[107] Padayatty S, Katz A, Wang Y, Eck P, Kwon O, Lee J, et al. Vitamin C as an antioxidant: Evaluation of its role in disease prevention. Journal of the American College of Nutrition. 2003;**22**:18-35. DOI: 10.1080/07315724.2003.10719272

[108] Popovic L, Mitic N, Miric D, Bisevac B, Miric M, Popovic B. Influence of vitamin C supplementation on oxidative stress and neutrophil inflammatory response in acute and regular exercise. Oxidative Medicine and Cellular Longevity. 2015:295497. DOI: 10.1155/2015/295497

[109] Bindhumol V, Chitra KC, Mathur PP. Bisphenol A induces reactive oxygen species generation in the liver of male rats. Toxicology. 2003;**188**:117-124. DOI: 10.1016/s0300-483x(03)00056-8

[110] Rouhier N, Lemaire SD, Jacquot JP. The role of glutathione in photosynthetic organisms: Emerging functions for glutaredoxins and glutathionylation. Annual Review of Plant Biology. 2008;**59**:143-166. DOI: 10.1146/annurev.arplant.59.032607.092811

[111] Kaźmierczak-Barańska J, Boguszewska K, Adamus-Grabicka A, Karwowski BT. Two faces of viamin C—Anti-oxidative and pro-oxidative agent. Nutrients. 2020;**12**:1501. DOI: 10.3390/nu12051501

[112] De Rosso VV, Mercadante AZ. Carotenoid composition of two Brazilian genotypes of acerola (*Malpighia punicifolia* L.) from two harvests. Food Research International. 2005;**38**:1073-1077. DOI: 10.1016/j.foodres.2005.02.023

[113] Prakash A, Baskaran R. Acerola, an untapped functional superfruit: A review on latest frontiers. Journal of Food Science and Technology. 2018;**55**:3373-3384. DOI: 10.1007/s13197-018-3309-5

[114] Belwal T, Devkota HP, Hassan HA, Ahluwalia S, Ramadan MF, Mocan A, et al. Phytopharmacology of acerola (*Malpighia* spp.) and its potential as functional food. Trends in Food Science and Technology. 2018;**74**:99-106. DOI: 10.1016/j.tifs.2018.01.014

[115] Motohashi N, Wakabayashi H, Kurihara T, Fukushima H, Yamada T, Kawase M, et al. Biological activity of Barbados cherry (acerola fruits, fruit of *Malpighia emarginata* DC) extracts and fractions. Phytotherapy Research. 2004;**18**:212-223. DOI: 10.1002/ptr.1426

[116] Hanamura T, Hagiwara T, Kawagishi H. Structural and functional characterization of polyphenols isolated from acerola (*Malpighia emarginata* DC.) fruit. Bioscience, Biotechnology, and Biochemistry. 2005;**69**:280-286. DOI: 10.1271/bbb.69.280

[117] Hanamura T, Mayama C, Aoki H, Hirayama Y, Shimizu M. Antihyperglycemic effect of polyphenols from Acerola (*Malpighia emarginata* DC.) fruit. Bioscience, Biotechnology, and Biochemistry. 2006;**70**:1813-1820. DOI: 10.1271/bbb.50592

[118] Dias FM, Leffa DD, Daumann F, Marques Sde O, Luciano TF, Possato JC, et al. Acerola (*Malpighia emarginata* DC.) juice intake protects against alterations to proteins involved in inflammatory and lipolysis pathways in the adipose tissue of obese mice fed a cafeteria diet. Lipids in Health and Disease. 2014;**13**:24. DOI: 10.1186/1476-511X-13-24

[119] Rezende YRRS, Nogueira JP, Narain N. Comparison and optimization of conventional and ultrasound assisted extraction for bioactive compounds and antioxidant activity from agro-industrial acerola (*Malpighia emarginata* DC) residue. Lebensmittel-Wissenschaft + Technologie. 2017;**85**:158-169. DOI: 10.1016/j.lwt.2017.07.020

[120] Betta FD, Nehring P, Seraglio SKT, Schulz M, Valese AC, Daguer H, et al. Phenolic compounds determined by LC-MS/MS and *in vitro* antioxidant capacity of Brazilian fruits in two edible ripening stages. Plant Foods for Human Nutrition. 2018;**73**:302-307. DOI: 10.1007/s11130-018-0690-1

[121] Carneiro APDG, Aguiar ALLD, Silva RBCD, Richter AR, Sousa PHMD, Silva LMRD, et al. Acerola by-product as a renewable source of bioactive compounds: Arabic gum and maltodextrin nanocapsules. Food Science and Technology. 2020;**40**(Suppl 2):466-474. DOI: 10.1590/fst.22819

[122] Righetto AM, Netto FM, Carraro F. Chemical composition and antioxidant activity of juices from mature and immature acerola (*Malpighia emarginata* DC). Food Science and Technology International. 2005;**11**:315-321. DOI: 10.1177/1082013205056785

[123] Mezadri T, Villano D, Fernandez-Pachon MS, Garcia-Parrilla MC, Troncoso AM. Antioxidant compounds and antioxidant activity in acerola (*Malpighia emarginata* DC.) fruits and derivatives. Journal of Food Composition and Analysis. 2008;**21**:282-290. DOI: 10.1016/j.jfca.2008.02.002

[124] Marques TR, Caetano AA, Simão AA, Castro FCDO, Ramos VDO, Corrêa AD. Methanolic extract of *Malpighia emarginata* bagasse: Phenolic compounds and inhibitory potential on digestive enzymes. Revista Brasileira de Farmacognosia. 2016;**26**:191-196. DOI: 10.1016/j.bjp.2015.08.015

[125] Mans DRA, Friperson P, Pawirodihardjo J, Djotaroeno M. Antioxidant activity of Surinamese medicinal plants with adaptogenic properties and correlation with total phenolic contents. Journal of Antioxidant Activity. 2020;**2**:11-28. DOI: 10.14302/issn.2471-2140.jaa-20-3478

[126] Almeida SDS, Alves WAL, Araujo SAD, Santana JCC, Narain N, Souza RRD. Use of simulated annealing

in standardization and optimization of the acerola wine production. Food Science and Technology Campinas. 2014;**34**:292-297. DOI: 10.1590/fst.2014.0037

[127] Naidu KA. Vitamin C in human health and disease is still a mystery? An overview. Nutrition Journal. 2003;**2**:7. DOI: 10.1186/1475-2891-2-7

[128] Singh DR, Singh S, Salim KM, Srivastava RC. Estimation of phytochemicals and antioxidant activity of underutilized fruits of Andaman Islands (India). International Journal of Food Sciences and Nutrition. 2012;**63**:446-452. DOI: 10.3109/09637486.2011.634788

[129] Wang L, Li F, He C, Dong Y, Wang Q. Antioxidant activity and melanogenesis inhibitory effect of acerola fruit (*Malpighia glabra* L.) aqueous extract and its safe use in cosmetics. Asian Journal of Chemistry. 2015;**27**:957-960. DOI: 10.14233/ajchem.2015.17771

[130] Anantachoke N, Lomarat P, Praserttirachai W, Khammanit R, Mangmool S. Thai fruits exhibit antioxidant activity and induction of antioxidant enzymes in HEK-293 cells. Evidence-based Complementary and Alternative Medicine: eCAM. 2016;**2016**:6083136. DOI: 10.1155/2016/6083136

[131] Dörmann P. Functional diversity of tocochromanols in plants. Planta. 2007;**225**:269-276. DOI: 10.1007/s00425-006-0438-2

[132] Jiang Q. Natural forms of vitamin E: Metabolism, antioxidant, and anti-inflammatory activities and their role in disease prevention and therapy. Free Radical Biology and Medicine. 2014;**72**:76-90. DOI: 10.1016/j.freeradbiomed.2014.03.035

[133] Niki E, Noguchi N, Tsuchihashi H, Gotoh N. Interaction among vitamin C, vitamin E, and beta-carotene. American Journal of Clinical Nutrition. 1995;**62**:1322S-1326S. DOI: 10.1093/ajcn/62.6.1322S

[134] Kowdley KV, Mason JB, Meydani SN, Cornwall S, Grand RJ. Vitamin E deficiency and impaired cellular immunity related to intestinal fat malabsorption. Gastroenterology. 1992;**102**:2139-2142. DOI: 10.1016/0016-5085(92)90344-x

[135] Wang X, Quinn PJ. The location and function of vitamin E in membranes (review). Molecular Membrane Biology. 2000;**17**:143-156. DOI: 10.1080/09687680010000311

[136] Bradford A, Atkinson J, Fuller N, Rand RP. The effect of vitamin E on the structure of membrane lipid assemblies. Journal of Lipid Research. 2003;**44**:1940-1945. DOI: 10.1194/jlr.M300146-JLR200

[137] Howard A, McNeil A, McNeil P. Promotion of plasma membrane repair by vitamin E. Nature Communications. 2011;**2**:597. DOI: 10.1038/ncomms1594

[138] Liu M, Wallmon A, Olsson-Mortlock C, Wallin R, Saldeen T. Mixed tocopherols inhibit platelet aggregation in humans: Potential mechanisms. American Journal of Clinical Nutrition. 2003;**77**:700-706. DOI: 10.1093/ajcn/77.3.700

[139] Brigelius-Flohé R, Traber MG. Vitamin E: Function and metabolism. FASEB Journal. 1999;**13**:1145-1155

[140] Li D, Saldeen T, Romeo F, Mehta JL. Different isoforms of tocopherols enhance nitric oxide

synthase phosphorylation and inhibit human platelet aggregation and lipid peroxidation: Implications in therapy with vitamin E. Journal of Cardiovascular Pharmacology and Therapeutics. 2001;**6**:155-1561. DOI: 10.1177/107424840100600207

[141] Rizvi S, Raza ST, Ahmed F, Ahmad A, Abbas S, Mahdi F. The role of vitamin E in human health and some diseases. Sultan Qaboos University Medical Journal. 2014;**14**:e157-e165

[142] Burton GW, Joyce A, Ingold KU. Is vitamin E the only lipid-soluble, chain-breaking antioxidant in human blood plasma and erythrocyte membranes? Archives of Biochemistry and Biophysics. 1983;**221**:281-290. DOI: 10.1016/0003-9861(83)90145-5

[143] Niki E. Role of vitamin E as a lipid-soluble peroxyl radical scavenger: In vitro and *in vivo* evidence. Free Radical Biology and Medicine. 2014;**66**:3-12. DOI: 10.1016/j.freeradbiomed.2013.03.022

[144] Niki E. Evidence for beneficial effects of vitamin E. Korean Journal of Internal Medicine. 2015;**30**:571-579. DOI: 10.3904/kjim.2015.30.5.571

[145] Ciarcià G, Bianchi S, Tomasello B, Acquaviva R, Malfa GA, Naletova I, et al. Vitamin E and non-communicable diseases: A review. Biomedicine. 2022;**10**:2473. DOI: 10.3390/biomedicines10102473

[146] Valentin HE, Qi Q. Biotechnological production and application of vitamin E: Current state and prospects. Applied Microbiology and Biotechnology. 2005;**68**:436-444. DOI: 10.1007/s00253-005-0017-7

[147] Carney JA, Rosomoff RN. In the Shadow of Slavery: Africa's Botanical Legacy in the Atlantic World. Berkeley: University of California Press; 2009

[148] Liu CL, Wang JM, Chu CY, Cheng MT, Tseng TH. *In vivo* protective effect of protocatechuic acid on tert-butyl hydroperoxide-induced rat hepatotoxicity. Food and Chemical Toxicology. 2002;**40**:635-641. DOI: 10.1016/s0278-6915(02)00002-9

[149] Mounnissamy VM, Kavimani S, Gunasegaran R. Antibacterial activity of gossypetin isolated from *Hibiscus sabdariffa*. The Antiseptic. 2002;**99**:81-82

[150] Abou AAA, Abu SFM, Abou AEA. Physicochemical properties of natural pigments (anthocyanin) extracted from roselle calyces (*Hibiscus subdariffa*). Journal of American Science. 2011;7:445-456

[151] Da-Costa-Rocha I, Bonnlaender B, Sievers H, Pischel I, Heinrich M. *Hibiscus sabdariffa* L.—A phytochemical and pharmacological review. Food Chemistry. 2014;165:424-443. DOI: 10.1016/j.foodchem.2014.05.002

[152] Ismail A, Ikram EHK, Nazri HSM. Roselle (*Hibiscus sabdariffa* L.) seeds—Nutritional composition protein quality and health benefits. Food. 2008;**2**:1-16

[153] Brunold C, Deters A, Knoepfel-Sidler F, Hafner J, Müller B, Hensel A. Polysaccharides from *Hibiscus sabdariffa* flowers stimulate proliferation and differentiation of human keratinocytes. Planta Medica. 2004;**70**:370-373. DOI: 10.1055/s-2004-818952

[154] Builders PF, Kabele-Toge B, Builders M, Chindo BA, Anwunobi PA, Isimi YC. Wound healing potential of formulated extract from *Hibiscus sabdariffa* calyx. Indian Journal of

Pharmaceutical Sciences. 2013;**75**:45-52. DOI: 10.4103/0250-474X.113549

[155] Khalil R, Yahya G, Abdo WS, El-Tanbouly GS, Johar D, Abdel-Halim MS, et al. Emerging approach for the application of *Hibiscus sabdariffa* extract ointment in the superficial burn care. Scientia Pharmaceutica. 2022;**90**:41. DOI: 10.3390/scipharm90030041

[156] Nkumah O. Phytochemical analysis and medicinal uses of *Hibiscus sabdariffa*. International Journal of Herbal Medicine. 2015;**2**:16-19

[157] Singh P, Khan M, Hailemariam H. Nutritional and health importance of Hibiscus sabdariffa: A review and indication for research needs. Journal of Nutritional Health and Food Engineering. 2017;**6**:1-4

[158] Al-Hashimi AG. Antioxidant and antibacterial activities of *Hibiscus sabdariffa* L. extracts. African Journal of Food Science. 2012;**6**:506-511. DOI: 10.5897/AJFS12.099

[159] Chikhoune A, Gagaoua M, Nanema KD, Souleymane AS, Hafid K, Aliane K, et al. Antioxidant activity of *Hibiscus sabdariffa* extracts incorporated in an emulsion system containing whey proteins: Oxidative stability and polyphenol-whey proteins interactions. Arabian Journal for Science and Engineering. 2017;**42**:2247-2260. DOI: 10.1007/s13369-017-2428-z

[160] Liu K-S, Tsao S-M, Yin M-C. *In vitro* antibacterial activity of roselle calyx and protocatechuic acid. Phytotherapy Research. 2005;**10**:942-945. DOI: 10.1002/ptr.1760

[161] Guardiola S, Mach N. Therapeutic potential of *Hibiscus sabdariffa*: A review of the scientific evidence. Endocrinología y Nutrición. 2014;**61**:274-295. DOI: 10.1016/j.endoen.2014.04.003

[162] Hirunpanich V, Utaipat A, Morales NP, Bunyapraphatsara N, Sato H, Herunsalee A, et al. Antioxidant effects of aqueous extracts from dried calyx of *Hibiscus sabdariffa* Linn. (Roselle) *in vitro* using rat low-density lipoprotein (LDL). Biological and Pharmaceutical Bulletin. 2005;**28**:481-484. DOI: 10.1248/bpb.28.481

[163] Subhaswaraj P, Sowmya M, Bhavana V, Dyavaiah M, Siddhardha B. Determination of antioxidant activity of *Hibiscus sabdariffa* and *Croton caudatus* in *Saccharomyces cerevisiae* model system. Journal of Food Science and Technology. 2017;**54**:2728-2736. DOI: 10.1007/s13197-017-2709-2

[164] Tsai PJ, McIntosh J, Pearce P, Camden B, Jordan BR. Anthocyanin and antioxidant capacity in roselle (*Hibiscus sabdariffa* L.) extract. Food Research International. 2002;**35**:351-356. DOI: 10.1016/S0963-9969(01)00129-6

[165] Ajiboye TO, Salawu NA, Yakubu MT, Oladiji AT, Akanji MA, Okogun JI. Antioxidant and drug detoxification potentials of *Hibiscus sabdariffa* anthocyanin extract. Drug and Chemical Toxicology. 2011;**34**:109-115. DOI: 10.3109/01480545.2010.536767

[166] Soetan KO, Olaiya CO, Oyewole OE. The importance of mineral elements for humans, domestic animals and plants: A review. African Journal of Food Science. 2010;**4**:200-222

[167] Quintaes KD, Diez-Garcia RW. The importance of minerals in the human diet. In: De la Guardia M, Garrigues S, editors. Handbook of Mineral Elements in Food. Hoboken: Wiley; 2015. pp. 1-21. DOI: 10.1002/9781118654316

[168] Zand N, Christides T, Loughrill E. Dietary intake of minerals. In: De la Guardia M, Garrigues S, editors. Handbook of Mineral Elements in Food. Hoboken: Wiley; 2015. pp. 23-39. DOI: 10.1002/9781118654316

[169] Hariharan S, Dharmaraj S. Selenium and selenoproteins: Its role in regulation of inflammation. Inflammopharmacology. 2020;**28**:667-695. DOI: 10.1007/s10787-020-00690-x

[170] Reddi AR, Jensen LT, Naranuntarat A, Rosenfeld L, Leung E, Shah R, et al. The overlapping roles of manganese and Cu/Zn SOD in oxidative stress protection. Free Radical Biology and Medicine. 2009;**46**:154-162. DOI: 10.1016/j.freeradbiomed.2008.09.032

[171] Kieliszek M, Błażejak. Selenium: Significance, and outlook for supplementation. Nutrition. 2013;**29**:713-718. DOI: 10.1016/j.nut.2012.11.012

[172] Kieliszek M. Selenium—Fascinating microelement, properties and sources in food. Molecules. 2019;**24**:1298. DOI: 10.3390/molecules24071298

[173] Bodnar M, Konieczka P, Namiesnik J. The properties, functions, and use of selenium compounds in living organisms. Journal of Environmental Science and Health, Part C: Environmental Carcinogenesis and Ecotoxicology Reviews. 2012;**30**:225-252. DOI: 10.1080/10590501.2012.705164

[174] Gupta M, Gupta S. An overview of selenium uptake, metabolism, and toxicity in plants. Frontiers in Plant Science. 2017;7:2074. DOI: 10.3389/fpls.2016.02074

[175] Navarro-Alarcon M, Cabrera-Vique C. Selenium in food and the human body: A review. Science of the Total Environment. 2008;**400**:115-1141. DOI: 10.1016/j.scitotenv.2008.06.024

[176] Rayman MP. Food-chain selenium and human health: Emphasis on intake. British Journal of Nutrition. 2008;**100**:254-268. DOI: 10.1017/S0007114508939830

[177] Kurokawa S, Berry MJ. Selenium. Role of the essential metalloid in health. Metal Ions in Life Sciences. 2013;**13**:499-534. DOI: 10.1007/978-94-007-7500-8_16

[178] Kiełczykowska M, Kocot J, Paździor M, Musik I. Selenium—A fascinating antioxidant of protective properties. Advances in Clinical and Experimental Medicine. 2018;**27**:245-255. DOI: 10.17219/acem/67222

[179] Rederstorff M, Krol A, Lescure A. Understanding the importance of selenium and selenoproteins in muscle function. Cellular and Molecular Life Sciences. 2006;**63**:52-59. DOI: 10.1007/s00018-005-5313-y

[180] Sunde RA. Selenium. In: Ross AC, Caballero B, Cousins RJ, Tucker KL, Ziegler TR, editors. Modern Nutrition in Health and Disease. 11th ed. Philadelphia: Lippincott Williams & Wilkins; 2012. pp. 225-237

[181] National Institutes of Health. Office of Dietary Supplements. Selenium. Fact Sheet for Health Professionals; 2021

[182] Rayman MP. Selenium and human health. Lancet. 2012;**379**:1256-1268. DOI: 10.1016/S0140-6736(11)61452-9

[183] Eliopoulos G, Eliopoulos I-P, Tsioubri M, Economou-Eliopoulos M. Distribution of selenium in the soil-plant-groundwater system: Factors controlling its bio-accumulation.

Minerals. 2020;**10**:795. DOI: 10.3390/min10090795

[184] Chen J. An original discovery: Selenium deficiency and Keshan disease (an endemic heart disease). Asia Pacific Journal of Clinical Nutrition. 2012;**21**:320-326

[185] Moreno-Reyes R, Mathieu F, Boelaert M, Begaux F, Suetens C, Rivera MT, et al. Selenium and iodine supplementation of rural Tibetan children affected by Kashin-Beck osteoarthropathy. American Journal of Clinical Nutrition. 2003;**78**:137-144. DOI: 10.1093/ajcn/78.1.137

[186] Dumont JE, Corvilain B, Contempre B. The biochemistry of endemic cretinism: Roles of iodine and selenium deficiency and goitrogens. Molecular and Cellular Endocrinology. 1994;**100**:163-166. DOI: 10.1016/0303-7207(94)90297-6

[187] Goldhaber SB. Trace element risk assessment: Essentiality vs. toxicity. Regulatory Toxicology and Pharmacology. 2003;**38**:232-242. DOI: 10.1016/s0273-2300(02)00020-x

[188] Lu J, Holmgren A. Selenoproteins. Journal of Biological Chemistry. 2009;**284**:723-727. DOI: 10.1074/jbc.R800045200

[189] Mehdi Y, Hornick JL, Istasse L, Dufrasne I. Selenium in the environment, metabolism and involvement in body functions. Molecules. 2013;**18**:3292-3311. DOI: 10.3390/molecules18033292

[190] Hadrup N, Ravn-Haren G. Absorption, distribution, metabolism and excretion (ADME) of oral selenium from organic and inorganic sources: A review. Journal of Trace Elements in Medicine and Biology. 2021;**67**:126801. DOI: 10.1016/j.jtemb.2021.126801

[191] Hatfield DL, Tsuji PA, Carlson BA, Gladyshev VN. Selenium and selenocysteine: Roles in cancer, health, and development. Trends in Biochemical Sciences. 2014;**39**:112-120. DOI: 10.1016/j.tibs.2013.12.007

[192] Ye R, Huang J, Wang Z, Chen Y, Dong Y. The role and mechanism of essential selenoproteins for homeostasis. Antioxidants. 2022;**11**:973. DOI: 10.3390/antiox11050973

[193] Tinggi U. Selenium: Its role as antioxidant in human health. Environmental Health and Preventive Medicine. 2008;**13**:102-108. DOI: 10.1007/s12199-007-0019-4

[194] Ju W, Li X, Li Z, Wu GR, Fu XF, Yang XM, et al. The effect of selenium supplementation on coronary heart disease: A systematic review and metaanalysis of randomized controlled trials. Journal of Trace Elements in Medicine and Biology. 2017;**44**:8-16. DOI: 10.1016/j.jtemb.2017.04.009

[195] Cai X, Wang C, Yu W, Fan W, Wang S, Shen N, et al. Selenium exposure and cancer risk: An updated meta-analysis and meta-regression. Scientific Reports. 2016;**6**:19213. DOI: 10.1038/srep19213

[196] Santos JR, Gois AM, Mendonça DM, Freire MA. Nutritional status, oxidative stress and dementia: The role of selenium in Alzheimer's disease. Frontiers in Aging Neuroscience. 2014;**6**:206. DOI: 10.3389/fnagi.2014.00206

[197] Yang J. Brazil nuts and associated health benefits: A review. LWT—Food Science and Technology. 2009;**42**:1573-1580. DOI: 10.1016/j.lwt.2009.05.019

[198] Chunhieng T, Pétritis K, Elfakir C, Brochier J, Goli T, Montet D. Study of selenium distribution in the protein

fractions of the Brazil nut, *Bertholletia excelsa*. Journal of Agricultural and Food Chemistry. 2004;**52**:4318-4322. DOI: 10.1021/jf049643e

[199] Chunhieng T, Hafidi A, Pioch D, Brochier J, Montet D. Detailed study of Brazil nut *(Bertholletia excelsa*) oil microcompounds: Phospholipids, tocopherols and sterols. Journal of the Brazilian Chemical Society. 2008;**19**:1374-1380. DOI: 10.1590/S0103-50532008000700021

[200] John JA, Shahidi F. Phenolic compounds and antioxidant activity of Brazil nut (Bertholletia excelsa). Journal of Functional Foods. 2010;**2**:196-209. DOI: 10.1016/j.jff.2010.04.008

[201] Kluczkovski AM, Martins M, Mundim SM, Simões RH, Nascimento KS, Marinho HA, et al. Properties of Brazil nuts: A review. African Journal of Biotechnology. 2015;**14**:642-648. DOI: 10.5897/AJB2014.14184

[202] Silva Junior EC, Wadt LHO, Silva KE, Lima RMB, Batista KD, Guedes MC, et al. Natural variation of selenium in Brazil nuts and soils from the Amazon region. Chemosphere. 2017;**188**:650-658. DOI: 10.1016/j.chemosphere.2017.08.158

[203] Thomson CD, Chisholm A, McLachlan SK, Campbell JM. Brazil nuts: An effective way to improve selenium status. American Journal of Clinical Nutrition. 2008;**87**:379-384. DOI: 10.1093/ajcn/87.2.379

[204] Da Silva A, Silveira BKS, de Freitas BVM, Hermsdorff HHM, Bressan J. Effects of regular Brazil nut (*Bertholletia excelsa* H.B.K.) consumption on health: A systematic review of clinical trials. Food. 2022;**11**:2925. DOI: 10.3390/foods11182925

[205] Cardoso BR, Duarte GBS, Reis BZ, Cozzolino SMF. Brazil nuts: Nutritional composition, health benefits and safety aspects. Food Research International. 2017;**100**:9-18. DOI: 10.1016/j.foodres.2017.08.036

[206] Eslami O, Shidfar F, Dehnad A. Inverse association of long-term nut consumption with weight gain and risk of overweight/obesity: A systematic review. Nutrition Research. 2019;**68**:1-8. DOI: 10.1016/j.nutres.2019.04.001

[207] Vasquez-Rojas WV, Martín D, Miralles B, Recio I, Fornari T, Cano MP. Composition of Brazil nut (*Bertholletia excelsa* HBK), its beverage and by-products: A healthy food and potential source of ingredients. Food. 2021;**10**:3007. DOI: 10.3390/foods10123007

[208] Schauss A, Wu X, Prior R, Ou B, Patel D, Huang D, et al. Phytochemical and nutrient composition of the freeze-dried Amazonian palm berry, *Euterpe oleraceae* Mart. (Açai). Journal of Agricultural and Food Chemistry. 2006;**54**:8598-8603. DOI: 10.1021/jf060976g

[209] Rosso VV, Hillebrand S, Montilla EC, Bobbio FO, Winterhalter P, Mercadante AZ. Determination of anthocyanins from acerola (*Malpighia emarginata* DC) and açai (*Euterpe oleracea* Mart.) by HPLC-PDA-MS/MS. Journal of Food Composition and Analysis. 2008;**21**:291-299. DOI: 10.1016/j.jfca.2008.01.001

[210] Panche AN, Diwan AD, Chandra SR. Flavonoids: An overview. Journal of Nutritional Science. 2016;**5**:e47. DOI: 10.1017/jns.2016.41

[211] Cesar LT, de Freitas CM, Maia GA, de Figueiredo RW, de Miranda MR, de Sousa PH, et al. Effects of clarification

on physicochemical characteristics, antioxidant capacity and quality attributes of açaí (*Euterpe oleracea* Mart.) juice. Journal of Food Science and Technology. 2014;**51**:3293-2300. DOI: 10.1007/s13197-012-0809-6

[212] Pina F, Oliveira J, de Freitas V. Anthocyanins and derivatives are more than flavylium cations. Tetrahedron. 2015;**71**:3107-3114. DOI: 10.1016/j.tet.2014.09.051

[213] Gallori S, Bilia AR, Bergonzi MC, Barbosa WLR, Vincieri FF. Polyphenolic constituents of fruit pulp of *Euterpe oleracea* Mart. (Açai palm). Chromatographia. 2004;**59**:739-743. DOI: 10.1365/s10337-004-0305-x

[214] Bichara CMG, Rogez H. Açai (*Euterpe oleracea* Martius). In: Yahia EM, editor. Postharvest Biology and Technology of Tropical and Subtropical Fruits. Vol. 2. Cambridge: Woodhead Publishing; 2011. pp. 1-27. DOI: 10.1533/9780857092762.1

[215] Laleh GH, Frydoonfar H, Heidary R, Jameei R, Zare S. The effect of light, temperature, pH and species on stability of anthocyanin pigments in four Berberis species. Pakistan Journal of Nutrition. 2006;**5**:90-92. DOI: 10.3923/pjn.2006.90.92

[216] West ME, Mauer LJ. Color and chemical stability of a variety of anthocyanins and ascorbic acid in solution and powder forms. Journal of Agricultural and Food Chemistry. 2013;**61**:4169-4179. DOI: 10.1021/jf400608b

[217] Contreras-Lopez E, Castañeda-Ovando A, González-Olivares LG, Añorve-Morga J, Jaimez-Ordaz J. Effect of light on stability of anthocyanins in ethanolic extracts of Rubus fruticosus. Food and Nutrition Sciences. 2014;**5**:488-494. DOI: 10.4236/fns.2014.56058

[218] Enaru B, Drețcanu G, Pop TD, Stănilă A, Diaconeasa Z. Anthocyanins: Factors affecting their stability and degradation. Antioxidants (Basel). 2021;**10**:1967. DOI: 10.3390/antiox10121967

Chapter 8

Antioxidant Activity of *Nigella sativa* Essential Oil

Kehinde Sowunmi and Zeenat Kaka

Abstract

Nigella sativa oils have anti-inflammatory, antibacterial, antifungal, antiparasitic and antiprotozoal, antiviral, cytotoxic, anticancer, neuro-, gastro-, cardio-, and hepatoprotective properties, making them potential treatments for a wide range of illnesses. *N. sativa* oil also suggests positive benefits on the immunological, respiratory, and reproductive systems in addition to diabetes mellitus (DM), fertility, breast cancer, dyspepsia, osmotic balance, and other conditions. Thymoquinone (TQ) is a suitable target for its potential antibacterial, antimicrobial, anti-inflammatory, chemopreventive, antitumoral, and other actions among the various isolated chemical moieties. The *N. sativa* oil has been shown in various non-clinical and clinical investigations to benefit health. On the other hand, TQ in several animal experiments is clear to generate no adverse modifications of the body biomarkers; rather, it enhanced health quality. This study presents a more mechanistic review of the constitutions and oil of *N. sativa*. In conclusion, research on Nigella oil may represent a health breakthrough.

Keywords: *Nigella sativa*, antioxidant, essential oils, potential treatment, thymoquinone (TQ)

1. Introduction

Nigella sativa L. is a short shrub of the Ranunculaceae botanical family. It is native to Southern Europe, North Africa, and Southeast Asia, and it is grown in a variety of nations across the world. Green leaves and 5–10 petalled rosaceous white, yellow, pink, pastel blue, or purple blooms. The mature fruit bears several small dark black seeds. The oil of *N. sativa* was widely utilised in traditional Asian and Middle Eastern medicines [1]. However, *N. sativa* has been used to treat a wide range of ailments affecting the respiratory system, digestive tract, cardiovascular system, kidney, liver, and immunological system. It has long been used to treat weariness and depression. Ailments such as asthma, bronchitis, rheumatism and associated inflammatory illnesses, indigestion, lack of appetite, diarrhoea, dropsy, amenorrhea, dysmenorrhea, worms, and skin eruptions are among the most prevalent traditional applications. It's both an antiseptic and a local anaesthetic [2].

Protein, fat, carbohydrates, crude fibre, total ash, volatile oil, fatty oil, cellulose, and moisture are all present in black seed oil [3]. The oil is also a good source of minerals including Ca, K, Se, Cu, P, Zn, and Fe, as well as several vitamins like A, B1, B2, and C. Additionally, seeds, roots, and shoots contain both carotenes and vanillic acid.

The primary unsaturated fatty acids include linolic acid, oleic acid, diomolinoleic acid, and eicosadienoic acid, which are found in fatty components. The two primary saturated fatty acids that palmitic acid and stearic acid are a part of our -sitosterol and stigmasterol [2]. According to Gharby et al. [4], other fatty acids include myristic acid, palmitoleic acid, linoleic acid, linolenic acid, arachidonic acid, cholesterol, campesterol, β-sitosterol, 5-avenasterol, and 7-avenasterol. The alkaloids in the oil are either imidazole ring-bearing alkaloids, pyrazole alkaloids, or isoquinoline alkaloids. Terpenes and saponins are also found in them. Evidence suggests that the most significant active ingredients in *N. sativa* include thymoquinone (TQ), thymohydroquinone, dithymoquinone, p-cymene, carvacrol, 4-terpineol, t-anethol, sesquiterpene longifolene, –pinene, and thymol, among others. Carvone, nigellicine, nigellone, citrostradienol,

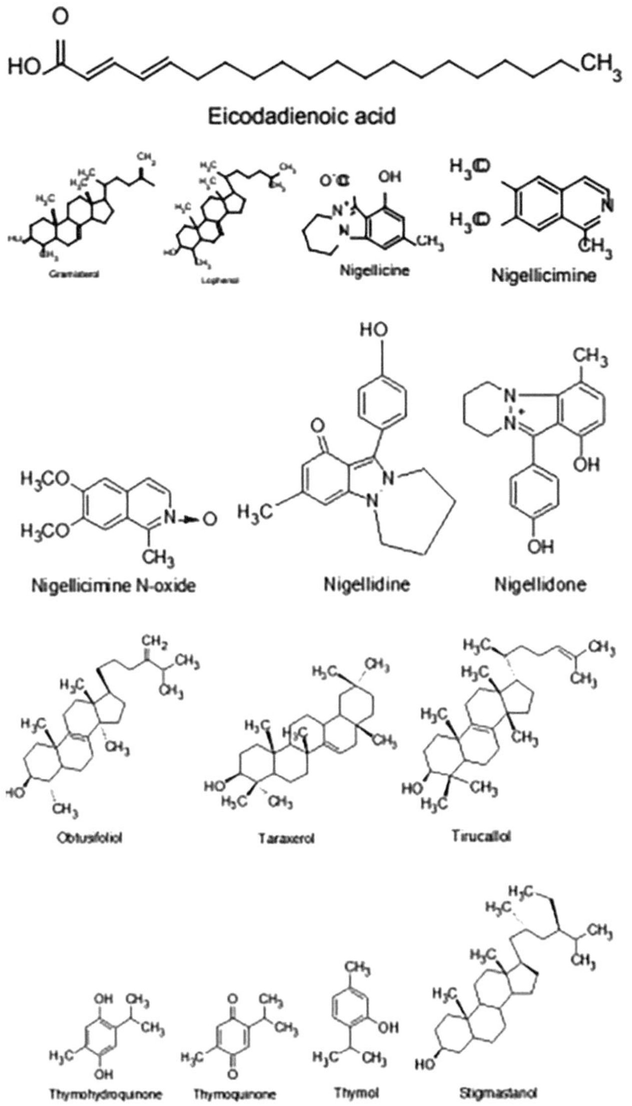

Figure 1.
Some important chemical moieties isolated from N. sativa.

cycloeucalenol, gramisterol, lophenol, ostusifoliol, stigmastanol, β -amyrin, butyrospermol, and cycloartenol are the other chemical components [2, 5] bitter principle, tannin, resin, reducing sugars, glycosidal saponin, hederagenin glycoside, esters of unsaturated fatty acids with C15 terpenoids, esters of dehydrostearic and linoleic acid, aliphatic alcohol, −unsaturated hydroxyl ketone, 3-O-[12-L-rhamnopyrasyl(12)-D-glucopyranosyl)-L-xylopyranosyl (12)] Stigma-5,22-dien-3-D-glucopyranoside, cycloart-23-methyl-7,20,22-triene-3, 25-diol, nigellidine-4-O-sulphite, 11-methoxy-16, 23-dihydroxy-28-methylolean-12-enoate, N. mines A1, A2, B1, and B2 in addition to A3, A4, and A5 [1, 6–16]. The chemical structures of some important chemical moieties are shown in **Figure 1**.

2. Activities of *N. sativa* oil

2.1 Antibacterial agent

According to reports, *N. sativa* has potent antibacterial activity against both gram-positive and gram-negative microorganisms. It has additive effects with spectinomycin, erythromycin, tobramycin, doxycycline, chloramphenicol, nalidixic acid, ampicillin, lincomycin, and co-trimoxazole and exhibits synergistic effects with streptomycin and gentamycin. It also functions similarly to topical mupirocin. It can combat resistant microorganisms, including many gram-positive and gram-negative bacteria that are multi-drug resistant [17]. Manju et al. [18] claim that an oil extract from Nigella can guard against *Vibrio parahaemolyticus* Dahv2 infection in Artemia spp. TQ has demonstrated anti-methicillin-resistant action in *Staphylococcus aureus*, according to Hariharan et al. [19].

2.2 Antiviral agent

It has been demonstrated that *N. sativa* increases the ratio of helper to suppressor T cells in people as well as the activity of natural killer (NK) cells. Otherwise, it is an effective inhibitor of murine CMV and HIV protease. In the latter instance, it was discovered that the generation of interferon-gamma (INF-) led to an increase in the quantity and functionality of M-phi and CD4 + ve T cells [7, 8, 17].

2.3 Antifungal activity

When used against Aspergillus niger, Fusarium solani, and Scopulariopsis brevicaulis, *N. sativa's* isolated chemical, TQ, was shown to be more efficient than griseofulvin and amphotericin-B. It also has antifungal action against *Candida albicans* and Madurella mycetomatis. The TQ also works well against Microsporum spp., Trichophyton spp., and Epidermophyton spp. Additionally, against a variety of clinical isolates, such as dermatophytes, moulds, and yeasts, thymohydroquinone and thymol also displayed an antifungal activity [9, 10, 20]. It is also obvious that black seed oil (10–200 g/mL) acts against *Saccharomyces cerevisiae* and C. utilise [21].

2.4 Effects on parasites

It has been demonstrated that *N. sativa* oil has potential against leishmaniasis, miracidia, cercariae, and *Schistosoma mansoni*. In the latter instance, co-treatment with praziquantel, a well-known anti-schistosomal and anthelmintic medicine for domestic animals, resulted in a potentiating effect from the oil of the black seed, which demonstrated high efficacy [13–16]. According to Simalango [22], ethanol extract of *N. sativa* (0.5–8%) exhibited anti-Ascaris suum action that was noticeably active.

2.5 Effect on wound infection

The ability of *N. sativa* oil to speed up the healing of wounds in mice, farm animals, and human gingival fibroblasts was examined. The accumulation result showed that the absolute difference in WBC counts, local infection and inflammation, bacterial growth and tissue damage, and free radical generation had all decreased. Additionally, transforming growth factor beta and basic fibroblast growth factor levels were found to be higher [17]. Studies using *N. sativa* extracts, seed oil, and TQ have been done on the antioxidant activity of Nigella. The research indicates that oxidative stress may have both potential anti-radical and inhibitory effects. Adenosine deaminase (ADA), catalase (CAT), myeloperoxidase (MPO), lipid peroxidase (LPO), reduced glutathione (GSH), glutathione-S-transferase (GSH-ST), glutathione peroxidase (GPx), superoxide dismutase (SOD), and nitric oxide were among the measures that TQ significantly altered (NO). In addition, it decreased levels of malonilealdehyde (MDA), conjugated diene (CGD), tumour necrosis factor-alpha (TNF-), interferon-gamma (IFN-), and prostaglandin (PGE2) rather than interleukin-10 (IL-10) and other pro-inflammatory mediators [2, 23].

2.6 Anti-inflammatory diseases

N. sativa extracts, seed oil, and TQ may have anti-inflammatory properties, according to research using several animal models. The lowering of NO synthesis, interleukin-1 (IL-1), cyclooxygenase-1 (COX-1), cyclooxygenase-2 (COX-2), histone deacetylase (HDAC), and other pro-inflammatory mediators, including IL-1, IL-6, TNF-, IFN-, and PGE2, is a function of this activity [1, 11]. In mice, topical TQ treatments increased the expression of heme oxygenase-1, NAD(P)H-quinone oxidoreductase-1, glutamate cysteine ligase, GSH-ST, and other enzymes, but rat seed oil inhibited COXs and 5-LPO in the pathways of arachidonate metabolism [17]. TQ has also been demonstrated to reduce nuclear translocation and nuclear factor-kappa-B (NF-B) DNA binding in mice by preventing I-phosphorylation Bs and subsequent degradation. TQ also reduced the phosphorylation of p38 mitogen-activated protein kinase, c-Jun-N-terminal kinase (c-JUNK), and protein kinase B (Akt) (MAPK–p38). The inactivation of caspase-1 was followed by the suppression of IL-1 and IL-18 in B16F10 mice whose expression of NLRP3 (NACHT, LRR, and pyrin domain-containing protein 3) was reduced. Additionally, the NLRP3 inflammasome was partially inactivated as a result of TQ's inhibitory action on NF-B and reactive oxygen species (ROS) [17, 23, 24].

2.7 Anticancer

The capacity of black seed oil to boost NK cells makes it potentially useful in immune treatment. Oil's constituents, however, may have a carcinogenic impact due to prooxidant effects caused by antioxidants. TQ was also evaluated on a variety of cancer cells generated from mice, indicating its capacity to stop G0/G1 phases of the cell cycle, which coincided with rapid increases in the expression of the cyclin-dependent kinase p16 (CDK-p16) and a drop in cyclin-d1 (dcl-1) protein expression in papilloma (SP-1) cell line, and G2/M arrest connected with an increase in the production. The chemopreventive potential of TQ may be attributed to its capacity to reduce cyclin-xl (bcl-xl) protein and enhance the ratio of apoptosis regulator (bcl-4)/ cyclin-2 (bax/bcl- 2) expression. Additionally, squamous cell carcinoma (SCC- VII), FsaR, and mouse tumour models of fibrosarcoma and SCC were found to exhibit TQ's anticancer efficacy. TQ significantly increased the sub-G1 population, live/dead cytotoxicity, chromatin condensation, DNA laddering, and Tunel-positive cells in A431 and Hep-2 cells, demonstrating substantial anticancer action through apoptosis. Caspase activation, cell proliferation, cleavage of poly ADP ribose polymerase, and a rise in the bax/bcl-2 ratio were also seen [17]. According to research, TQ caused p53-independent apoptosis in human colon cancer cells, as well as p21 expression, and stopped the S phase of the cell cycle [25]. TQ is a potent down-regulator of NF-B and MMP-9 in Panc-1 cells as well as bcl-2 and an up-regulator of caspase-3 and caspase-9 in gastric cancer cells. It is also an anticancer drug for several cell lines, including MCF-7/Topo breast carcinoma cells. The antitumor action of certain TQ derivatives, including 6-menthoxybutyryl, 6-hencosahexanyl conjugate, 4-acyl hydrazones, and 6-alkyl derivatives, is also visible in cancer cell lines [2].

2.8 Effect on diabetes mellitus

In rats, *N. sativa* was discovered to be crucial in the lowering of blood glucose levels with an increase in insulin and C-peptide levels. TQ lowers tissue MDA levels, DNA damage, mitochondrial vacuolization, and fragmentation, and by acting as an antioxidant, it protects the integrity of pancreatic beta-cells. According to a study, TQ clearly raises insulin and Hb levels while also significantly lowering glucose and HbA1c levels. In T2 D rats, *N. sativa* improved bone mass, connection, biomechanical behaviour, and strength in a synergistic manner with parathyroid hormone [26, 27]. Additionally, it is clear that the black seeds are an effective treatment for those with dyslipidemia and the insulin resistance syndrome. Diabetes patient *Meriones Shawi* treated with *N. sativa* likewise had an insulin-sensitization effect through increased ACC phosphorylation (primarily MAPK signalling pathway) and muscle GLUT4 content as well as gradual restoration of glycemia [1, 28]. In rats with diabetic mellitus (DM) brought on by streptozotocin, lipid and volatile fractions decreased toxicological and unfavourable effects [29]. Additionally, Heshmati et al. [30] reported that therapy with oil at 3 g three times per day might improve glycemic status and lipid profiles in DM patients ($n = 72$). When TQ was tested in clonal beta-cells and rodent islets, it had a protective effect with normalisation of chronic malonyl CoA accumulation and elevation of acetyl CoA carboxylase (ACC), fatty acid synthase (FAS), and fatty acid binding proteins (FABPs) following chronic glucose overload, suggesting a modification in beta-cell redox circuitry and enhancing the sensitivity of beta-cell metabolic pathways to glucose and glucose-stimulated insulin secretion (GSIS) under both normal conditions and hyperglycemia [31]. Otherwise, MAPK controls several transcriptional variables, the alteration of which disrupts the cell cycle. Therefore, *N. sativa* and TQ may be effective treatments for both type 1 and type 2 DM patients, as maintaining beta-cell integrity and secreting enough insulin to support glycogenesis and the phosphorylation of elevated blood glucose levels are essential in this context. Otherwise, oxidative stress, illness, and trauma are the other variables that raise blood sugar levels in addition to eaten meals. Therefore, the antioxidant, antibacterial, cytotoxic, and anti-inflammatory properties of *N. sativa* and TQ may be related to each other. Otherwise, lowering HbA1c levels is one of the treatments for retinopathy, nephropathy, and cardiovascular disease.

2.9 Effect on the immune system

N. sativa is a demodulator of the production of numerous pro-inflammatory mediators, with an increase in the release of Th2 vs. Th1 cytokines in splenocytes, along with NK antitumor activity. Black seed extracts can regain resistance against granulocyte-dependent *C. albicans*. According to research conducted by the oil, the immunosuppressive cytotoxic impact of typhoid immunisation may result in a decrease in antibody production. Additionally, it is clear that the oxytetracycline (OXT)-induced imbalances in leukocyte, lymphocyte, heterophil: lymphocyte, lysosomal enzyme activity, and reticuloendothelial system function need to be addressed. When pigeons received continuous antibiotic therapy, nevertheless, it had an immuno-protective effect. The black seed oil also has radioprotective properties against the oxidative and immunosuppressive effects of ionising radiation. In addition, *N. sativa* oil administration resulted in a rise in IFN- levels and a considerable reduction in the pathological alterations in the guinea pigs' lungs. Additionally, it works well for allergic diarrhoea [1, 23, 24]. Recent research reveals that seed oil can shield the jejunal mucosa from harm caused by -radiation [26]. After 6 weeks of therapy, Nigella EO in hens at doses between 5 and 20 g/kg (oral feed) enhanced FCR, plasma lipid profile, and antibody-mediated immunity [32]. Additionally, in individuals with Hashimoto's thyroiditis, nigella oil decreased thyroid stimulating hormone (TSH) and anti-thyroid peroxidase antibodies [12, 33].

2.10 Effect on the nervous system (NS)

The methanolic extract of *N. sativa* is an effective analgesic and antidepressant. Additionally, rat brains showed anxiolytic action by elevating serotonin (5-HT) and lowering hydroxy indole acetic acid (5-HIAA) levels [20]. Rats showed improved learning and memory associated with an increase in 5-HT secretion. It may aid in the treatment of anxiety since it increased the levels of tryptophan [20, 23]. In contrast, TQ decreased the generation of NO and MDA while still having a GABA-mediated calming effect in mice [1]. Due to its antioxidant, free radical scavenging, and anti-inflammatory properties, it may have neuroprotective properties.

2.11 Effect on the gastrointestinal tract (GIT) system

TQ is gastroprotective because it increases the quantity and activity of gastric mucin, GSH, total nitric oxide (TNO), and SOD while decreasing stomach acid secretion, acid output (AO), pepsin, mucosal lipid peroxidase (LPO), the proton (H+) pump, MPO, and ulcer index (UI). Prostaglandin (PGD)-mediated and/or via antioxidant and ant secretion pathways were hypothesised to reduce ulcer severity in rats. Rats also showed a decrease in LPO and lactate dehydrogenase (LDH), MPO, MDA, and an increase in GSH, SOD, GPx, and GSH-ST without changing stomach CAT. TQ was discovered to have considerable benefits on inflammatory bowel illnesses, anti-*Helicobacter pylori*, body weight reduction, colitis, and diarrhoea [2].

2.12 Effect on the hepatic system

The hepatoprotective action of *N. sativa* is shown by its effects on the enzymes alanine aminotransferase (ALT), aspartate aminotransferase (AST), LDH, total antioxidant capacity (TAC), CAT, MPO, total oxidative status (TOS), and oxidative stress index (OSI). Additionally, GSH and TQ enhanced protein carbonyl content, which reduced protein oxidation and improved the cellular fraction's decreased antioxidant levels [1]. Hepatocytes in mouse TIB-73 cells were shielded against N-acetyl-p-aminophenol (APAP)-induced hepatotoxicity and metabolic abnormalities by *N. sativa* oil at a concentration of 25–100 g/mL [34]. With an aqueous extract of *N. sativa*, a comparable activity was also seen by Hamza and Salem Al-Harbi [35]. This activity was assumed to be related to enhancing antioxidant capacity and inhibiting both lipid peroxidation and ROS formation [34]. It is also clear that black seed oil, when administered to rats receiving cisplatin (CP), at a dosage of 2 mg/kg, has hepatoprotective effects via enhancing energy metabolism and fortifying antioxidant defence mechanisms [36].

2.13 Effect on the urinary system

N. sativa with ascorbic acid (Vitamin C) reduced serum creatinine (CK), blood urea nitrogen (BUN), and antioxidant activity in rabbits, resulting in a nephroprotective effect. Otherwise, TQ had an impact on the renal expression of organic ion transporters and proteins linked to multidrug resistance in rats. Rats showed lower expression of OAT1, OAT3, OCT1, and OCT2 and increased protein levels of the efflux transporters MRP2 and MRP4. Along with lowering the tubular necrosis score, *N. sativa* is effective at lowering levels of CK, urea, MDA, NO, ROS, OSI, and TOS in kidney tissue and blood while increasing TAC, SOD, and GPx. The gentamicin (GM)-induced change in blood CK, BUN, thiobarbituric acid substances (TBARS), and total bilirubin is reversed by TQ. The black seed ethanol extracts showed considerable nephroprotective effect against paracetamol-induced nephrotoxicity in female Wistar Albino rats at doses of 250-100 mg/kg [37]. Otherwise, Erboga et al. [38] have shown that Cd-induced nephroprotective is also detectable in rats.

2.14 Effect on the pulmonary system

Leukotriene-d4 (LT4) is inhibited by both nigellone and TQ in the trachea, where the activity of the former was determined by mucociliary clearance. The peribronchial inflammatory cell infiltration, alveolar septal infiltration, alveolar edema, alveolar exudates, alveolar macrophages, intestinal fibrosis, granuloma, necrosis formation, NOS, and an increase in surfactant protein D in the pulmonary system were all significantly decreased by *N. sativa*. It is also clear that *N. sativa* protects the lungs from damage brought on by hypoxia and lung injury. *N. sativa* puffs have also been shown to have a bronchodilatory impact on PFT values, frequency of asthma symptoms/weakness, chest wheezing, and asthma symptoms [1].

2.15 Effect on the reproductive system

TQ reduced the levels of TAC and MPO in C57BL/6 male mice. Additionally, TQ warned of methotrexate-related occurrences such as intestinal space enlargement, edema, disruption of the somniferous epithelium, and smaller seminiferous tubule diameter. Treatment of 34 infertile men for two months with 2.5 mL black seed oil enhanced their abnormal semen quality without having any negative effects [39]. Black seed oil is a promising therapy for treating male infertility, according to Mahdavi et al. [28] In Sprague-Dawley male and female rats, *N. sativa* extracts in hexane and methanol significantly reduced fertility. In contrast, *N. sativa* prevented the contraction of uterine smooth muscle in rats and guinea pigs [1, 28]. TQ reduced the number of polycystic ovaries in rats by reducing their exposure to olive oil [40].

2.16 Effect on dyspepsia

A substantial reduction in dyspepsia was seen in individuals (n = 70) with functional dyspepsia who received treatment with 5 mL of Nigella oil (p.o.) daily for 8 weeks [41]. In osmotic balance: Nigella It was determined that black seed oil (22.6 g/25 l) should be used as an alternate therapy to isotonic sodium chloride (0.9% NaCl) solution for the elderly patients (n = 42) after they received treatment for two weeks (**Table 1**) [43].

Chemicals	Dose	Activity	References
Essential oil	Antioxidant assays: 5–50 g/L, antimicrobial assays: 0.2–2.0 g/mL	Produced antioxidant activity and shielded Artemia species following experimental *Vibrio parahaemolyticus* Dahv2 infection.	Manju et al. [42]
Oil	—	Decreased levels of TG, LDL, and total cholesterol; higher levels of HDL.	Sahebkar et al. [27]
Oil	400 mg/kg (i.g.) in Wistar albino rats	Reduced glutathione peroxidase (GSH-Px) and superoxide dismutase (SOD) activity were increased and reduced glutathione aldehyde (MDA) levels were decreased in intestinal tissue samples.	Orhon et al. [26]
Oil	Oil 2 mg/kg (p.o.) in cisplatin (CP) treated mice	improved energy metabolism and strengthened antioxidant defence mechanisms to produce hepatoprotective effects.	Kehinde et al. [20]
Oil	Patients with functional dyspepsia 5 ml (p.o.)	Lowered dyspepsia	Mohtashami et al. [41]
Oil	—	Antioxidant, immunomodulatory, and anti-inflammatory properties. a viable therapy option for male infertility. Potential to combat diabetes mellitus. Interaction with hepato- and kidney protection	Kehinde et al. [20]
TQ	In β–cells and rodent islets	During chronic glucose overload, a protective activity linked to the stabilisation of chronic malonyl CoA buildup and increase of acetyl CoA carboxylase (ACC), fatty acid synthase (FAS), and fatty acid binding proteins (FABPs). Thus, in both normal circumstances and hyperglycemia, the modified cell redox circuitry and enhanced sensitivity of the metabolic pathways to glucose and glucose-stimulated insulin secretion (GSIS) are present.	Grey et al. [31]

Table 1.
Several new research findings on nigella recipes.

3. Conclusion

One of the potential sources of drugs comes from plants, specifically shrubs. It's interesting to note that people worldwide are paying a lot of attention to herbal medicines today. Otherwise, traditional medicines continue to rule a certain kingdom of remedies. The excitement for drug researchers comes from the possible and varied activities of a trustworthy source. According to earlier research, *N. sativa* generated notable pharmacological actions, mainly through the use of TQ and its derivatives, nigellone, −hederin, and linoleic acid. Additionally, a few human clinical applications imply that *N. sativa* and its genetic makeup have a safety record. *N. sativa* and its derivatives may be chemically modified to produce useful results for the drug library. It is been found to be safe and healthy in several clinical applications, particularly in anti-fertility studies. Fixed oil of black seed was found to have LD50 values of 26.2–31.6 mg/kg in mice when administered intraperitoneally (i.p.) and orally (p.o.). TQ was found to be more tolerable than the *N. sativa* extract. They may be effective sources of cytoprotective agents due to their substantial antioxidant activity through antiradical, including ROS, direct reduction of oxidizable substrates, and stimulation of cellular antioxidant molecules. Antibiotics or radiation therapy can be used in conjunction with *N. sativa* oil to counteract its cytotoxic, immunosuppressive, and carcinogenic effects. TQ fits within this category, while further research is needed to determine its genotoxic and mutagenic potential.

Author details

Kehinde Sowunmi[1]* and Zeenat Kaka[2]

1 Department of Cell Biology and Genetics, University of Lagos, Akoka, Lagos, Nigeria

2 Department of General Education, Government Technical College, Ikorodu, Lagos, Nigeria

*Address all correspondence to: sowunmikehinde111@gmail.com

References

[1] Ahmad A, Husain A, Mujeeb M, et al. A review on therapeutic potential on Nigella sativa: A miracle herb. Asian Pacific Journal of Tropical Biomedicine. 2013;**3**(5):337-352

[2] Karna SKL. Phytochemical screening and gas chromatography–mass spectrometry and analysis of seed extract of Nigella sativa Linn. International Journal of Chemistry Studies. 2013;**1**(4):183-188

[3] Heshmati J, Namazi N. Effects of black seed (Nigella sativa) on metabolic parameters in diabetes mellitus: A systematic review. Complementary Therapies in Medicine. 2015;**23**(2):275-282

[4] Gharby S, Harhar H, Guillaume D, et al. Chemical investigation of Nigella sativa L. seed oil produced in Morocco. Journal of the Saudi Society of Agricultural Sciences. 2015;**14**(2):172-177

[5] Periasamy VS, Athinarayanan J, Alshatwi AA. Anticancer activity of an ultrasonic nanoemulsion formulation of Nigella sativa L. essential oil on human breast cancer cells. Ultrasonics Sonochemistry. 2016;**31**:449-455

[6] Huseini HF, Kianbakht S, Mirshamsi MH, et al. Effectiveness of topical Nigella sativa seed oil in the treatment of cyclic Mastalgia: A randomized, triple–blind, active, and placebo-controlled clinical trial. Planta Medica. 2016;**82**(4):285-288

[7] Ahlatci A, Kuzhan A, Taysi S, et al. Radiation–modifying abilities of Nigella sativa and Thymoquinone on radiation-induced nitrosative stress in the brain tissue. Phytomedicine. 2014;**21**(5):740-744

[8] Hobbenaghi R, Javanbakht J, Sadeghzadeh S, et al. Neuroprotective effects of Nigella sativa extract on cell death in hippocampal neurons following experimental global cerebral ischemia-reperfusion injury in rats. Journal of the Neurological Sciences. 2014;**337**(1-2):74-79

[9] Fahmy HM, Noor NA, Mohammed FF, et al. Nigella sativa as an anti-inflammatory and promising remyelinating agent in the cortex and hippocampus of experimental autoimmune encephalomyelitis–induced rats. The Journal of Basic & Applied Zoology. 2014;**67**(5):182-195

[10] Omar NM. Nigella sativa oil alleviates ultrastructural alterations induced by tramadol in the rat's motor cerebral cortex. Journal of Microscopy and Ultrastructure. 2015;**4**(2):76-84

[11] Bin Sayeed MS, Shams T, Fahim Hossain S, et al. Nigella sativa L. seeds modulate mood, anxiety, and cognition in healthy adolescent males. Journal of Ethnopharmacology. 2014;**152**(1):156-162

[12] Sahebkar A, Beccuti G, Simental–Mendía LE, et al. Nigella sativa (black seed) effects on plasma lipid concentrations in humans: A systematic review and meta-analysis of randomized placebo-controlled trials. Pharmacological Research 2016;**106**:37-50

[13] Al–Attass SA, Zahran FM, Turkistany SA. Nigella sativa and its active constituent thymoquinone in oral health. Saudi Medical Journal. 2016;**37**(3):235-244

[14] Irwin ML, Smith AW, Mc Tiernan A, et al. Influence of pre–and

postdiagnosis physical activity on mortality in breast cancer survivors: The health, eating, activity, and lifestyle study. Journal of Clinical Oncology. 2008;**26**(24):3958-3964

[15] Gupta SC, Hevia D, Patchva S, et al. Upsides and downsides of reactive oxygen species for cancer: The roles of reactive oxygen species in tumorigenesis, prevention, and therapy. Antioxidants & Redox Signaling. 2012;**16**(11):1295-1322

[16] Martindale JL, Holbrook NJ. Cellular response to oxidative stress: Signaling for suicide and survival. Journal of Cellular Physiology. 2002;**92**(1):1-15

[17] Aljabre SHM, Alakloby OM, Randhawa MA. Dermatological effects of Nigella sativa. Journal of Dermatology & Dermatologic Surgery. 2015;**19**(2):92-98

[18] Manju S, Malaikozhundan B, Vijayakumar S, et al. Antibacterial, antibiofilm and cytotoxic effects of Nigella sativa essential oil coated gold nanoparticles. Microbial Pathogenesis. 2016;**91**:129135

[19] Hariharan P, Paul-Satyaseela M, Gnanamani A. In vitro profiling of antimethicillin–resistant Staphylococcus aureus activity of thymoquinone against selected type and clinical strains. Letters in Applied Microbiology. 2016;**62**(3):283-289

[20] Sowunmi K, Modupeola AS, Lawal AA, Ayomikun KE, Kaur G. Evaluation of biochemical, hematological and antioxidant properties in mice exposed to a Triherbal (*Nigella sativa, Carica papaya, and Boswellia sacra*) Formular. Cell Biology. 2021;**9**(1):7-15

[21] Nadaf NH, Gawade SS, Muniv AS, et al. Exploring anti-yeast activity of Nigella sativa seed extracts. Industrial Crops and Products. 2015;77:624-630

[22] Simalango DM, Utami NV. In–vitro Antihelminthic effect of ethanol extract of black seeds (Nigella sativa) against Ascaris suum. Procedia Chemistry. 2014;**13**:181-185

[23] Amin B, Hosseinzadeh H. Black cumin (Nigella sativa) and its active constituent, Thymoquinone: An overview on the analgesic and anti-inflammatory effects. Planta Medica. 2016;**82**(1-2):8-16

[24] Gholamnezhad Z, Keyhanmanesh R, Boskabady MH. Anti-inflammatory, antioxidant, and immunomodulatory aspects of Nigella sativa for its preventive and bronchodilatory effects on obstructive respiratory diseases: A review of basic and clinical evidence. Journal of Functional Foods. 2015;**17**:910-927

[25] Khalife R, Hodroj MH, Fakhoury R, et al. Thymoquinone from Nigella sativa seeds promotes the antitumor activity of noncytotoxic doses of Topotecan in human colorectal cancer cells in vitro. Planta Medica. 2016;**82**(4):312-321

[26] Orhon ZN, Uzal C, Kanter M, et al. Protective effects of Nigella sativa on gamma radiation-induced jejunal mucosal damage in rats. Pathology, Research and Practice. 2016;**212**(5):437-443

[27] Shahraki S, Khajavirad A, Shafei MN, et al. Effect of total hydroalcoholic extract of Nigella sativa and its n-hexane and ethyl acetate fractions on ACHN and GP–293 cell lines. Journal of Traditional and Complementary Medicine. 2016;**6**(1):89-96

[28] Mahdavi R, Heshmati J, Namazi N. Effects of black seeds (Nigella sativa) on male infertility: A systematic review. Journal of Herbal Medicine. 2015;**5**(3):133-139

[29] Sultan MT, Butt MS, Karim R, et al. Toxicological and safety evaluation of Nigella sativa lipid and volatile fractions in streptozotocin-induced diabetes mellitus. Asian Pacific Journal of Tropical Disease. 2014;**4**(2):S693-S697

[30] Heshmati J, Namazi N, Memarzadeh MR, et al. Nigella sativa oil affects glucose metabolism and lipid concentrations in patients with type 2 diabetes: A randomized, double-blind, placebo-controlled trial. Food Research International. 2015;**70**:87-93

[31] Gray JP, Burgos DZ, Yuan T, et al. Thymoquinone, a bioactive component of Nigella sativa, normalizes insulin secretion from pancreatic β–cells under glucose overload via regulation of malonyl–CoA. American Journal of Physiology. Endocrinology and Metabolism. 2016;**310**(6):E394-E404

[32] Ghasemi HA, Kasani N, Taherpour K. Effects of black cumin seed (Nigella sativa L.), a probiotic, a prebiotic and a synbiotic on growth performance, immune response and blood characteristics of male broilers. Livestock Science. 2014;**164**:128-134

[33] Tajmiri S, Farhangi MA, Dehghan P. Nigella sativa treatment and serum concentrations of thyroid hormones, transforming growth factor β (TGF-–β) and interleukin 23 (IL–23) in patients with Hashimoto's thyroiditis. European Journal of Integrative Medicine. 2016;**8**(4):576-580

[34] Adam GO, Rahman MM, Lee SJ, et al. Hepatoprotective effects of Nigella sativa seed extract against acetaminophen-induced oxidative stress. Asian Pacific Journal of Tropical Medicine. 2016;**9**(3):221-227

[35] Hamza RZ, Al–Harbi MS. Amelioration of paracetamol hepatotoxicity and oxidative stress on mice liver with silymarin and Nigella sativa extract supplements. Asian Pacific Journal of Tropical Biomedicine. 2015;**5**(7):521-531

[36] Farooqui Z, Afsar M, Rizwan S, et al. Oral administration of Nigella sativa oil ameliorates the effect of cisplatin on membrane enzymes, carbohydrate metabolism, and oxidative damage in rat liver. Toxicology Reports. 2016;**3**:328-335

[37] Canayakin D, Bayir Y, Kilic Baygutalp N, et al. Paracetamol–induced nephrotoxicity and oxidative stress in rats: The protective role of Nigella sativa. Pharmaceutical Biology. 2016;**54**(10):2082-2091

[38] Erboga M, Kanter M, Aktas C, et al. Thymoquinone ameliorates cadmium–induced nephrotoxicity, apoptosis, and oxidative stress in rats is based on its anti–apoptotic and anti–oxidant properties. Biological Trace Element Research. 2016;**170**(1):165-172

[39] Kolahdooz M, Nasri S, Modarres SZ, et al. Effects of nigella satiVA L. seed oil on abnormal semen quality in infertile men: A randomized, double-blind, placebo-controlled clinical trial. Phytomedicine. 2014;**21**(6):901-905

[40] Arif M, Thakur SC, Datta K. Implication of thymoquinone as a remedy for polycystic ovary in the rat. Pharmaceutical Biology. 2016;**54**(4):674-685

[41] Mohtashami R, Huseini HF, Heydari M, et al. Efficacy and safety of honey-based formulation of Nigella sativa seed oil in functional dyspepsia: A double-blind randomized controlled clinical trial. Journal of Ethnopharmacology. 2015;**175**:147-152

[42] Manju S, Malaikozhundan B, Withyachumnarnkul B, et al. Essential oils of Nigella sativa protects Artemia from the pathogenic effect of Vibrio parahaemolyticus Dahv2. Journal of Invertebrate Pathology. 2016;**136**:43-49

[43] Oyu C, Tosun A, Yilmaz HB, et al. Topical nigella sativa for nasal symptoms in elderly. Auris, Nasus, Larynx. 2014;**41**(3):269-272

Chapter 9

Bioactive Compounds and Antioxidant Activity of Essential Oil of Species of the Genus Tagetes

Rosa Huaraca Aparco, María del Carmen Delgado Laime, Fidelia Tapia Tadeo, Henrry Wilfredo Agreda Cerna, Edwin Mescco Cáceres, Juan Alarcón Camacho, Hans Yuri Godoy Medina, Calixto Cañari Otero, Martha Teresa Ecos Ramos, Victor Raul Ochoa Aquije, Rosa Nelida Ascue Ruiz, Grecia Valverde Mamani and Niki Franklin Flores Pacheco

Abstract

This study investigated the bioactive compounds and antioxidant activity of the essential oil of two species of the genus Tagetes (*Tagetes minuta L.* and *Tagetes elliptica Sm*). The essential oil was obtained by steam distillation, and its extraction performance, relative density, refractive index, and solubility in ethanol (70% v/v) were determined. The chemical components were evaluated by gas chromatography coupled to mass spectrometry (GC-MS). Antioxidant activity was determined by the free radical 2,2-diphenyl-1-picrylhydrocyl (DPPH) method and the trapping capacity of the ABTS*+ radical cation. In the essential oils of the species Tagetes, it was possible to identify 26 chemical components for the species *Tagetes elliptica* Sm. and 16 for *Tagetes minuta* L., both species presented as main components monoterpenes (61%) and sesquiterpenes (44%). The compounds found were β-myrcene, trans-tagetone, β-trans-ocimene, and β-caryophyllene. Essential oils showed a variation in extraction yields and density. The refractive index was higher in the species *Tagetes elliptica* Sm., finding a high solubility in both species. A variation was found between 1.77 and 2.56 mg/mL of antioxidant activity by the DPPH method and 21.02–41.06 mg/mL for ABTS*+. The essential oils of the species *Tagetes elliptica* Sm.y and *Tagetes minuta* L. have bioactive components with antimicrobial and antioxidant potentialities for use for food preservatives.

Keywords: chromatography, density, monoterpenes, sesquiterpenes, solubility

1. Introduction

Peru is one of the 12 countries with the greatest biological diversity, with approximately 10% of the world's flora, estimated at 25,000 species, 30 of which are endemic [1]. There is a growing interest in bioactive compounds and the antioxidant properties of substances from natural sources that can potentially be used in food industries. Essential oils from aromatic and medicinal plants are known to possess biological activity [2, 3]. Essential oils are natural plant products that contain a complex mixture and therefore have multiple antimicrobial properties [4]. To be the constituents of the most important groups of raw materials for the food, pharmaceutical, perfumery, and related industries [5]. Most of these compounds are derived from oxygenated terpenoids, particularly phenolic terpenes, phenylpropanoids, and alcohols [6, 7]. Tagetes species were originally used as a source of essential oils that were extracted from leaves, stems, and flowers, being applied as flavorings in the food industry; in addition, their pigments have potential as a natural food colorant.

Tagetes is an important genus belonging to the family Asteraceae [8], aromatic, native to Central and South America with a cosmopolitan distribution due to anthropic activities [9]. *Tagetes minuta* L. is an aromatic plant with a broad spectrum of biological activity that has medicinal, antioxidant, and antimicrobial properties [10]. The great importance of Tagetes is due to the presence of essential oil in almost all parts of its plants, except in the stem [11]. It has biological activities such as antibacterial, antifungal, antiviral, antioxidant, anticancer, acaricide, nematicide, insecticidal, and allelopathic activities [12]. The growing interest in the food, flavor, and perfumery industries contributes to the investigation of environmental conditions affecting qualitative composition and yield [13].

Tagetes minuta L. is known by the common name of "huacatay" in Peru; in Mexico, it is known as "Mexican marigold" [14]. It is a species that accumulates a long world history of uses such as food, therapeutics, and aromatherapy that are inherent in the unique chemistry of the plant, its composition, and bioactivities. According to the research background review on bioactive metabolites and antioxidant activity of the aromatic species *Tagetes minuta* L. and *Tagetes elliptica* Sm., no publications are reported in our country; however, there are many reports on essential oils of these species in other countries [15].

Despite their importance as food species, research on the species *Tagetes minuta* L. and *Tagetes elliptica* Sm. in terms of chemical composition, genetic diversity, and biological properties is limited. Therefore, the objective was to determine the physical properties and identify the bioactive components and antioxidant activity of the essential oils of both species of the genus Tagetes that grow wild and are adapted to moderate-altitude ecosystems of the Andean region of Peru.

2. Materials and methods

2.1 Plant matter and botanical identification

The sheets of *Tagetes minuta* L. and *Tagetes elliptica* Sm were used. The samples were collected from the high Andean zone of the district of José María Arguedas (13°42 S.73°24 W at an altitude of 2935 m above sea level) belonging to the province of Andahuaylas, Apurimac region. With climate Cwd according to Koppens with average annual rainfall around 1000 mm/year, average relative humidity of 50% and temperature of –5 to 21°C, with moderate incidence of frost. The sample sheets were collected during the months of February to March 2019. The plants were identified and authenticated by Dra. María del Carmen Delgado Laime and deposited in the botany laboratory of the Basic Sciences pavilion of the José María Arguedas National University.

2.2 Essential oil extraction

For the extraction of essential oils, fresh leaves of *Tagetes minuta* L. were selected and *Tagetes elliptica Sm.*; 2.5 kg of fresh leaves of each species were used and subjected to extraction by distillation by dragging water vapor at a pressure of 10 psi. Once distilled, the essential oils were separated by difference in densities using a graduated Florentine decanter. Then dried in anhydrous sodium sulfate and stored at 4°C until the time of analysis, extraction yields were evaluated according to (Eq. 1).

$$\%P = \frac{Masafinaldeaceiteesencial\left(g\right)}{Masainicialdemuestraofollaje\left(g\right)} * 100 \tag{1}$$

2.3 Determination of the physical properties of the essential oil

In the essential oils obtained from each species, the relative density at 20°C was determined according to the Peruvian technical standard: NTP 3129.081:1974; refractive index in the ABBE refractometer; optical rotation in polarimeter and solubility in ethanol. For the latter, a 70% solution was used taking 100 μL of essential oil.

2.4 Determination of chemical compounds by gas chromatography coupled to mass spectrometry (GC-MS)

The analysis of the chemical composition of essential oils was identified by gas chromatography coupled to mass spectrometry (GC-MS) at the natural products research center of the Universidad Peruana Cayetano Heredia.

For the analysis of each sample, 20μL of essential oil in 980 μL of dichloromethane was used, which was injected into the gas chromatograph coupled to a selective mass detector. The compounds were separated in a mixture by an apolar capillary column DB-5MS (60 m × 250 μm × 0.25 μm) (J and W Scientific of 5% phenyl-polymethylsiloxane).

The temperature of the injector was maintained at 250°C with an injection in Split mode (50:1), the programming of the furnace temperature was: initial temperature 50°C, maintained for 5 mins; then increasing to 10°C/min to reach 100°C and finally to 10°C/min to 270°C, maintaining the final temperature for 1 min. The execution time was 77.8 mins, helium was used as a drag gas at a constant flow of 1 ml/min. The compounds of Tagetes oils *minute* L. and *Tagetes elliptica* Sm. were identified using software provided by Agilent; MSD chemstation (verse EO2.00.493), by comparing the mass spectra of each peak with those of the mass spectra library of the flavor databases and the National Institute of Standards and Technology (NIST, 08).

2.5 Evaluation of the antioxidant activity of essen0tial oils

For the determination of the antioxidant activity of the essential oils of the species of the genus Tagetes, two methodologies were used:

2.5.1 DPPH radical method

Aqueous ethanol dilutions of hydroalcoholic extracts were prepared to obtain concentrations of 0.0–150.0 μg/mL. About 1.0 mL of each dilution was combined with 0.5 mL of a 0.3 mM solution of DPPH in ethanol and allowed to react at room temperature for 30 mins, then the absorbance of the mixtures at 517 nm was measured in the spectrophotometry equipment. The percentage of antioxidant activity of each sample was calculated according to the following (Eq. 2):

$$Actividad\ Antioxidante\,(\%) = \frac{MAC - AM - AB(g)}{AC} X\,100 \tag{2}$$

AM: is the absorbance of the sample + DPPH,
AB: is the absorbance of the target (sample + ethanol),
AC: is the absorbance of the reactant target (DPPH + ethanol).

The concentration of the hydroalcoholic extract was neutralized at 50% of the DPPH radicals (EC_{50}, mean effective concentration) and was obtained directly by drawing the line between the percentage of antioxidant activity, compared with the concentration of the sample of essential oils mg/mL.

2.5.2 Radical method ABTS+*

The $ABTS^+$ free radical scavenging activity was determined by the method developed by Re et al. (1999), with some modifications.

About 3.5 mM of ABTS was reacted with 1.25 mM of potassium persulfate. The samples were incubated at temperatures of 2–8°C for 16–24 h in darkness. The formed ABTS*+ radical is diluted with ethanol to an absorbance of 0.7+ minus 0.05 to 734 nm. At a volume of 190 μL dilution of the ABTS*+ radical A, 10 μL of the AE sample was added and incubated at room temperature for 5 mins. After the time it took to determine by means of the spectrophotometer equipment at 734 nm in the Themoscientific microplate reader. For the positive control of the absorption of A radicals ABTS*+, ascorbic acid (4 μg/mL) was used.

2.6 Statistical analysis

The analyses were performed in triplicate, for the statistical evaluation, the completely randomized design (DCA) was used; The analysis of variance was worked with 0.05 significance; upon finding a significant difference, the Fisher's mean comparison test (LSD) was performed at a level of $\alpha = 0.05$. The data were processed with the help of the statistical programs Centurion XVII and the Microsoft Excel 2016 spreadsheet.

3. Results

3.1 Performance and physical properties of essential oils

The determination of the physicochemical properties allows us to know the quality control and purity in essential oils.

Table 1 shows the percentage of extraction yield and the physical properties of the essential oils of both species of the genus Tagetes. Where:, a is different from b.

3.2 Chemical composition of essential oils of two species of the genus Tagetes

The main components of the essential oils of both species of the genus Tagetes are shown in **Table 2**.

Retention time (TR) and relative abundance (%) of essential oils, Not detected (ND).

In the analysis of the chemical composition, a total of 26 chemical compounds were detected and quantified in the essential oil of *Tagetes elliptica* Sm., with main fraction in monoterpenes in (61.00%) and 16 chemical compounds for the essential oil of *Tagetes minuta* L. being found as the main fraction to the monoterpenes (50.0%); between both species, a standard deviation below 5% was obtained between the percentages of each analyte in both columns used. They were identified as bioactive compounds in essential oils in species of the genus Tagetes to β-trans-ocimene, trans-tagelone, cis-tagelone, β-myrcene, and β-caryophyllene.

Analysis	*Tagetes minuta* L.	*Tagetes elliptica* Sm.
Performance (%)	0.05 ± 0.002^{to}	0.048 ± 0.001^{to}
Density (g/mL) at 24°C	0.900 ± 0.0004^{to}	0.882 ± 0.0043^{B}
Refractive index at 24°C	1.93 ± 0.05^{to}	1.482 ± 0.04^{to}
EtOH solubility 70% (v/v)	Positive	Positive
Specific gravity at 20°C	$0.872^{to} \pm 0.01$	0.945 ± 0.034^{b}

Table 1.
Performance and physical properties of the essential oils of Tagetes minuta *L. and* Tagetes elliptica *Sm.*

Compound	% relative abundance, (TR. %)	
	Tagetes minuta L.	*Tagetes elliptica* Sm.
β-transocimeno	21.07 (25.03)	16.5 (11.45)
β-Myrcene	ND	15.01 (2.78)
β-Linalool	ND	18.56 (1.18)
Cis-Tagetone	25.6 (3.5)	20 (16.27)
M-tert-butyl-phenol	ND	22.6 (1.44)
Trans-Tagetona	25.94 (51.37)	20.22 (10.25)
β-caryophyllene	36.39 (0.48)	28.21 (1.17)
Guaiol	41.96 (1.25)	ND
Apiol	42.45 (3.28)	33.41 (0.43)
α-Bisabolol	44.29 (1.1)	ND

Table 2.
Main components detected in the essential oils of Tagetes minuta *L. and* Tagetes elliptica *Sm.*

Essential oil	Methods	
	DPPH IC $_{50}$ (mg/mL)	ABTS IC_{50} (mg/mL)
Tagetes minuta L.	1.77 ± 0.02	21.02 ± 0.14
Tagetes elliptica Sm.	2.56 ± 0.12	0.06 ± 41.23

Table 3.
Antioxidant activity by DPPH and ABTS methods.

3.3. Antioxidant activity of AE of *Tagetes minuta* L. and *Tagetes elliptica* Sm

The antioxidant activity of the essential oil, evaluated by the DPPH and ABTS methods, is shown in **Table 3**.

Significant differences were found in the antioxidant activity of both Tagetes samples as shown in **Table 3**. According to the DPPH methodology, CI_{50} varied from 1.77 to 2.56 mg/mL; however, the CI_{50} of ABTS*+ varied from 21.02 to 41.06 mg/mL, finding a higher antioxidant activity the value of CI $_{50}$ 41.06 mg/mL. *Tagetes* essential oil had a lower CI_{50} of 1.77 mg/mL, respectively, exhibited considerable DPPH radical scavenging activity compared with ABTS*+ method A.

4. Discussion

The essential oils of *Tagetes minuta* L. and T*agetes elliptica* Sm. did not show significant differences in the percentage of performance. The yield of the essential oil depends on the plant and the district where it is grown [16]. According to the results of the physical properties of the essential oil, the density showed a variation for both species of the genus Tagetes; however, the refractive index did not show a variation between both species. The presence of a lower refractive index and density value is related to an amount of phenols [17].

The refractive index of both species presented high values, which indicate the presence of high-molecular-weight compounds such as sesquiterpenes and diterpenes and eventually oleoresins in high concentrations [18], being also indicative of essential oils of higher quality and purity.

According to the results of specific gravity of the essential oils of both species, significant differences were found with a presence of higher quality (0.945 ± 0.034) in the essential oil of *Tagetes elliptica* Sm., finding similar values obtained according to previous studies [19].

The analysis of the chemical components in the essential oils of the species *Tagetes minuta* L. *and Tagetes elliptica* Sm. showed mainly the presence of the following compounds: Trans-Tagetone, β-trans-Ocimene, Cis-Tagetone, β-Caryophyllene, and Apiol.

The essential oils of the species *Tagetes spp*. are rich in monoterpene hydrates (Ocimenes, limonene, terpinene, myrcene, and acyclic monoterpene ketones (tagetone, dihydrotagetone, and tagetenone), which are the main odors in addition to smaller amounts of sesquiterpene hydrocarbons oxygenated compounds [20].

According to the results of the study in species *of Tagetes patula*, strong bioactivity was found in its essential oils against pathogenic test organisms, which is attributed to the presence of terpinolene, E-karyophene, Z-tagetone, E-tagetone, Caryophene oxide, and Germacrene D.

Regarding its bioactivities of the species family of the genus Tagetes, strong-to-mild antibacterial activity was found against strains of large-positive and large-negative bacteria tested in the study [4].

Regarding its applications of the essential oil according to the presence of metabolites, it was found that the metabolites synthesized by plants of the genus Tagetes show significant effects as antioxidants, enzyme inhibitors, precursors of toxic substances, and pigments. The activity of secondary metabolites in species of the genus Tagetes is thought to be related to their composition, concentration, and environmental conditions affecting their content.

Essential oils obtained from different parts of the plant may show different biological capabilities and can therefore be used in a variety of industries, such as cosmetics, pharmaceuticals, or food production [21].

According to [22], I report the antimicrobial activity of the essential oils of *Tagetes minuta* L. against phytopathogenic bacteria, *Pseudomonas savastanoi* pv, and *Phaseoli axonopodis* pv, which are responsible for different plant diseases.

The results indicated that *Tagetes spp*. plays a role of great importance for the preparation and preservation of food, considered as an excellent source of food spice. Even from a traditional point of view, the nature of *Tagetes spp*. and its composition affect the quantity and quality of extracts [23]. Despite the promising results obtained in vitro, more detailed studies of the mechanisms of action of the extracts and essential oils of *Tagetes spp*. would be beneficial to reach its potential in biotechnology. It was documented that the components of essential oils, especially terpenoids such as dihydrotagetones, tagetones, and ocymenones, were sufficient to explain the observed antimicrobial activity [24].

The difference in antioxidant activity between the two samples could be attributed to the presence of monoterpenes in their polyphenolic compounds, and oxygenated monoterpenes lead to increased antioxidant, antibacterial, and antifungal activities [25–27].

5. Conclusions

In this study, it was possible to determine the bioactive metabolites of the essential oils of the species of *Tagetes minuta* L. and *Tagetes elliptica* Sm., finding greater abundance of the bioactive metabolites: β-trans-ocimene, trans-tagelota, cis-tagelone, β-myrcene, and β-caryophyllene being the monoterpenic acyclicos, with significant effects as antioxidants, enzyme inhibitors, precursors of toxic substances, and pigments beneficial to reach their potential in biotechnology. The abundance in monoterpenes leads to antioxidant activities, being in the study greater presence of antioxidants in the species of *Tagetes elliptica* L. The physical properties of both species of the genus Tagetes were found in the quality ranges of essential oils.

Acknowledgements

The authors thank the Natural Products Research Laboratory of the Universidad Peruana Cayetano Heredia and the Universidad Nacional José María Arguedas.

Author details

Rosa Huaraca Aparco[1*], María del Carmen Delgado Laime[1], Fidelia Tapia Tadeo[1], Henrry Wilfredo Agreda Cerna[1], Edwin Mescco Cáceres[1], Juan Alarcón Camacho[2], Hans Yuri Godoy Medina[2], Calixto Cañari Otero[2], Martha Teresa Ecos Ramos[1], Victor Raul Ochoa Aquije[3], Rosa Nelida Ascue Ruiz[4], Grecia Valverde Mamani[1] and Niki Franklin Flores Pacheco[5]

1 José María Arguedas National University, Andahuaylas, Apurimac, Perú

2 Universidad Tecnología de los Andes, Andahuaylas, Apurimac, Peru

3 Autonomous University of Peru, Andahuaylas, Apurimac, Peru

4 Universidad Nacional José María Arguedas, Andahuaylas, Apurímac, Perú

5 National University Micaela Bastidas of Apurimac, Andahuaylas, Apurimac, Perú

*Address all correspondence to: rhuaraca@unajma.edu.pe

References

[1] Vásquez-Ocmín P, Cojean S, Rengifo E, Suyyagh-Albouz S, Guerra CAA, Pomel S, et al. Antiprotozoal activity of medicinal plants used by Iquitos-Nauta road communities in Loreto (Peru). Journal of Ethnopharmacology. 2018;**210**:372-385

[2] Chrysargyris A, Mikallou M, Petropoulos S, Tzortzakis N. Profile of components of essential oils and polyphenols to determine their antioxidant activity of medicinal and aromatic plants grown under different environmental conditions. Agronomy. 2020;**10**(5):727

[3] Tajkarimi M, Ibrahim S, Cliver D. Antimicrobial herbs and spice compounds in food. Food Control. 2010;**21**:1199-1218

[4] Safar AA, Ghafoor AO, Dastan D. Chemical Composition, Antibacterial and Antioxidant Activities of the essential oil of Tagetes patula L. grown in Erbil, Iraq. Journal of Reports in Pharmaceutical Sciences 9.1 2020:59. DOI: 10.4103/jrptps.JRPTPS_68_19

[5] Oliveira-Everton G, Pereira-Araújo RJ, da Silva dos Santos AB, Serra-Rosa PV, de Oliveira-Carvalho Junior RG, Teles AM, et al. Caracterização química, atividade antimicrobiana e toxicidade dos óleos essenciais da Pimenta dioica L. (pimenta da Jamaica) e Citrus sinensis L. Osbeck (laranja doce). Revista colombiana de ciencias quimico-farmaceuticas. 2020;**49**(3):641-655

[6] Bassolé IH, Juliani HR. Essential oils in combination and their antimicrobial properties. Molecules. 2012;**17**:3989-4006. Back to quoted text No. 23

[7] Burt S. Essential oils: Their antibacterial properties and possible applications in food: A review. International Journal of Food Microbiology. 2004;**94**:223-253

[8] Marotti M, Piccaglia R, Biavati B, Marotti I. Characterization and evaluation of the performance of essential oils of different *species of tagetes*. Journal of Essential Oil Research. 2004;**16**:440-444

[9] Ojeda MS, Torkel Karlin UO, Martinez GJ, Massuh Y, Ocaño SF, Torres LE, et al. Models of Aromatic and Medicinal Plants for Domestication, Production and Sustainable Uses. Ed. Córdoba, Argentina: UNC; 2015

[10] Kyarimpa CM, Böhmdorfer S, Wasswa J, Kiremire BT, Ndiege IO, Kabasa JD. Essential oil and composition of *Tagetes minuta* from Uganda. Larvicidal activity in Anopheles gambiae. Industrial Crops and Products. 2014;**62**:400-404

[11] Singh V, Singh B, Kaul VK. Domestication of wild marigold (*Tagetes minuta* L.) as a potential economic crop in the western Himalayas and northern plains of India. Economic Botany. 2003;**57**:535-544

[12] Gakuubi MM, Wanzala W, Wagacha JM, Dossaji SF. Bioactive properties of *Tagetes minuta* L. essential oils (Asteraceae): A review. American Journal of Essential Oils and Natural Products. 2016a;**4**:27-36

[13] Swati W, Srijana M, Vinod B, Rakshak K, Rakesh K. Variability in Chemical Composition and Antimicrobial Activity of Tagetes Minute L. Essential Oil Collected from Different Locations in the Himalayas. Vol. 112449. New Delhi, India: Academy of Scientific and Innovative Research; 2020

[14] Wanzala, Wycliffe, et al. Bioactive properties of essential oils from *Tagetes minuta* L. (Asteraceae): A review. American Journal of Essential Oils and Natural Products. AJEONP; 2016;**4**(2):27-36

[15] Santillán MPR, Coico FRM. Plants used in traditional medicine for viral respiratory conditions. Rebiol. 2020;**40**(1):109-130

[16] Preedy, Victor R, editors. Essential oils in food preservation, flavor and safety. Academic Press. 2015. ISBN: 978-0-12-416641-7. Available from: https:// store.elservier.com/

[17] Hüsnü K, Başer C, Demirci F. Chemistry of essential oils. Flavors and Fragrances. 2007;**1**:43-86

[18] Simard S, Hachey JM, Collin GJ. Variations in the composition of the essential oil during the extraction process. The case of Thuja occidentalis L. and Abies balsamea (L.) mill. Journal of Wood Chemistry and Technology. 1988;**8**:561-573

[19] Chalchat JC, Garry RP, Muhayimana A. Essential oil of *Tagetes minuta* from Rwanda and France: Chemical composition according to place of collection, stage of growth and part of the plant extracted. Journal of Essential Oil Research. 1995;**7**(4):375-386

[20] Salehi B, Valussi M, Morais-Braga MFB, Carneiro JNP, Leal A, Coutinho HDM, et al. *Tagetes* spp. essential oils and other extracts: Chemical characterization and biological activity. Molecules. 2018;**23**:2847

[21] Santos DCD, Schneider LR, da Silva Barboza T, Diniz Campos Â, Lund RG. Systematic review and technological overview of the antimicrobial activity of *tagetes minuta and* future prospects. Journal of Ethnopharmacology. 2017;**208**:8-15

[22] Gakuubi MM, et al. Chemical composition and antibacterial activity of essential oils of Tagetes minuta (Asteraceae) against selected plant pathogenic bacteria. International Journal of Microbiology. 2016;**2016**. Available from: https://doi. org/10.1155/2016/7352509

[23] Wanjala W, Wanzala W. Oils from Tagetes (Tagetes minuta). Essential oils in the preservation, flavor and safety of food. Academic Press. 2016. p. 791-802. DOI: 10.1016/ B978-0-12-416641-7.00090-0

[24] Senator F, Neapolitan F, Mohamed MAH, Harris PJC, Minkeni PNS, Henderson J. Antibacterial activity of minute tagetes L. essential oil (Asteraceae) with different chemical composition. Flavour and Fragrance Journal. 2004;**19**:574-578

[25] Rostaei M, Fallah S, Lorigooini Z, Abbasi Surki A. Crop productivity and chemical compositions of black cumin essential oil in single cultivation and intercropping with soybeans under contrasting fertilization. Industrial Crops and Products. 2018b;**125**:622-629. DOI: 10.1016/j.indcrop. 09.044

[26] Deba F, Xuan TD, Yasuda M, Tawata S. Chemical composition and antioxidant, antibacterial and antifungal activities of Bidens pilosa Linn essential oils. Var. Radiata. Food Control. 2008;**19**:346-352

[27] Tohidi B, Rahimmalek M, Arzani A. Composition of essential oils, total phenolic content, flavonoids and antioxidant activity of thymus species collected from different regions of Iran. Food Chemistry. 2017;**220**:153-161. DOI: 10.1016/j.foodchem.2020.127268

Chapter 10

Organic Culture Media for Sustainable Carotenoid Production from Microalgae

Wa Iba, Nur Illyin Akib, Ilham, La Ode Muhammad Jumardin, Bolo Arif, Nursainuddin, Sendry Yosalina and Jumtrisnanda Asmin Andas

Abstract

Antioxidants, particularly those carotenoid produced in microalgae, can be increased by induced stress, including light, nutrients, and salinity. Nutrient stress can be achieved by using imbalanced nutrients to boost antioxidant production without compromising the growth, that is, biomass. Culture media is an important factor in microalgae production because it is affecting growth and biomass production, as well as the biochemical content of microalgae. Synthetic or conventional culture media is considerably expensive for mass culture and the supply is limited, especially for developing countries. Therefore, there is a need for cheap and easily available culture media. This chapter discusses the use of organic media to culture several species of microalgae and cyanobacteria (*Arthrospira platensis*) for antioxidant production, particularly of those total carotenoids and beta carotene. The antioxidant content data mainly comes from our research with several organic culture media, such as fermented water hyacinth biomass, soybean processing waste, and Acadian Marine Plant Extract Powder (AMPEP). Carotenoid can be used for pharmaceuticals, including for anticancer, anti-inflammatory, and anti-obesity. Also, they can be used in aquaculture to increase cultured animals' health and immunity. Using organic media that may also serve as waste stream microalgae, which is aiding in a sustainable microalgae culture. Additional data presented in this chapter come from literature reviews of similar research topics.

Keywords: carotenoid, microalgae, organic, culture media

1. Introduction

Microalgae are microscopic organisms that are known to have very efficient photosynthesis capabilities. These organisms in nature are generally phytoplankton that acts as constituents of secondary metabolites in the form of natural pigments [1]. These natural pigments play an important role in microalgae photosynthesis and growth both for light harvesting and cell protection from stress, thus as an

 IntechOpen

antioxidant. Antioxidant compounds contained in microalgae can be pigments, such as chlorophyll, phycobilin protein, and carotenoids [2]. Microalgae produce different types of carotenoids, more than 40 carotene and xanthophylls have been isolated and characterized. Carotenoid compounds are natural pigments found in bacteria, algae, fungi, and plants but are not produced by animals.

Carotenoids are formed from eight isoprene molecules, so that they have 40 carbon atoms. In general, carotenoids are grouped into carotene (pure hydrocarbon carotenoids, having no oxygen atoms) and xanthophyll (oxygen atom-carrying carotenoids) [3]. Carotenoids have several types, including α-carotene, β-carotene, astaxanthin, lycopene, lutein, zeaxanthin, β-cryptoxanthin, and fucoxanthin [4–6]. Carotenoids also have perishable or degradable properties caused by light, heat, and oxygen, and prolonged exposure to those factors decreases the content of carotenoids in the biomaterial [7]. Carotenoids are organic pigments found in chloroplasts and chromoplasts of plants and other groups of organisms. Carotenoid compounds provide several health functions for the body, especially as antioxidants, that may protect the body from free radicals. Because of these functions, carotenoids are also applied to nutraceutical products [8]. These pigments are found in almost all classes of microalgae and can be used as pharmaceutical or health products because they can reduce the risk of developing cancer, vitamin A precursor for good vision and eye health, a strong immune system, and the health of the skin and mucus membranes. In the food industry, β-carotene is used as a pigment in food, in the pharmaceutical industry, β-carotene acts as a tablet coloring agent, and in the cosmetic industry, it is used as a bioactive ingredient in creams, which protects the skin from exposure to UV radiation [2–4].

Microalgae can be propagated by culture or cultivation in controlled closed photobioreactors or open ponds and raceways. Algae culture activities are one of the efforts to develop and meet the needs of carotenoid-producing microalgae. Microalgae in the process of their growth require macroelements of N and P and various other microelements to increase the growth rate and produce maximal nutrient content. The complete nutrient composition and proper concentration of nutrients determine biomass production and nutritional content of microalgae [9, 10]. Synthetic culture media commonly used for microalgae culture include Walne, Bold Basalt Medium (BBM), Conway, and F/2 media [9]. Meanwhile, organic media that have been used as microalgae culture media include seaweed waste [11], fermented water hyacinth [12], chicken manure [13], and brown seaweed extract [14]. Conventional culture media tend to be expensive and limited in availability for mass culture of microalgae, especially in developing countries. Using organic media is considered more sustainable and cheaper, particularly for the mass culture of microalgae. Also, culturing microalgae in organic media can be used as a bioremediation strategy and waste stream microalgae. Therefore, alternative culture media continues to be researched and developed. More importantly, organic media is considered as nutrient imbalances media, particularly of those N and P, and therefore may induce nutrient stress in microalgae that may lead to high production of carotenoid. This chapter discussed the use of several organic culture media, such as Acadian Marine Plant Extract Powder (AMPEP), fermented water hyacinth biomass, and soybean processing waste from tempeh production. These media were used to culture several species of microalgae in our lab, such as *Chlorella vulgaris, Dunaliella salina, Nannochloropsis* sp., *Tetraselmis* sp., and *Arthrospira (Spirulina) platensis,* that has been experimented in our lab for carotenoids, including β-carotene production.

2. Carotenoid biosynthesis in microalgae

Microalgae produce a variety of beneficial compounds, such as anticancer, anti-inflammatory compounds, antioxidants, vitamins, minerals, omega-3 fatty acids, and pigments [15]. One of the antioxidant compounds in microalgae is carotenoids, including β-carotene. Carotenoids exhibit biological activity as antioxidants, influencing cell growth regulation and modulating gene expression and immune responses. Carotenoids are natural pigments found in plant chloroplasts together with chlorophyll. Carotenoids act as additional pigments that help chlorophyll in absorbing light energy. The formation of carotenoids in microalgae increases in physiological conditions that are not balanced in cells caused by various environmental pressures, including nutrient content in nonoptimal media. This response is modulated by the phytoene synthase (PSY), an enzyme responsible for carotenoid biosynthesis in the photosynthetic organism. It is suggested that different PSY genes family is responsible for microalgae development and cell defense under environmental stress [3, 16]. Also, the composition and combination of nutrient content in the medium (C:N:P ratio) can affect the content of carotenoids in microalgae [17].

Carotenoids are synthesized in plastids through phytoene to lycopene synthesis and resulting in α- and β-carotene. The most common carotenoid used in several industries is β-carotene, which is a yellow, orange, or red organic pigment that occurs naturally in photosynthetic plants. β-Carotene can be fat-soluble, insoluble in water, and easily damaged by oxidizing at high temperatures. β-Carotene can be useful as a natural food coloring, antioxidant, and pro-vitamin A source for humans and can be beneficial in treating and preventing tumors and cancer [2–4]. β-Carotene can be commercially synthesized from natural source extraction. β-Carotene was found to accumulate in oil globules in thylakoids present in chloroplasts and consisted of two isomers, all-trans, and 9-cis β-carotene [18] (**Figure 1**).

β-Carotene biosynthesis begins with head-tail condensation on two molecules of C20 geranylgeranyl pyrophosphate (GGPP), resulting in C40 phytoene catalyzed by phytoene synthase (PSY). Phytoene is further modified gradually into β-carotene, neurosporent, lycopene by phytoene desaturase (PDS), β-carotene desaturase (ZDS), and carotenoid isomerase (CRTISO). There is an increase in the number of conjugated double bonds at each stage. The terminal structure of isoprene on lycopene molecules is further cyclized by lycopene β-cyclase (LCYB) and forms β-carotene (**Figure 2**). GGPP, PDS, ZDS, CRTISO, and LCYB coding genes are found in all terrestrial plants and algae. The path of carotenoid biosynthesis to the β-carotene stage has been conserved in these organisms [4, 19, 20]. Many other important carotenoid types are β-carotene derivatives, such as astaxanthin, zeaxanthin, and dinoxanthin (**Figure 2**).

Almost all types of carotenoids (**Figure 3**) are found in microalgae, but distribution is varied among classes and species. Carotenoids in algae contain allene

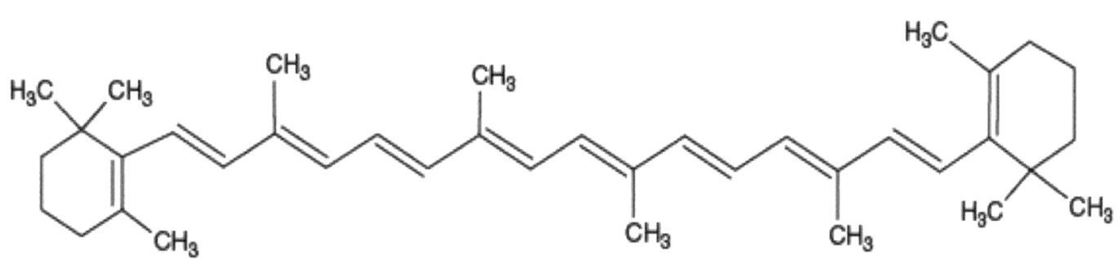

Figure 1.
Chemical structure of β-carotene [19].

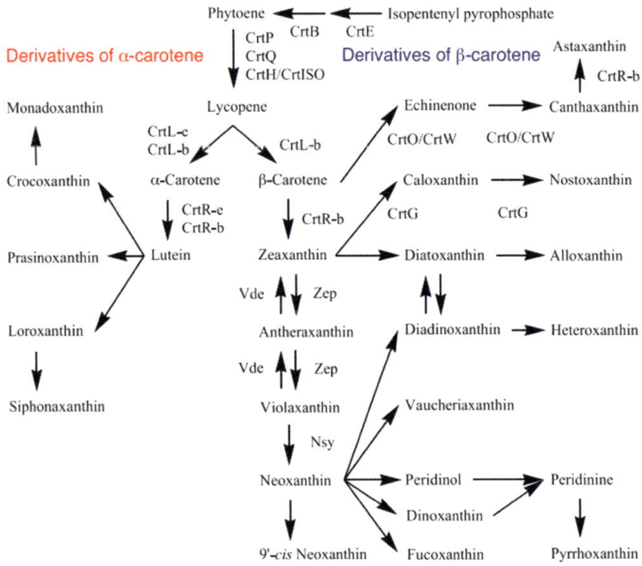

Figure 2.
Carotenoid biosynthesis in microalgae [4].

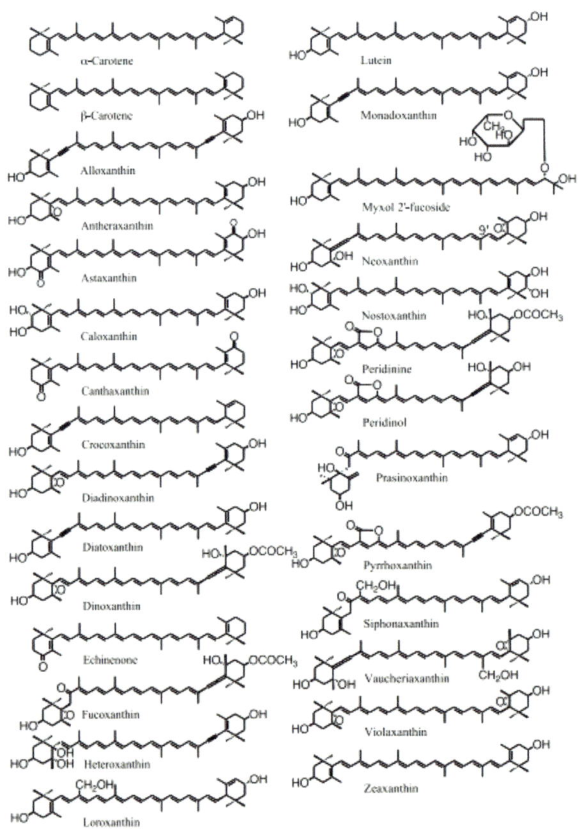

Figure 3.
Carotenoid structure found in microalgae [4].

(C=C=C) and acetylene (C≡C) bounds. Allenic carotenoids found in algae include fucoxanthin in brown algae and diatoms, 19′-acyloxyfucoxanthin in Haptophyta and Dinophyta, peridinin only in dinoflagellates, and 9′-cis neoxanthin in green algae. Whereas acetylenic carotenoids, such as alloxanthin, crocoxanthin, and monadoxanthin, are found in Cryptophyta, and diadinoxanthin and diatoxanthin in Heterokontophyta, Haptophyta, Dinophyta, and Euglenophyta. Acetylated carotenoids (-O-CO-CH3), such as fucoxanthin, peridinin, and dinoxanthin, are also mainly found in algae, such as Heterokontophyta, Haptophyta, and Dinophyta. Many cyanobacteria contain β-carotene, zeaxanthin, echinenone, and myxol pentosides (myxoxanthophyll), while some species lack part of these and some contain additional carotenoids, such as nostoxanthin, canthaxanthin, and oscillol dipentoside [4]. Several microalgae species are known to produce abundant carotenoid, and therefore commercially cultured include *Haematococcus pluvialis*, *Dunaliella salina*, *Chlorella vulgaris, Nannochloropsis* sp., and *Arthrospira (Spirulina)* sp.

3. Effect of organic culture media on carotenoid production in microalgae

The growth and carotenoid production in microalgae are affected by culture media through the availability of nutrients. The nutrient ratio of C/N/P is an important regulator in carotenoid production. Different concentrations of N and P are found in organic media as shown in our studies. This concentration was higher compared to Walne, a commercially available culture media commonly used for culturing microalgae and cyanobacteria (**Table 1**).

Optimal utilization of nutrients produces maximum growth indicated by high cell number and biomass one culture cycle, thus may affect carotenoid content. Media composition plays a role in nutrient utilization and pigment production of microalgae [25], including carotenoids [26]. A growth medium depleted in phosphorus content has a positive effect on the synthesis of β-carotene. The P element has a role in the process of energy metabolism, but the response to P stress in culture media is different for each microalgae species. Depleted P content in the microalgae growth medium of *Tetraselmis marina* increases its carotenoid content [27]. Conversely, the β-carotene content in *Oocystis* sp. can be improved by giving excess P nutrients. The highest β-carotene content in the microalgae *Oocystis* sp. was detected in induction treatment with a fivefold addition of KH_2PO_4 [28].

Some organic media that have been successfully used as microalgae culture media for carotenoid production are green bean sprouts extract for growth and carotenoid content of *D. salina* [29], lamtoro leaf extract medium for growth and contains carotenoids *Dunaliella* sp. [30] and fermented water hyacinth for the growth and carotenoids of *C. vulgaris*. We found that organic media from fermented hyacinths with a concentration of 0.1% was able to produce maximum *C. vulgaris* growth on the sixth day with a culture volume of 150 mL with a density value of 66.7×10^4 sel mL^{-1} with the highest carotenoid content of *C. vulgaris* obtained at a 1% organic media concentration of 0.545 μg mL^{-1} [31].

Other organic culture media that was experimented in our lab is brown seaweed extract or commercially sold as AMPEP. This is derived from extracts of brown algae (*Ascophyllum nodosum*), which have been used to increase the productivity of agricultural crops and have the potential to be used as a microalgae culture medium for the production of carotenoids. The experiment of microalgae grown for 7 days without the addition of *A. nodosum* extract was able to increase the cell density of *C. vulgaris*

Media	N (mg L^{-1})	P (mg L^{-1})	Reference
1	*2*	*3*	*4*
AMPEP	1.040	0.930	Our lab
Walne	0.00001	0.0002	Our lab
F/2	12.353	1.125	[21]
Fermented water hyacinth	0.67	190,143	[22]
Liquid hotel waste	13.35	0.43	[23]
Soybean processing waste (tofu)	8.74	1.06	[24]
Soybean processing waste (tempeh)	1.95	1.07	Our lab

Table 1.
N and P concentration in organic and synthetic culture media.

and *Scenedesmus* sp., whereas the addition of *A. nodosum* extract at concentrations of 3 and 4% inhibited the growth and antioxidant activity of *C. vulgaris* and *Scenedesmus sp*., although it was able to improve protein synthesis. Conversely, the addition of *A. nodosum* extract at low concentrations (1 and 2%) was able to increase the growth and antioxidant activity of *C. vulgaris* and *Scenedesmus* sp. [14]. Therefore, low doses of *A. nodosum* extract can be applied for the acceleration of microalgae cultivation and the production of antioxidants, particularly of those carotenoids. The use of AMPEP in low concentrations will be very profitable in terms of the cost and productivity of microalgae cultures for carotenoid production.

Our studies with 10 ppm AMPEP concentration for culturing *D. salina,* resulting in high biomass and *β-carotene* production at 418.1 × 10^4 cells mL^{-1} and 0.3545 μg mL^{-1}, respectively. Similar trends were found in our experiment when *Spirulina* sp. was cultured in the same AMPEP concentration, although the growth and carotenoid content were lower compared to *D. salina*. The growth and carotenoid content of *Arthrospira* (*Spirulina*) was also the highest in 0.1% of tempeh processing waste and 25% of moringa leaf extract [32]. Conversely, the lowest growth of *C. vulgaris* was found at 10 ppm AMPEP culture media but with the highest carotenoid content at 0.267 μg mL^{-1}. Our study indicated that different species responded differently in terms of growth and carotenoid content when using the same concentration of AMPEP (**Tables 2** and **3**). It seems that cyanobacteria *Arthrospira* sp. adapted well in different organic culture media except for AMPEP with good growth and considerably high carotenoid content (**Table 4**).

No	Culture media	S	L	T	D (10^4)	C	References
1.	Green bean sprout extract	30–35	16.2	20–23	477	0.97	[29]
2.	Lamtoro leaf extract	30	20.25	26	470	1.07	[30]
3.	Moringa leaf extract	30	27	25	1073	1.39	[32]
4.	AMPEP	30	16.2	29–30	418	0.36	Our Lab
5.	*Walne*	30	16.2	29–30	347	0.17	Our Lab

Notes: S = salinity (ppt), L = light intensity (μmoles m^{-2} s^{-1}), T = temperature (°C), D = cells density (cells mL^{-1}), and C = β-carotene (carotenoid) = μg mL^{-1}.

Table 2.
β-Carotene and carotenoid content of D. salina cultured in various organic culture media.

No.	Media	Culture condition					Carotenoid (μg mL^{-1})	Reference
		V	P	S	pH	I		
1.	AMPEP	1.000	12:12	32	8	19	0.27	Our lab
2.	Walne	18.000	12:12	30	8	1.49	0.24	[33]
3.	F/2	150	12:12	30	7	10	0.52	
4.	Fermented water hyacinth	149.85	12:12	30	7	10	0.54	Our Lab
5.	BG-11	18.000	12:12	30	8	1.49	0.33	[33]
6.	Beneck	18.000	12:12	30	8	1.49	0.31	[33]

Notes: V = culture volume (mL), P = photoperiod (dark: light), S = salinity (psu), and I = light intensity (μmol photon $m^{-1} s^{-2}$).

Table 3.
Carotenoid content of C. vulgaris cultured in various organic media.

No.	Culture media	P	V	B	L	S	Sh	C	References
1.	*Walne*	12:12	2	Glass beaker	40.48	30	20–30	0.00183	Hanani et al., [34]
2.	Hearing waste	12:12	1	Glass beaker	25.64	30	25–29	0.5459	Pramusinta et al. [26]
3.	*Zarrouk*	12:12	0.4	Erlenmeyer	53.97	15	29	5.346	Fakhri et al. [35]
4.	*Walne*	12:12	0.2	Plastic bottle	13.49	29–30	28–30	0.98	
5.	Tempeh processing waste	12:12	0.2	Plastic bottle	13.49	29–30	28–30	0.80–1.70	
6	AMPEP	12:12	0.3	Plastic bottle	13.49	29–30	28–30	0.0691	
7	*Walne*	12:12	0.3	Plastic bottle	13.49	29–30	28–30	0, 1354	

Note: *P = photoperiod (jam), V = culture volume (L), B = bioreactor, I = intensitas cahaya (μmol photon s^{-1} m^{2}), S = salinitas (psu/ppt), Sh = Suhu (°C), C = karotenoid (μg mL^{-1}).*

Table 4.
Carotenoid content of A. platensis *cultured in various media.*

The content of carotenoids in microalgae is highly dependent on the species cultured and the media used. In addition, cell density, culture volume, bioreactor, light intensity, salinity, and temperature also affect the carotenoid content (**Tables 3** and **4**). The difference in carotenoid content from each study is thought to be due to differences in nutrient content in each medium used as well as supporting factors that affect such as light, salinity, pH, and temperature. All such factors must be in optimum conditions for maximum microalgae cell growth and carotenoid content.

In our lab, the standard culture condition for carotenoid production in microalgae is 28–30°C, salinity of 29–30 psu, pH 7–8, and light intensity of 16.2 μmoles m^{-2} s^{-1} [31]. Besides organic culture media, these conditions have been proven to induce stress during microalgae culture, thus the carotenoid content in cultured species.

4. Conclusion

Organic culture media, such as fermented water hyacinth, tempeh processing waste, and AMPEP, can be used to culture several microalgae species, including D. salina and C. vulgaris, and cyanobacteria *A. platensis*. However, AMPEP is not ideal for culture *A. platensis* for carotenoid production and may need some adjustment to its N and P content.

Author details

Wa Iba[1*], Nur Illyin Akib[2], Ilham[3], La Ode Muhammad Jumardin[4], Bolo Arif[4], Nursainuddin[4], Sendry Yosalina[4] and Jumtrisnanda Asmin Andas[4]

1 Faculty of Fisheries and Marine Sciences, Aquaculture Department, University of Halu Oleo, Kendari, South East Sulawesi, Indonesia

2 Faculty of Pharmacy, Pharmacy Department, University of Halu Oleo, Kendari, South East Sulawesi, Indonesia

3 Fisheries Resources Section, Directorate General of Capture Fisheries, Ministry of Marine Affairs and Fisheries, Jakarta, Indonesia

4 Faculty of Mathematics and Life Sciences, Biotechnology Department, University of Halu Oleo, Kendari, South East Sulawesi, Indonesia

*Address all correspondence to: wa.iba@uho.ac.id

References

[1] Rafaelina M, Rustam Y, Amini S. Growth and antioxidant activity of microalgae *Porphyridium cruentum* and *Chlorella* sp. (in Indonesian). Jurnal Bioma. 2015;**12**:12-21. DOI: 10.21009/bioma11(1).2

[2] Fabrowska J, Leska B, Schroeder G, Messyasz B, Pikosz M. Biomass and extracts of algae as material for cosmetics. In: Se-Kwon K, Katarzyna C, editors. Marine Algae Extracts: Processes, Products and Applications. Weinheim, Germany: Wiley-VCHVerlag GmbH & Co.; 2015. pp. 681-706

[3] Kiokias S, Proestos C, Varzakas T. A review of the structure, biosynthesis, absorption of carotenoids-analysis and properties of their common natural extracts. Current Research in Nutrition and Food Science. 2016;**4**:25-37

[4] Takaichi S. Carotenoids in algae: Distributions, biosyntheses and functions. Marine Drugs. 2011;**9**:1101-1118. DOI: 10.3390/md9061101

[5] Wrolstad RE, Culver CA. Alternatives to those artificial FD & C food colorants. Annual Review of Food Science and Technology. 2012;**3**:59-77. DOI: 10.1146/annurev-food-022811-101118

[6] Rodriguez-Amaya DB. Structures and analysis of carotenoid molecules. Sub-Cellular Biochemistry. 2016;**79**:71-108. DOI: 10.1007/978-3-319-39126-7_3

[7] Mertz C, Brat P, Caris-Veyrat C, Gunata Z. Characterization and thermal lability of carotenoids and vitamin C of tamarillo fruit (*Solanum betaceum* Cav.). Food Chemistry. 2010;**119**:653-659

[8] Honda M. Nutraceutical and pharmaceutical applications of carotenoids. In: Jacob-Lopes E, Queiroz M, Zepka L, editors. Pigments from Microalgae Handbook. Cham: Springer; 2020. pp. 449-469. DOI: 10.1007/978-3-030-50971-2_18

[9] Iba W, Rice MA, Wikfors G.H. Microalgae in eastern pacific white shrimp, Litopenaeus vannamei (Boone 1931) hatcheries: A review on roles and culture environments. Asian Fisheries Science Journal. 2014;**27**: 212-233. DOI: 10.33997/j.afs.2014.27.3.005

[10] Iba W, Rice MA, Maranda L, Wikfors GH. Growth characteristics of newly isolated Indonesian microalgae under different salinity. Indonesian Aquaculture Journal. 2018;**13**:71-81. DOI: 10.15578/iaj.13.2.2018.71-81

[11] Komarawidjaja W. Study on utilization of solid waste from seaweed processing industry as culture Media of *Chlorella* sp (In Indonesian). Jurnal Teknologi Lingkungan. 2011;**12**:241-250. DOI: 10.29122/jtl.v12i3.1232

[12] Iba W, Utami C, Balubi AM. The growth of *Chlorella vulgaris* cultured in liquid organic fertilizer of water hyacinth (*Eichhornia crassipes*) at different salinities. Aquacultura Indonesiana. 2019;**20**:117-126. DOI: 10.21534/ai.v20i2.158

[13] Padang CY. Potential of Chicken Manure as Culture Media of *Chlorella vulgaris* Beyerinck [Beijerinck], (1890) for Single Cell Protein Production (In Indonesian). South East Sulawesi: University of Halu Oleo; 2021

[14] Shi P, Geng S, Feng T, Wu H. Effects of *Ascophyllum nodosum* extract on growth and antioxidant Defense Systems of two Freshwater Microalgae. Journal of Applied Phycology. 2018;**30**:851-859. DOI: 10.1007/s10811-017-1287-z

[15] Novoveská L, Ross ME, Stanley MS, Pradelles R, Wasiolek V, Sassi JF. Microalgal carotenoids: A review of production, current markets, regulations, and future direction. Marine Drugs. 2019;**17**:1-21. DOI: 10.3390/md17110640

[16] Paniagua-Michel J, Olmos-Soto J, Ruiz MA. Pathways of carotenoid biosynthesis in bacteria and microalgae. Methods in Molecular Biology. 2012;**892**:1-12. DOI: 10.1007/978-1-61779-879-5_1. PMID: 22623294

[17] Suárez-Quintana WH, García-Rico RO, García-Martínez JB, Urbina-Suarez NA, López-Barrera GL, Barajas-Solano AF, et al. Enhancement of metabolite production in high-altitude microalgal strains by optimized C/N/P ratio. Applied Sciences. 2022;**12**:6779. DOI: 10.3390/app12136779

[18] Kleinegris MMD, Janssen M, Brandenburg WA, Wijffels HR. Continuous production of carotenoids from *Dunaliella salina*. Enzyme and Microbial Technology. 2011;**48**:253-259. DOI: 10.1016/j.enzmictec.2010.11.005

[19] Marino T, Casella P, Sangiorgio PV, Ferraro A, Hristoforou E, Molino A, et al. Natural beta-carotene: A microalgae derivate for nutraceutical applications. Chemical. Engineering Transactions. 2020;**79**:103-108. DOI: 10.3303/CET2079018

[20] Ye ZW, Jiang JG, Wu H. Biosynthesis and regulation of carotenoids in *Dunaliella*: Progresses and prospects. Biotechnology Advances. 2008;**25**:352-360. DOI: 10.1016/j.biotechadv.2008.03.004

[21] El Nabris KJA. Development of cheap and simple culture medium for the microalgae *Nannochloropsis* sp. based on agricultural grade fertilizers available in the local market of Gaza Strip (Palestine). Journal of Al Azhar University-Gaza (Natural Sciences). 2012;**14**:61-76

[22] Goa S, Iba W, Indrayani. Effect of organic fertilizer water hyacinth (*Eichhornia crassipes*) dosages on the growth of *Chlorella vulgaris* (In Indonesian). Jurnal Media Akuatika. 2019;**4**:68-76

[23] Wahid AR. The Potential of Microalgae *Chlorella vulgaris* to Decrease the Pollutants Concentration in Liquid Hotel Waste. South East Sulawesi: University of Halu Oleo; 2020

[24] Dianursanti RBT, Gumelar MT, Abdullah TH. Industrial tofu wastewater as a cultivation medium of microalgae *Chlorella vulgaris*. Energy Procedia. 2014;**47**:56-61. DOI: 10.1016/j.egypro.2014.01.196

[25] Sujatha K, Nagarajan P. Optimization of growth conditions for carotenoid production from *Spirulina platensis* (Geitler). International Journal of Current Microbiology and Applied Science. 2013;**10**:325-328. Available from: http://ijcmas.com/vol-2-10/

[26] Pramusinta G, Masithah D, Rahardja S. Effect of waste liquid hearing fish fertilizer of *Spirulina platensis* carotenoid content (in Indonesian). Journal of Marine and Coastal Science. 2012;**1**:91-100

[27] Moussa IDB, Chtourou H, Karray F, Sayadi M, Dhouib A. Nitrogen or phosphorus repletion strategies for enhancing lipid or carotenoid production from *Tetraselmis marina*. Bioresource Technology. 2017;**238**:325-332

[28] Elfiza WN, Dharma A, Nasir N. Screening of carotenoid producing microalgae and study of the effect of nitrogen and phosphorus stress on the production of β-carotene in microalgae

Oocystis sp (in Indonesian). JPB Kelautan dan Perikanan. 2019;**14**:9-20. DOI: 10.15578/jpbkp.v14i1.598

[29] Dianita I, Hasibuan S, Syafriadiman. Effect of green bean (*Phaseolus radiatus*) sprouts fertilizer on density and carotenoid content of *Dunaliella salina* (in Indonesian). Jurnal Perikanan Dan Kelautan. 2020;**25**:18-26

[30] Mahardani D, Putri B, Hudaidah S. Effect of different salinity on the growth and carotenoids content of *Dunaliella* sp. in Lamtoro (*Leucaena leucocephala*) Leaf Extract Media (in Indonesian). Jurnal Perikanan Dan Kelautan. 2017;**7**:50-58

[31] Iba W, Nur I, Suryani A, Jumardin L, Nurani G. Culture method of microalgae (*Chlorella vulgaris*) in liquid fertilizer from fermented water hyacinth (*Eichornia Crassipes*) for carotenoid production (In Indonesian, Patent). Registered in Indonesia no. IDS000005004. 2022

[32] Wahyuni N, Rahardja BS, Azhar MH. The effect of giving combination concentration of leaves of *Moringa oleifera* with Walne fertilizer in culture media on the growth and content of carotenoids in *Dunaliella salina*. Journal of Aquaculture Science. 2019;**4**:37-49. DOI: 10.31093/joas.v4i1.67

[33] Wijoseno T. The Effect of Culture Media Variations on Growth Rate and Content of Proteins, Lipids, Chlorophyll, and Carotenoids in *Chlorella vulgaris* Buitenzorg Microalgae. Jakarta: Universitas Indonesia; 2011

[34] Hanani T, Ita W, Susanto AB. Beta carotene content of spirulina platensis cultured under different period of light intensity (in Indonesian). Buletin Oseanografi Marina. 2020;**1**:55-58. DOI: 10.14710/buloma.v9i1.24681

[35] Fakhri M, Prive W, Antika, Arning WE, Nasrullah BA. Growth, pigment and protein production of spirulina platensis under different $Ca(NO_3)_2$ concentrations (in Indonesian). Journal of Aquaculture and Fish Health. 2020;**1**:38-47. DOI : 10.20473/jafh.v9i1. 15769

Section 3

Applications of Antioxidants from Natural Origin

Chapter 11

Elaboration of a Purple Corn Drink with Maximum Retention of Anthocyanins

Genaro Christian Pesantes Arriola, Víctor Alexis Higinio Rubio, Carlos Enrique Chinchay Barragán, Enrique Gustavo García Talledo, César Ángel Durand Gonzales and Wilmer Huamani Palomino

Abstract

In the present work, the anthocyanin extraction process was characterized during the elaboration of a purple corn drink, using the response surface analysis method with temperature intervals between 47.57 and 132.43°C, and times from 11, 36 at 138.64 minutes. In addition, with the stationary point technique, the maximum retention of anthocyanin (33.99 mg/g) was determined at a temperature of 98.39°C at a time of 105.89 minutes of extraction. Since this time is too long and to reduce production costs, without resorting to considerable losses of anthocyanins, canonical analysis was used, redefining the optimal extraction parameters at a temperature of 100°C for 60 minutes with a reduction of the anthocyanin content of 2.49% (33.14 mg/g) concerning the maximum, a value that is within the optimum area of performance of the process. With the extract obtained under optimal conditions, a drink was prepared and, using the differential pH method and Student's t-test ($p = 0.05$), its anthocyanin content was quantified and compared with that of a commercial drink with typical characteristics. Similar, observing that the elaborated drink presents higher contents, whose difference varies within the range of 2.79 and 4.72 mg/mL. Finally, using a satisfaction test with a nine-point hedonic scale, it was determined that the beverage was "very well liked" by a semi-trained sensory panel.

Keywords: purple corn, anthocyanin, optimization, response surface, canonical analysis

1. Introduction

The cultivation of purple corn is of growing economic importance in Peru, mainly for producers in the mountains who have few possibilities of generating economic income from the sale of agricultural products that they produce on their plots. In recent years, the consumption of purple corn has intensified, in the country and abroad, because the purple pigment that this type of corn has (anthocyanins) prevents diseases such as colon cancer, and reduces obesity and diabetes, among other diseases; likewise, it is a natural colorant for the industry. Among the anthocyanins of purple corn, cyanidin-3-glucoside is found in greater quantity, constituting a powerful natural antioxidant [1].

Purple corn is a vegetable resource native to Andean Peru and to which an interesting biological activity as an antioxidant is attributed, due to the type of bioactive compounds it contains. Due to the increased demand for this plant resource and its derivatives in the national and international market, efforts have been made in the country to expand the cultivation areas and introduce improved varieties of purple corn that can be adapted to these new cultivation areas. and that they improve the production and commercialization of this resource [2].

Antioxidants are responsible for stabilizing free radicals by transferring electrons and hydrogen atoms, and they also have the ability to inhibit oxidative degradation such as lipoperoxidation. For this reason, they play an important role in the prevention of various degenerative diseases such as cancer, diabetes, obesity, high blood pressure [3–5].

Within this group of antioxidants are anthocyanins, natural dyes that belong to the group of flavonoids, because they have a characteristic structure of C6-C3-C6 (**Figure 1**). Its basic structure is the flavylium group (2-phenylbenzopyrylium). These pigments are responsible for giving the pink, red, blue, mauve and violet color of flowers, fruits and vegetables, they are polar compounds, which allows them to be soluble in ethanol and water. Anthocyanins are glycosides that have a sugar in position 3 linked by the ß-glycosidic bond that, when broken, forms the aglycone, known as anthocyanidin, the most common being: pelargonidine, cyanidin, delphinidin, peonidin, malvidin and petunidin [6–10]. On the other hand, pelargonidin-3-glucoside, peonidin-3-glucoside, cyanidin-3-glucoside and the acylated forms of each of them were found in purple corn from the Andean region of Peru [11].

In the Peruvian market, two commercial beverages based on purple corn are offered; however, the industry has prioritized the sanitary quality of the product before the beneficial effect on health provided by anthocyanins due to their antioxidant capacity and the phenolic compounds present in their chemical structure [12].

The extraction of anthocyanins depends on the temperature and extraction time, being favored by the 20% ethanolic medium and pH between 1 and 4 [13]. While, used solutions as solvents hydroalcoholic (ethanol or methanol) acidified with acetic acid, concluding that the acid methanol is more effective for extraction, although its toxicity prevents it from being used when the extracted substances will be used for human consumption [8]. On the other hand, recommend using water, methanol, or

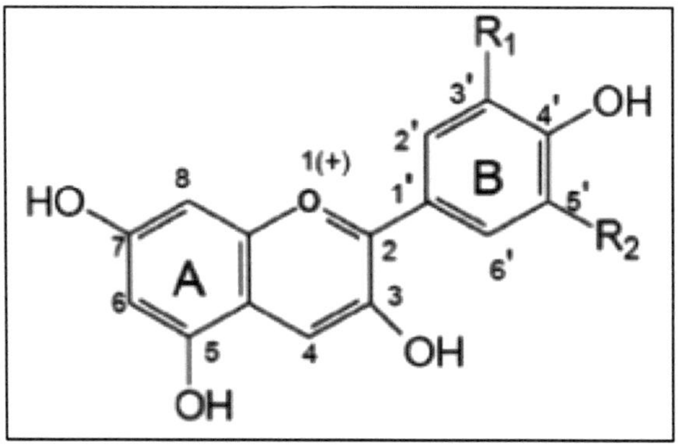

Figure 1.
Basic structure of anthocyanins.

ethanol acidified with hydrochloric acid at a pH between 4 and 5 at a temperature between 70 and 100°C as solvents, to avoid pigment degradation [14]. The extraction using an ethanolic solution as solvent acidified with hydrochloric acid by immersion for 15 minutes in an ultrasound bath; finally, the appropriate extraction conditions take place in an aqueous medium with a contact time of 120 minutes and a limit temperature of 50°C [15, 16]. All the aforementioned extraction techniques were carried out under laboratory conditions using inorganic acids as acidifying agents and alcoholic solutions as solvents; conditions that cannot be reproduced on an industrial scale due to the high toxicity of said compounds.

In this sense, the present work aims to determine the optimal physical parameters of time and temperature for the extraction of anthocyanins from corn earns to fortify a commercial purple corn drink.

2. Materials and method

A Central Composite Rotational Design (DCCR) was carried out with 4 factorial points, 4 axial points, and 5 repetitions in the central points, having a total of 13 treatments. The independent variables or "Factors" of the design were factor A (X1): Temperature, with a low level at 60°C, a high level at 120°C, the central point at 90°C and axial points at 47.57°C and 132.43°C); and factor B (X2): Time, with a low level at 30 min, high level at 120 min, a central point at 75 min and its axial points at 11.36 min and 138.64 min as shown in **Table 1**.

The purple corn cobs used came from the Majes district of the department of Arequipa, Peru, located between 200 and 800 meters above sea level, with an average annual temperature between 14 and 32°C.

Natural Variables		Coded Variables	
Factor A: Temperature	**Factor B: Time**	**X1**	**X2**
60	30	−1	−1
120	30	+1	−1
60	120	−1	+1
120	120	+1	+1
90	75	0	0
90	75	0	0
90	75	0	0
90	75	0	0
90	75	0	0
132.43	75	$\sqrt{2}$	0
47.57	75	$-\sqrt{2}$	0
90	138.64	0	$\sqrt{2}$
90	11.36	0	$-\sqrt{2}$

Source: self made.

Table 1.
Design of Experiments Matrix.

The present research work was carried out in the Food Technology laboratories of the Chucuito Pilot Plant, of the Faculty of Fisheries and Food Engineering of the National University of Callao, and Bromatology of the Faculty of Pharmacy and Biochemistry of the University Inca Garcilaso de la Vega.

2.1 Obtaining the anthocyanin extract

The ears were selected to discard those that have symptoms of deterioration or perceptible damage, then they were shelled to remain only with the shelled ears in the next stage of the process, later they were rolled in a circular shape with an approximate thickness of 3 mm and dried. in an oven at a temperature of 65°C for 2 hours, until reaching an approximate humidity of 8%.

The shelled and dehydrated cobs were ground with a manual mortar and diluted in a ratio of 2.5 g. in 100 mL of extraction solution (treated water adjusted to pH 2 with citric acid), applying the times and temperatures as indicated in **Table 1**, to develop the experimental model.

Subsequently, the temperature of the extract was brought below 30°C to filter it through a 1 mm diameter mesh.

2.2 Anthocyanin quantification

The quantification of the content of anthocyanins was expressed as mg of cyanidin 3-glucoside/g of shelled cob, was used, where an aliquot of 0.3 ml of extract was diluted in 2.7 mL of buffer solution of potassium chloride (pH 1) and sodium acetate (pH 4.5), separately, leaving it to stand for 20 minutes [17]. Finally proceeding to read their respective absorbances as indicated in the following expression:

$$\text{Total anthocyanins}\left(\text{mg}/\text{L}\right) = \text{A x PM x FD x 1000}/\left(\text{n x l}\right)$$

Where:

TA = cyanidin 3-glucoside content; A = (A510 – A700) pH 1 - (A510 – A700) Ph 4.5; MW = molecular weight; DF = dilution factor; 1000 = conversion factor from grams to milligrams; ϵ = molar extinction factor (26900) for cyanidin 3-glucoside; l = cell length.

Subsequently, the data were analyzed to obtain the response surface, identifying the point of maximum performance through the stationary point methodology,

2.3 Response surface methodology

The response surface methodology was applied to the response variable using the commercial statistical software Design Expert Version 5.0 (Stat-Ease, Minneapolis, USA). Second-order polynomials were fitted to the data to obtain regression equations for the response variables analyzed. The graph of the response surfaces, the variance analysis, and the determination coefficients (R^2) was generated with the same software. Then, the canonical analysis of the data was performed to adjust the optimal point of the process.

2.4 Preparation of the drink and comparison of the anthocyanin content with that of a commercial drink

For this, the purple corn drink was prepared, for which the purple corn extract obtained using the optimal parameters determined in the previous point was diluted with treated water at a temperature of 78°C in a volumetric ratio of 2 of treated water and 1 of extract. Subsequently, the drink was standardized until it reached a pH of 3, an acidity content of 0.2% citric acid, and 13°Brix. The mixture was pasteurized at 72°C for 10 minutes and then bottled in glass bottles with a capacity of 250 mL, amber color, and screw cap.

Finally, the anthocyanin content was determined in triplicate, in the drink made under the aforementioned conditions, and in a commercial purple corn drink. The mean values were compared using the t-Student test ($p = 0.05$).

2.5 Satisfaction degree test

It was carried out with 50 students of the eighth cycle of the Professional School of Food Engineering of the National University of Callao, who had completed the Sensory Analysis of Food subject, following the methodology [18].

3. Results and discussion

3.1 Anthocyanin quantification and application of the response surface methodology

The yield of anthocyanins in the extracts obtained with the different treatments tested is shown in **Table 2**.

To determine if the anthocyanin extraction levels were within the region of maximum yield, the fit was made to a second-order polynomial model [19] (**Table 3**).

Based on the fact that the Fc of the lack of fit is much lower than the Ft, for a significance level of 0.5%, it can be concluded with a statistical significance level

Natural Variables		Anthocyanin Content (mg/g)
Factor A: Temperature	Factor B: Time	
60	30	25.856
120	30	31.056
60	120	28.918
120	120	32.802
90	75	32.761
90	75	33.012
90	75	33.405
90	75	33.212
90	75	34.219
132.43	75	29.642
47.57	75	25.971
90	138.64	33.489
90	11.36	29.969

Source: self made.

Table 2.
Design of Experiments Matrix.

Source of Variation	**Degrees of freedom**	**Sum of squares**	**Middle Square**	F_c	F_t
Model	5	93.34	18.67	60.49	22.46
Factor A	1	25.47	25.47	82.55	31.33
Factor B	1	11.97	11.97	38.79	31.33
Factor A^2	1	54.30	54.30	175.94	31.33
Factor B^2	1	4.75	4.75	15.39	31.33
Interaction AB	1	0.43	0.43	1.40	31.33
Residual	7	3.26	0.45		
Lack of Adjustment	3	1.92	0.64	2.08	31.33
Mistake	4	1.23	0.31		
Total	12	96.49			

Table 3.
Analysis of variance table for a second order model.

of 99.5% that the second-order model is an adequate approximation to the actual behavior of the experiment. Therefore, the second-order equation was established to predict anthocyanin yields when the food matrix is subjected to the extraction factors that are the object of this study. The analysis of the yields of anthocyanins obtained with the Desing Expert Version 5.0 software, allowed us to calculate the values of the regression coefficients that are presented in **Table 4**.

The equation obtained to predict the content of anthocyanins was:

$$Y = -3.07 + 0.64X1 + 0.11X2 - 0.00024X1X2 - 0.003X12 - 0.82X22$$

Where: Y = yield of anthocyanins in mg of cyanidin 3-glucoside/g of shelled cob; X1 = temperature in °C; X2 = time in minutes. This corroborates that the established mathematical model describes the anthocyanin extraction process very closely to reality under the pre-established experimental conditions and within the study region.

Coefficients	**Anthocyanin content (mg/g)**
Constant β_o	−3.07
Linear	
β_1 (Temperature)	0.64
β_2 (Time)	0.11
Interaction	
β_3 (Time*Temperature)	−0.00024
Quadratic	
β_4 (Time*Time)	−0.003
β_5 (Temperature*Temperature)	−0.82
R^2	0.96
Source: self made.	

Table 4.
Values of the regression coefficients obtained in the anthocyanin extraction process.

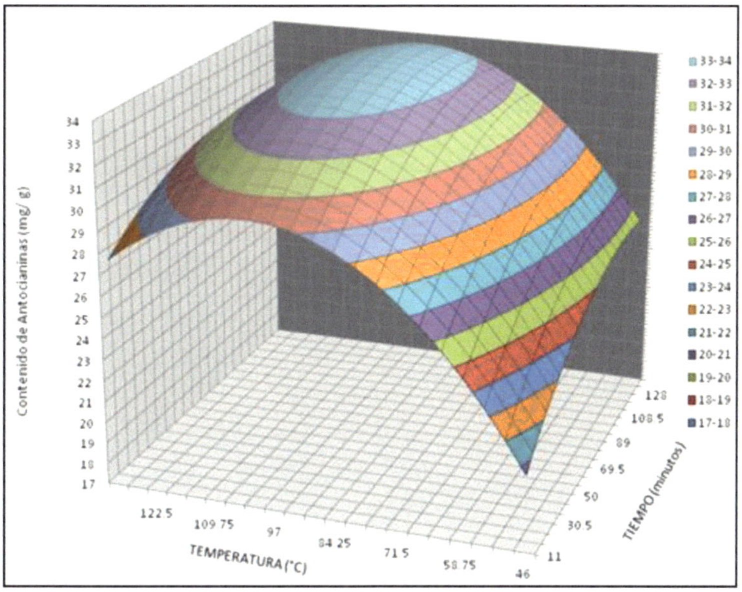

Figure 2.
Response surface of the experiment.

This is important to highlight, since the equation obtained should not be used for extrapolate data outside the study range or for conditions other than those pre-established in the design. With this equation, we proceeded to characterize the response surface shown in **Figure 2**, for this the adjusted data of the experiment were used.

Figure 2 shows the behavior of the process against the factors of temperature and time, where overexposure to high temperatures and times causes a decrease in | performance by degradation of anthocyanins. The auxiliary graph or contour graph was also made to facilitate the interpretation of the response surface and the region of the maximum performance of the process, which can be seen in green in **Figure 3**.

With the use of the stationary point methodology, it was obtained that the highest yield of anthocyanins (33.99 mg/g) is obtained at a temperature of 98.39°C and 105.89 minutes of extraction, maintaining preset pH values and the shelled cob/solvent ratio. However, a time of approximately 106 minutes is excessive and represents high power consumption. From the analysis of **Figure 3**, it was deduced that the extraction process has a greater dependence on temperature than on extraction time, so it was decided to reduce the time to the minimum possible without leaving the zone of maximum yield and using parameters of the time and temperature variables that present operational ease in a process at an industrial level. For this reason, the canonical analysis of the results was performed, obtaining an extraction yield of 33.08 mg/g for a temperature of 96.29°C and a time of 59.50 min. These new extraction parameters are very advantageous compared to those with higher yields, however, in an industrial process, they are difficult to maintain constant and even to achieve exactly, so it was decided to explore the neighborhood of the new parameters obtained, in the order to establish as optimal points of the process, those that are also easy to operationalize.

Based on the results in **Table 5**, it was decided to operate the extraction process at a temperature of 100°C for 60 minutes, reaching an anthocyanin yield of 33,144 mg/g. Comparing these parameters with the highest yield initially obtained, it can be seen

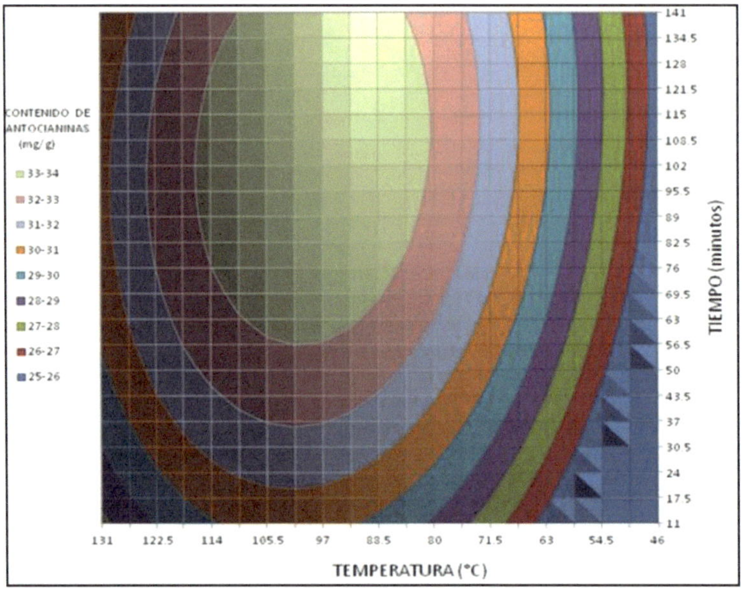

Figure 3.
Contour plot of the response surface of the experiment.

Natural variables		Performance (mg/g)
Temperature (X_1)	Time (X_2)	
95	55	32,860
100	55	32.950
95	60	33.061
100	60	33.144

Source: self made.

Table 5.
Exploration of the optimal point of the extraction process.

that with a temperature increase of 2°C the extraction time was reduced by 45% with only a 2.49% decrease in the yield of anthocyanins.

3.2 Comparison of the anthocyanin content of the beverage made with a commercial beverage

Table 6 shows the average values and standard deviation of the anthocyanin content in the samples evaluated. The difference test showed that the elaborated beverage had a significantly higher average anthocyanin content ($p = 0.05$) than that of the commercial beverage, this difference is found in a range between 2.79 and 4.72 mg/mL.

3.3 Satisfaction degree test

According to the hedonic scale of acceptability, the attribute color and flavor obtained average ratings of 8.28 and 7.64 (**Figure 4**), which is equivalent to saying

Nomenclature	Variable	Value
Average content of anthocyanins of the beverage made with the optimal parameters (mg/mL)	Y_1	33.138
Average anthocyanin content of the commercial beverage (mg/mL)	Y_2	29.380
Estimation of the sample variance	S_p^2	1.4250
Sample size of the brewed beverage	n_1	13
Commercial drink sample size	n_2	13
Significance level	A	0.05
Calculated statistical variable	T_c	8.0246
Tabulated statistical variable	T_t	2.064

Source: self made.

Table 6.
Summary of the comparison of means test.

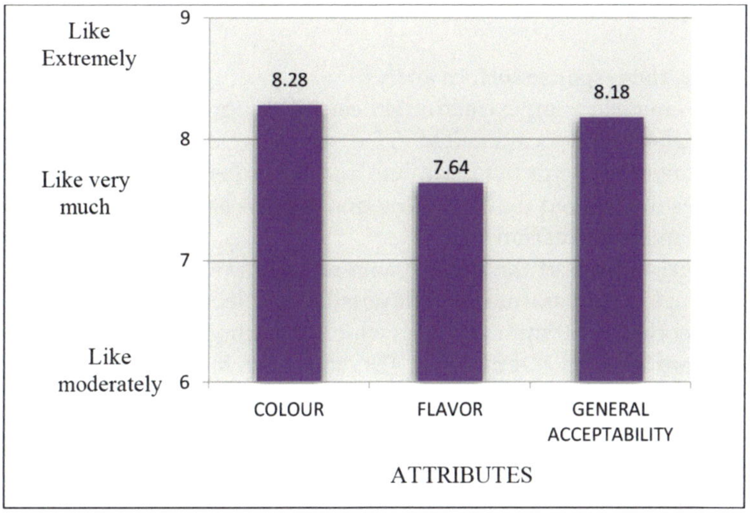

Figure 4.
Degree of satisfaction with the drink.

that the color was "liked a lot" and the flavor "liked a lot", respectively. The average of the general acceptability was 8.18, that is, "liked a lot", which indicated that the flavor attribute does not significantly affect ($p = 0.05$) the general acceptability of the beverage made with the optimal parameters.

4. Discussions

Carried out the extraction of anthocyanins from shelled ears of purple corn at different pH, solvents, temperatures, and times, observing that for a process at pH 2, and using water as the solvent, a maximum yield was obtained (33.509 mg/g) at a temperature of 90°C and a time of 240 minutes, yield very similar to that obtained in the present work (33.14 mg/g), using the same pH and solvent, but at a temperature of 100°C and a time of 60 minutes [13]. That is, by increasing the extraction temperature by 10°C, it is possible to reduce the process by 3 hours, which allows for increasing the production volumes of a purple corn drink and a significant reduction in the cost of producing the product.

On the other hand, it has been shown that the anthocyanin extraction process depends mainly on the temperature, rather than on the extraction time; because in recent works, an anthocyanin content of 22.68 mg/g in an extract obtained from the same raw material (shelled cobs), using water as a solvent, but at a temperature of 50°C with contact times of 120 minutes [16].

An important factor to consider is the type of statistical treatment used in the study of the extraction process only carried out the variance analysis of the different factors considered, which allowed to select the best combination of the different levels of the tested factors; while in the present study the response surface analysis was carried out, the same one that allows characterizing the entire process within the range under study and optimizing it [13, 16].

5. Conclusion

In this study, the response surface analysis was a useful technique to forecast a hight anthocyanin yield in an extraction process of this molecule from earns corn. We obtained the highest anthocyanin yield (33.99 mg/g) at 98.39°C after 105.89 minutes of extraction, maintaining preset pH values and the hulled ears/solvent ratio. In addition, the results showed that the extraction process has a higher dependence on temperature than the extraction time.

The canonical analysis of the anthocyanin retention results in the vicinity of the maximum retention temperature made it possible to select an extraction temperature of 100°C for a period of 60 minutes, with which an anthocyanin yield of 33.144 mg/g (2.49% below optimal yield), but with a 45% reduction in extraction time.

Author details

Genaro Christian Pesantes Arriola[1*], Víctor Alexis Higinio Rubio[1], Carlos Enrique Chinchay Barragán[1], Enrique Gustavo García Talledo[1], César Ángel Durand Gonzales[1] and Wilmer Huamani Palomino[2]

1 National University of Callao, Callao, Perú

2 Facultad de Ingenieria Pesquera y de Aiimentos, Universidad Nacional del Callao, Lima, Perú

*Address all correspondence to: gcpesantesa@unac.edu.pe

References

[1] Ccaycca A. Compuestos bioactivos y actividad antioxidante del maíz morado *Zea Mays L*. procedente de tres regiones del Perú. [Tesis de maestría. Universidad Nacional Mayor de San Marcos; 2020

[2] MINAGRI. Guía de Producción Comercial de Maíz morado [Internet]. 2016. Available from: http://repositorio.minagri.gob.pe/.

[3] Drago M, López M, Sainz T. Componentes bioactivos de alimentos funcionales de origen vegetal. Revista Mexicana de Ciencias Farmacéuticas. 2006;**37**(4):58-68

[4] Lagouge M, y Larsson, N. The role of mitochondrial DNA mutations and free radicals in disease and ageing. Journal of Internal Medicine. 2013;**273**(6):529-543. DOI: 10.1111/joim.12055

[5] Sánchez V, Méndez N. Estrés oxidativo, antioxidantes y enfermedad. Revista de Investigación Médica Sur México. 2013;**20**(3):161-168

[6] Cuevas, E., Antezana, A., y Winterhalter, P. (2008). Análisis y caracterización de Antocianinas en diferentes variedades de Maíz Morado (*Zea Mays* L.) boliviano. Memorias del Encuentro Final Red-Alfa Lagrotech. 79-95.

[7] Guillén, J., Mori, S., y Paucar, L.M. (2014). Características y propiedades funcionales del maíz morado (*Zea mays* L.) var. Subnigroviolaceo. Revista Scientia Agropecuaria; 5, 211-217. DOI: 10.17268/sci.agropecu.2014.04.05

[8] Salinas Y, Rubio D, y Díaz, A. Extracción y uso de pigmentos del grano de maíz (*Zea mays* L.) como colorantes en yogur. Archivos Latinoamericanos de Nutrición. 2005;**55**(3):293-298

[9] Garzón GA. Las antocianinas como colorantes naturales y compuestos bioactivos. Acta Biológica Colombiana. 2008;**13**(3):27-36

[10] Arroyo J, Raez E, Rodríguez M, Chumpitaz M, Burga J, De la Cruz W, et al. Reducción del colesterol y aumento de la capacidad antioxidante por el consumo crónico de maíz morado (*Zea mays* L.) en ratas hipercolesterolémicas. Revista Peruana de Medicina Experimental y Salud Pública. 2007;**24**(2):157-162

[11] Pedreschi R, y Cisneros, L. Phenolics profiles of andean purple corn (*Zea mays* L.). Food Chemical. 2007;**100**:956-963. DOI: 10.1016/j.foodchem.2005.11.004

[12] Pesantes G, Paucar J, Franco J. Elaboración de una bebida de maíz morado con máxima retención de antocianinas. Revista Alpha Centauri. 2021;**2**(1):52-61. DOI: 10.47422/ac.v2i1.29

[13] Gorriti, A; Quispe, F; Arroyo, J; Córdova, A; Jurado, B; Santiago, I y Taype, E. Extracción de antocianinas de las corontas de *Zea mays* L. "Maíz Morado", Revista de Ciencia e Investigación de la Facultad de Farmacia y Bioquímica de la UNMSM. 2009; 12 (2):64-74. DOI: 10.15381/ci.v12i2.3395

[14] Elías, J. y Gamero, D. Obtención de colorante a partir del maíz morado. [Tesis de pregrado, Universidad Nacional de Ingeniería]. 1988.

[15] Mendoza C. Las antocianinas del maíz: su distribución en la planta y producción. [Tesis de maestría. Colegio de Posgraduados, Campus Montecillo; 2012

[16] Almeida J. Extracción y caracterización del colorante natural del maíz negro

(*Zea mays* L.) y determinación de su actividad. [Tesis de pregrado. Escuela Politécnica Nacional; 2012

[17] Giusti M, Wrolstad R. Characterization and measurement of anthocyanins by UV-visible spectroscopy. Current Protocols in Food Analytical Chemistry. 2001;(1):F1-2. DOI: 10.1002/0471142913.faf0102s00

[18] Anzaldúa-Morales A. La evaluación sensorial de los alimentos en la teoría y en la práctica. Editorial Acribia; 1994

[19] Montgomery D. Diseño y análisis de experimentos (2da edición). Editorial Limusa; 2002

Chapter 12

Antioxidant Strategies to Improve Female Reproduction

Tarique Hussain

Abstract

Animals are only productive once their reproductive cycle is continuously flown. There are several causes of stresses which interrupt animal physiology and make animal less productive. All factors involved in stress could eventually generate reactive oxygen species (ROS). Limited production of these reactive species performs several functions to maintain redox homeostasis. When these reactive oxidative metabolites are overwhelmed, it may generate oxidative stress. Disruption in oxidant/antioxidant mechanism leads to cause oxidative stress. Naturally, the body system is equipped with an antioxidant defense system. Once this system is broken-down due to the overproduction of ROS, it may have a detrimental effect on lipids, proteins, DNA, and carbohydrates and eventually influence animal fertility and productivity. Antioxidants available in nature are of two types: natural and synthetic. These compounds endowed several properties in the mitigation of various animal stresses, starting from physiology to molecular level. This chapter elucidates oxidative stress, natural and synthetic antioxidants, and particular focus are emphasized that how antioxidant supplementation can help to improve animal fertility and productivity. Moreover, the mechanism by which antioxidants produce fruitful effects will also be highlighted.

Keywords: reactive oxygen species, oxidative stress, animal fertility, productivity, antioxidants

1. Introduction

Oxidative stress is the condition in which the overproduction of free radicals is produced and the antioxidant system unable to neutralize them [1]. Limited quality of free radicals is compulsory to maintain physiological function, and accelerated production may lead to damage lipids, DNA, and proteins [2]. The efficacy of oxidative metabolites in female reproduction depends upon the site, amount and exposing levels to oxidant molecules [3].

In livestock, the appearance of the disease causes a reduction in the antioxidant status of the animals [4]. Oxidative stress is observed in several pathological conditions that influence animal health, welfare, and productive performance [5]. Indeed, in some productive phases, animals experience physiological alteration, such as farrowing and lactation, weaning, high temperature, and different stresses, that may decline antioxidant status [6–8].

Oxidative stress may influence physiological function of various reproductive events which thus involved in problems associated with pregnancy [9]. Antioxidants are chemical compounds is known to suppress autoxidation *via* reduction in free radicals' production using several different mechanisms. They can be categorized as primary antioxidants, chelators, $O_2^{\bullet-}$ quenchers, oxygen scavengers, and antioxidant regenerators [10]. The purpose of this chapter is to exploit the beneficial effect of antioxidant compounds various aspects of female reproduction and also discuss how antioxidant approaches improve animal productive performance and well-being.

2. Reactive oxygen species

Reactive oxygen species (ROS) encompasses of superoxide anion, hydrogen peroxide and hydroxyl radical. Their production is possible due to natural oxygen leakage [11]. Other origin of ROS production are metabolic reactions that are sustainable for life, the exogenous sources include X-rays, ozone, cigarette smoking, air pollutants, certain drugs and pesticides, and industrial chemicals [12]. The endogenous site of free radicals' production may be from mitochondria, xanthine oxidase, peroxisomes, inflammation, phagocytosis, arachidonate pathways, exercise, and ischemia/reperfusion injury [13]. Interestingly, the reactions of consists of enzymatic and nonenzymatic reactions within the body also produce free radicals. Many enzymatic reactions prevail in the respiratory chain, phagocytosis, prostaglandin synthesis, and cytochrome P-450 system [14], although nonenzymatic reactions are based on oxygen with organic compounds and ionizing reactions also generate free radicals [15].

ROS are comprised of oxygen ions, free radicals and peroxides. High level of ROS or reduce concentration of antioxidants induce oxidative stress that trigger cellular damage of macromolecules utilizing different ways. It has responsible for causing chronic diseases by interacting with molecular signaling pathways which alters gene expression [16]. The interaction between chemicals and signaling molecules are necessary to understand the involvement of ROS role in pathogenesis. Redox interaction with various proteins residues and ROS is the key component of inter-processes. Further reaction yields to produce reactive sulfenic acid and sulfonamide. Oxidation of these molecules leads to cause ultra-structural changes or functional alteration [17].

Pregnancy is a physiological phenomenon in which an ample amount of energy is required to balance the body's condition and combat fetal requirements. Thus, for this purpose more oxygen is required which in turn causes the overproduction of ROS. So, it is very crucial to maintain the balance between oxidative stress and the antioxidant system for perfect functioning of the body [18].

3. Antioxidants

Antioxidants are substances that overcome adverse effect of oxidative damages. They are available as natural and synthetic compounds. Natural antioxidants are derived from natural sources like food, cosmetics, and pharmaceutical industries. While the synthetic one is created artificially through chemical reactions [19].

The antioxidant system consists of enzymatic and non-enzymatic. The first one is also referred as natural antioxidants. They consist of superoxide dismutase (SOD) catalase and glutathione peroxidase (GSH-Px). Antioxidant enzymes are endowed to protect living cells against oxidant products. The SOD is an enzyme district superoxide anion radical into hydrogen peroxide. Another enzyme called catalase is in charge of catalysing the breakdown of hydrogen peroxide into water and oxygen. GSH-Px employs glutathione as a co-substrate and is composed of selenium. An enzyme found in the cytoplasm, it excludes hydrogen peroxide. However, in comparison with catalase, it has various ranges of substrates comprising lipid peroxides. The prime function of the Glutathione peroxidase is to decontaminate low levels of hydrogen peroxide in the cell.

Non-enzymatic antioxidants include dietary supplements or synthetic antioxidants. The complex nature of the body antioxidant system is impaired by consumption of dietary antioxidant such as vitamins and minerals [20]. Vitamin C, vitamin E, plant polyphenol, carotenoids, and glutathione are non-enzymatic antioxidants, they causes inhibition of free radicals reactions. Antioxidants can be classified as water-soluble or lipid-soluble depending on how potent they are. A water-soluble vitamin called vitamin C is found in cellular fluids such the cytosol and cytoplasmic matrix.

Antioxidants can be divided into small-molecule and large-molecule antioxidants depending on their size. The small one neutralizes ROS through scavenging process. The example includes Vitamin C, vitamin E, carotenoids, and glutathione (GSH). A large size of the molecule antioxidants comprises SOD, CAT, and GPx and albumin that captivate ROS and the attack form essential proteins. The mechanism by which antioxidants are utilized which offer protection against inhibition of free radical formation, scavenging free radicals, involved in repair-damage via free radicals, help to establish an environment that is conducive for the antioxidants to function effectively [21].

4. Synthetic antioxidants

Synthetic antioxidants are phenolic compounds responsible for eliminating free radicals and suppressing chain-reaction. They consist of butylated hydroxyl anisole (BHA), butylated hydroxyltoluene (BHT), propyl gallate (PG), metal chelating agent (EDTA), tertiary butyl hydroquinone (TBHQ), and nordihydroguaiaretic acid (NDGA) [21].

5. Oxidative stress and selenium

In commercial dairy and beef farming, various stresses influence economic benefit that is linked with declined productive and reproductive performance in cattle. It has been observed that diverse endogenous and exogenous sources of ROS lead to stresses that cause over generation of free radicals and eventually result in oxidative stress [22, 23]. It is well recognized that the consequences of oxidative stress have deleterious effects on immune system reproductive function, animal growth, development, and on general health [24, 25]. Hence, the antioxidant network is responsible for the preservation and maintenance of animal redox status in cells and tissues and is thus responsible for neglecting the harmful effect of stresses. In animals' body, the antioxidant system work either individually or in combination to exert particular function. Considering this mechanism, selenium has its own importance [26, 27]. It is noted that 25 selenoproteins have been identified in animal tissues; most of them are contributed in the conservation of body redox balance and antioxidant defense [27]. A deep theoretical knowledge of Se uptake toward the body/cells is required and its particular utilization for the balance of animal health. It is well-recognized in some animal species that the bioavailability of the Se relies on the dietary source of Se provided [28–30]. The Se integration relies on the rumen environment, which gradually declines depending upon the particular source of Se [31]. Selenium is present in two forms, inorganic and organic [32]. These forms may be a vital source of selenium [33].

It has been known that Se supplementation enhances female fertility but the exact mechanism is still not unknown. The progesterone hormone derived from the corpus luteum is a dominant hormone of pregnancy. This hormone is synthesized from cholesterol *via* several enzymatic reactions in which molecular oxygen is utilized for its reactions. These reactions generate oxygen radicals and different peroxides which are detrimental to cells [34]. In *in vivo* study, indicated that the inclusion of luteinizing hormone in luteal cells culture concurrently enhanced progesterone level in the medium and also the lipid peroxides in cells [35]. For luteal regression, the accretion of H_2O_2 [36] or lipid peroxides [37] in the corpus luteum has been documented. These findings show that corpus luteum requires antioxidant defense toward peroxides to stabilize normal functions. The significance of the corpus luteum has also been projected by Ref. [38]. Moreover, the inclusion of Se in luteal cells reduced the concentration of lipid peroxides in a cell [35]. Se as the part of glutathione peroxidase may destroy peroxides, in connection with superoxide dismutase, vitamin E, and beta-carotene.

6. Oxidative stress during pregnancy and antioxidants

Pregnancy is a normal mechanism in which overburden metabolic rate disrupts antioxidant status and energy balance. During first phase of pregnancy, 25% of the embryos die or reabsorbed within two weeks of pregnancy before implantation [39]. Once the zona pellucida is separated from the embryo, it enhances the production of ROS [40]. The imbalance between oxidant/antioxidant systems during early pregnancy may lead to disturbances in molecules which eventually compromise growth and development of embryo [41].

The nutritional requirement during early pregnancy is increased to maintain animal health and pregnancy, which is in turn generation of oxidative stress [42]. Although, malnutrition is also common around the globe in small ruminants because of the high price of the feed, especially in developing countries. Hence, small ruminants are easy to keep due to several reasons [43]. Malnutrition during pregnancy has deleterious effect on the conception rate and on fetus development [44]. Animal supplementation in a diet with plant source have sufficient nutrition and has been assumed to be the potential source of antioxidants to attenuate early pregnancy stress in goats [45, 46]. The plant compounds exert diverse nutrition comprises of rich source of antioxidants and immune-modulatory properties, which act as a potential feed supplement for ruminants [47, 48].

Moringa oleifera (MO) is a multifaceted medicinal tree with high nutritional values [49]. Its leaves are rich sources of several nutritious compounds, such as proteins, amino acids, minerals, and vitamins [50]. Apart of that, MO is also a rich source of antioxidant compounds, such as phenolic acids, vitamin E, vitamin C, selenium, zinc, and β carotene. These compounds have more robust antioxidant potential than synthetic ones [51]. The basal diet supplemented with 3.2% MOLP increased antioxidant index and blood biochemical in early pregnancy in Beetal goats. It also promoted progesterone profile, improved conception rate, and attenuated ROS production in early pregnancy of goats.

In another study, by Ref. [52] reported the use of herbal antioxidants during pregnancy and their effect on piglet performance. The supplementation profoundly enhanced number of live-born piglets, total litter weight, and reducing the chance of low-weight piglets. Moreover, supplementation declined MDA levels in sows and piglets. The mothers who had supplementation showed a higher trend of weaning weight. The results conclude from 1000 pregnancies that offering maternal supplementation with herbal antioxidants in pregnancy profoundly enhanced reproductive efficiency, litter traits, and piglet performance.

7. Oxidative stress during lactation and antioxidants

Reproductive performance is a main indicator related to maternal nutrition. The periparturient period causes reduced feed intake, and endocrine and metabolic alterations which disrupt energy balance and antioxidant index [22, 53]. In this period, increased nutritional requirements, such as digestion rate, mammary development, and fetus growth have been reported [54]. Pasture grazing and feeding on crop residues have a diverse nutritional profile and feeding on such sources is not adequate to meet the energy requirement of lactating animals [55]. In this scenario, pregnant animals are vulnerable to oxidative stress [56], which threatens to biomolecules and eventually affect productive and reproductive parameters [57]. Colostrum is the composition of immunoglobulins, minerals and other biological substances which transfer form colostrum to the young ones [58]. The quality of the colostrum depends upon maternal nutrition [59, 60]. The diet supplemented with phytobiotics has been assumed to be the main source of managing nutrition-induced oxidative stress in pregnancy and lactation in livestock [45, 46, 61]. In a recent study by Ali et al., (2022) using 2% and 3.5% *M. oleifera* leaf powder (MOLP) during periparturient period. He reported the increased biochemical and antioxidant indices of colostrum and milk. The milk yield, weight gain of the kids, and reproductive performance were enhanced with 2 and 3.5% MOLP. Further, the findings suggested that the diet supplemented with 3.5% MOLP promotes antioxidant index, milk yield, and reproductive performance in goats.

8. Effect of oxidants and antioxidants on embryo production

The *in vitro* embryo production (IVEP) technique is employed to combat infertility-related problems in mammalian species [62]. This tool has been known to be utilized for the production of large scale offspring from elite animals. The IVM prognosis relies on diverse factors consisting of oocyte quality and culture conditions [63]. The source of antioxidants from female organs has been reported to reduce ROS production [64]. The main hurdle which decides the fate of oocyte success during IVM is oxidative stress [64]. Accelerated ROS production might result in oocyte death and embryonic loss [65, 66]. An antioxidant approach during IVM has been proposed to govern oocytes from the deleterious effect of oxidative stress by maintaining a basal level of ROS [67, 68]. Presently, different antioxidants are utilized during IVM to confirm balanced intracellular redox status, resulting in good-quality of oocytes [69, 70]. The inclusion of antioxidants, such as thiols, polyphenols, melatonin, carotenoids, resveratrol, and vitamins C and E, to the IVM medium has been verified in different studies to increase oocyte quality and attenuate exceeding ROS damage [71, 72].

Previous evidence has reported that the balance amount of antioxidants and ROS in IVEP media which may be favorable for embryonic development [73, 74]. At present, the widely employed antioxidant in IVEP is cysteamine; its efficiency is mostly associated with the stage of IVM. It has been found to stimulate the embryonic process and secreting of glutathione (GSH), which is prevalent in male and female gametes from harmful effect of ROS [75]. Moreover, cysteine and glutathione have been implied in IVEP protocols with good results [73, 76]. The application of quercetin (2 μM), resveratrol (2 μM), vitamin C (50 μg/mL), carnitine (0.5 mg/mL), and cysteamine (100 μM) were determined to prove the vibrant antioxidant toward deleterious effects of ROS during IVM of bovine oocytes [71]. The positive effect of antioxidants is illustrated in **Table 1**.

Antioxidants	Dose	Animal species	Maturation vs. control rate	References
Melatonin	10^{-9} M 10^{-7} M 10^{-6} M	Bovine Sheep Mouse	82.3 (65.7) * 85.3 (75.3) * 85 (64) *	[77–79]
Lycopene	2×10^{-7} M	Bovine	76 (66.3) *	[80]
Beta-Mercaptoethanol (β-ME)	2×10^{-5} M	Buffalo	76.2 (66.7)ns	[81]
Cystamine	10^{-5} M	Mouse	80.1 (57.7) *	[82]
Vitamin C	2.3×10^{-3} M (1 mg/mL)	Bovine	~80 (~80)ns	[83]
Vitamin E	2.3×10^{-3} M (1 mg/mL)	Bovine	~80 (~80)ns	[83]
Vitamin E; Selenium (SeMet)	10^{-3} M; 2.5×10^{-8} M	Porcine	85.1 (67.6) *	[84]
Resveratrol	10^{-6} M	Bovine	93.4 (87.9) *	[85]
Quercetin	10^{-5} M	mouse	86.6 (79.7) *	[86]
Retinoic acid	10^{-8} M 2×10^{-5} M	Goat Camel	78.7 (65.1) * 69.4 (52.9) *	[87, 88]
Coenzyme Q10	5×10^{-5} M	Human	82.6 (63.0) *	[89]

**Shows the significant effects.*

Table 1.
The beneficial effect of antioxidant supplementation in different animal species.

Author details

Tarique Hussain
Animal Sciences Division, Nuclear Institute for Agriculture and Biology College (NIAB-C), Pakistan Institute of Engineering and Applied Sciences (PIEAS), Faisalabad, Pakistan

*Address all correspondence to: drtariquerahoo@gmail.com

IntechOpen

References

[1] Sies H, Berndt C, Jones DP. Oxidative stress. Annual Revicw of Biochemistry. 2017;**86**:715-748

[2] Rahal A, Kumar A, Singh V, Yadav B, Tiwari R, Chakraborty S, et al. Oxidative stress, prooxidants, and antioxidants: The interplay. BioMed Research International. 2014;**2014**:19. Article ID 761264

[3] Aruoma OI, Halliwell B. Superoxide-dependent and ascorbate-dependent formation of hydroxyl radicals from hydrogen peroxide in the presence of iron. Are lactoferrin and transferrin promoters of hydroxyl-radical generation? Biochemical Journal. 1987;**241**:273-278

[4] Lykkesfeldt J, Svendsen O. Oxidants and antioxidants in disease: Oxidative stress in farm animals. The Veterinary Journal. 2007;**173**:502-511

[5] Buchet A, Belloc C, Leblanc-Maridor M, Merlot E. Effects of age and weaning conditions on blood indicators of oxidative status in pigs. PLoS One. 2017;**12**:e0178487

[6] Rossi R, Pastorelli G, Cannata S, Corino C. Effect of weaning on total antiradical activity in piglets. Italian Journal of Animal Science. 2009;**87**:2299-2305

[7] Berchieri-Ronchi C, Kim S, Zhao Y, Correa C, Yeum K-J, Ferreira A. Oxidative stress status of highly prolific sows during gestation and lactation. Animal. 2011;**5**:1774-1779

[8] Guo Z, Gao S, Ouyang J, Ma L, Bu D. Impacts of heat stress-induced oxidative stress on the milk protein biosynthesis of dairy cows. Animals. 2021;**11**:726

[9] Mbah C, Orabueze I, Okorie N. Antioxidant Properties of Natural and Synthetic Chemical Compounds: Therapeutic Effects on Biological System. Telangana, India; 2019;**3**(6):28-42

[10] Augustyniak A, Bartosz G, Čipak A, Duburs G, Horáková LU, Łuczaj W, et al. Natural and synthetic antioxidants: An updated overview. Free Radical Research. 2010;**44**:1216-1262

[11] Zhang X, Wang G, Gurley EC, Zhou H. Flavonoid apigenin inhibits lipopolysaccharide-induced inflammatory response through multiple mechanisms in macrophages. PLoS One. 2014;**9**:e107072

[12] Jhang J-J, Lu C-C, Ho C-Y, Cheng Y-T, Yen G-C. Protective effects of catechin against monosodium urate-induced inflammation through the modulation of NLRP3 inflammasome activation. Journal of Agricultural and Food Chemistry. 2015;**63**:7343-7352

[13] Ellis LZ, Liu W, Luo Y, Okamoto M, Qu D, Dunn JH, et al. Green tea polyphenol epigallocatechin-3-gallate suppresses melanoma growth by inhibiting inflammasome and IL-1β secretion. Biochemical and Biophysical Research Communications. 2011;**414**:551-556

[14] Han SG, Han S-S, Toborek M, Hennig B. EGCG protects endothelial cells against PCB 126-induced inflammation through inhibition of AhR and induction of Nrf2-regulated genes. Toxicology and Applied Pharmacology. 2012;**261**:181-188

[15] Tang B, Chen G-X, Liang M-Y, Yao J-P, Wu Z-K. Ellagic acid prevents monocrotaline-induced pulmonary artery hypertension via inhibiting NLRP3 inflammasome activation in rats.

International Journal of Cardiology. 2015;**180**:134-141

[16] Hussain T, Tan B, Yin Y, Blachier F, Tossou MC, Rahu N. Oxidative stress and inflammation: What polyphenols can do for us? Oxidative Medicine and Cellular Longevity. 2016;**2016**:9. Article ID 7432797

[17] Ray PD, Huang B-W, Tsuji Y. Reactive oxygen species (ROS) homeostasis and redox regulation in cellular signaling. Cellular Signalling. 2012;**24**:981-990

[18] Toboła-Wróbel K, Pietryga M, Dydowicz P, Napierała M, Brązert J, Florek E. Association of oxidative stress on pregnancy. Oxidative Medicine and Cellular Longevity. 2020;**2020**:12. Article ID 6398520

[19] Mahmoud AM, Wilkinson FL, Lightfoot AP, Dos Santos JM, Sandhu MA. The Role of Natural and Synthetic Antioxidants in Modulating Oxidative Stress in Drug-Induced Injury and Metabolic Disorders 2020. Hindawi; 2021

[20] Shakir HM. Antioxidant and infertility. In: Antioxidants-Benefits, Sources, Mechanisms of Action. London, UK: IntechOpen; 2021. DOI: 10.5772/intechopen.95791

[21] Aziz MA, Diab AS, Mohammed AA. Antioxidant Categories and Mode of Action. London, UK, London, UK: IntechOpen; 2019

[22] Abuelo A, Hernández J, Benedito JL, Castillo C. Redox biology in transition periods of dairy cattle: Role in the health of periparturient and neonatal animals. Antioxidants. 2019;**8**:20

[23] Roth Z. Effect of heat stress on reproduction in dairy cows: Insights into the cellular and molecular responses of the oocyte. Annual Review of Animal Biosciences. 2017;**5**:151-170

[24] Rolland M, Le Moal J, Wagner V, Royère D, De Mouzon J. Decline in semen concentration and morphology in a sample of 26 609 men close to general population between 1989 and 2005 in France. Human Reproduction. 2013;**28**:462-470

[25] Sengupta P, Dutta S, Krajewska-Kulak E. The disappearing sperms: Analysis of reports published between 1980 and 2015. American Journal of Men's Health. 2017;**11**:1279-1304

[26] Sikka SC. Relative impact of oxidative stress on male reproductive function. Current Medicinal Chemistry. 2001;**8**:851-862

[27] Agarwal A, Prabakaran SA. Mechanism, Measurement, and Prevention of Oxidative Stress in Male Reproductive Physiology. New Delhi, India; 2005;**43**(11):963-974

[28] Rakhit M, Gokul SR, Agarwal A, du Plessis SS. Antioxidant strategies to overcome OS in IVF-embryo transfer. In: Studies on Women's Health. NewYork, USA: Springer; 2013. pp. 237-262

[29] Barazani Y, Katz BF, Nagler HM, Stember DS. Lifestyle, environment, and male reproductive health. Urologic Clinics. 2014;**41**:55-66

[30] Sullivan LB, Chandel NS. Mitochondrial reactive oxygen species and cancer. Cancer & Metabolism. 2014;**2**:1-12

[31] Darbandi S, Darbandi M. Lifestyle modifications on further reproductive problems. Cresco Journal of Reproductive Science. 2016;**1**:1-2

[32] Sunde R. Selenium. In: Bowman BA, Russell RM, editors. Present knowledge in nutrition. 9th ed. Washington, DC: ILSI Press; 2006. pp. 480-497

[33] Brand and A. Schade. Selenium and the Metallic Metal

[34] Larroque C, Lange R, Maurin L, Bienvenue A, van Lier JE. On the nature of the cytochrome P450scc "ultimate oxidant": Characterization of a productive radical intermediate. Archives of Biochemistry and Biophysics. 1990;**282**:198-201

[35] Kamada H, Ikumo H. Effect of selenium on cultured bovine luteal cells. Animal Reproduction Science. 1997;**46**:203-211

[36] Riley JC, Behrman HR. In vivo generation of hydrogen peroxide in the rat corpus luteum during luteolysis. Endocrinology. 1991;**128**:1749-1753

[37] Sawada M, Carlson JC. Rapid plasma membrane changes in superoxide radical formation, fluidity, and phospholipase A2 activity in the corpus luteum of the rat during induction of luteolysis. Endocrinology. 1991;**128**:2992-2998

[38] Carlson JC, Sawada M, Boone DL, Stauffer JM. Stimulation of progesterone secretion in dispersed cells of rat corpora lutea by antioxidants. Steroids. 1995;**60**:272-276

[39] Spencer TE, Johnson GA, Bazer FW, Burghardt RC. Implantation mechanisms: Insights from the sheep. Reproduction. 2004;**128**:657-668

[40] Al-Gubory KH, Faure P, Garrel C. Different enzymatic antioxidative pathways operate within the sheep caruncular and intercaruncular endometrium throughout the estrous cycle and early pregnancy. Theriogenology. 2017;**99**:111-118

[41] Eick SM, Barrett ES, Erve TJ, Nguyen RH, Bush NR, Milne G, et al. Association between prenatal psychological stress and oxidative stress during pregnancy. Paediatric and Perinatal Epidemiology. 2018;**32**:318-326

[42] Nawito M, Abd El Hameed AR, Sosa A, Mahmoud KGM. Impact of pregnancy and nutrition on oxidant/antioxidant balance in sheep and goats reared in South Sinai, Egypt. Veterinary World. 2016;**9**:801

[43] Härter C, Lima L, Silva H, Castagnino D, Rivera A, Resende K, et al. Energy and protein requirements for maintenance of dairy goats during pregnancy and their efficiencies of use. Journal of Animal Science. 2017;**95**:4181-4193

[44] Sharma D, Shastri S, Sharma P. Intrauterine growth restriction: Antenatal and postnatal aspects. Clinical Medicine Insights Pediatrics. 2016;**10**:S40070

[45] Kholif A, Morsy T, Gouda G, Anele U, Galyean M. Effect of feeding diets with processed Moringa oleifera meal as protein source in lactating Anglo-Nubian goats. Animal Feed Science and Technology. 2016;**217**:45-55

[46] Abou-Elkhair R, Mahboub H, Sadek K, Ketkat S. Effect of prepartum dietary energy source on goat maternal metabolic profile, neonatal performance, and economic profitability. Journal of Advanced Veterinary and Animal Research. 2020;**7**:566

[47] Bampidis V, Christodoulou V, Christaki E, Florou-Paneri P, Spais A. Effect of dietary garlic bulb and garlic husk supplementation on performance and carcass characteristics of growing lambs. Animal Feed Science and Technology. 2005;**121**:273-283

[48] Patra AK, Amasheh S, Aschenbach JR. Modulation of

gastrointestinal barrier and nutrient transport function in farm animals by natural plant bioactive compounds–a comprehensive review. Critical Reviews in Food Science and Nutrition. 2019;**59**:3237-3266

[49] Padayachee B, Baijnath H. An updated comprehensive review of the medicinal, phytochemical and pharmacological properties of Moringa oleifera. South African Journal of Botany. 2020;**129**:304-316

[50] Abbas R, Elsharbasy F, Fadlelmula A. Nutritional values of moringa oleifera, total protein: Amino acid, vitamins, minerals, carbohydrates, total fat and crude fiber, under the semi-arid conditions of Sudan. Journal of Microbe Biochemica Technology. 2018;**10**:56-58

[51] Saleem A, Saleem M, Akhtar MF. Antioxidant, anti-inflammatory and antiarthritic potential of Moringa oleifera lam: An ethnomedicinal plant of Moringaceae family. South African Journal of Botany. 2020;**128**:246-256

[52] Parraguez VH, Atlagich M, Araneda O, García C, Munoz A, De los Reyes M, et al. "Effects of antioxidant vitamins on newborn and placental traits in gestations at high altitude: Comparative study in high and low altitude native sheep." Reproduction, Fertility and Development. 2011;**23**:285-296

[53] Sordillo L. Nutritional strategies to optimize dairy cattle immunity. Journal of Dairy Science. 2016;**99**:4967-4982

[54] Berchieri-Ronchi CB, Presti PT, Ferreira ALA, Correa CR, Salvadori DMF, Damasceno DC, et al. Effects of oxidative stress during human and animal reproductions: A review. International Journal of Nutrology. 2015;**8**:006-011

[55] Idamokoro EM, Muchenje V, Afolayan AJ, Hugo A. Comparative fatty-acid profile and atherogenicity index of milk from free grazing Nguni, Boer and non-descript goats in South Africa. Pastoralism. 2019;**9**:1-8

[56] Obrador E, Liu-Smith F, Dellinger RW, Salvador R, Meyskens FL, Estrela JM. Oxidative stress and antioxidants in the pathophysiology of malignant melanoma. Biological Chemistry. 2019;**400**:589-612

[57] Vitale SG, Capriglione S, Peterlunger I, La Rosa VL, Vitagliano A, Noventa M, et al. The role of oxidative stress and membrane transport systems during endometriosis: A fresh look at a busy corner. Oxidative Medicine and Cellular Longevity. 2018;**2018**:14. Article ID 7924021

[58] Hernández-Castellano LE, Morales-delaNuez A, Sánchez-Macías D, Moreno-Indias I, Torres A, Capote J, et al. The effect of colostrum source (goat vs. sheep) and timing of the first colostrum feeding (2 h vs. 14 h after birth) on body weight and immune status of artificially reared newborn lambs. Journal of Dairy Science. 2015;**98**:204-210

[59] Zachwieja A, Szulc T, Potkański A, Mikuła R, Kruszyński W, Dobicki A. Effect of different fat supplements used during dry period of cows on colostrum physicochemical properties. Biotechnology in Animal Husbandry. 2007;**23**:67-75

[60] Hyrslova I, Krausova G, Bartova J, Kolesar L, Curda L. Goat and bovine colostrum as a basis for new probiotic functional foods and dietary supplements. Journal of Microbial and Biochemical Technology. 2016;**8**:56-59

[61] Kekana TW, Nherera-Chokuda V, Baloyi JJ, Muya C. Immunoglobulin G response and performance in Holstein calves supplemented with garlic powder and probiotics. South African Journal of Animal Science. 2020;**50**:263-270

[62] Baldassarre H. Laparoscopic ovum pick-up followed by in vitro embryo production and transfer in assisted breeding programs for ruminants. Animals. 2021;**11**:216

[63] Mikkelsen AL, Smith S, Lindenberg S. Possible factors affecting the development of oocytes in in-vitro maturation. Human Reproduction. 2000;**15**:11-17

[64] Choi H-y, Cho K-H, Jin C, Lee J, Kim T-H, Jung W-S, et al. Exercise therapies for Parkinson's disease: A systematic review and meta-analysis. Parkinson's Disease. 2020;**2020**:22. Article ID 2565320

[65] Guérin PE, Menezo Y. Oxidative stress and protection against teactive oxygen species in the pre implantation embryo and its surroundings. Human Reproduction Update. 2001;**7**:175

[66] Khazaei M, Aghaz F. Reactive oxygen species generation and use of antioxidants during in vitro maturation of oocytes. International Journal of Fertility & Sterility. 2017;**11**:63

[67] Takahashi M. Oxidative stress and redox regulation on in vitro development of mammalian embryos. Journal of Reproduction and Development. 2012;**58**:1-9

[68] Silva E, Greene AF, Strauss K, Herrick JR, Schoolcraft WB, Krisher RL. Antioxidant supplementation during in vitro culture improves mitochondrial function and development of embryos from aged female mice. Reproduction, Fertility and Development. 2015;**27**:975-983

[69] Morado SA, Cetica PD, Beconi MT, Dalvit GC. Reactive oxygen species in bovine oocyte maturation in vitro. Reproduction, Fertility and Development. 2009;**21**:608-614

[70] Romero S, Pella R, Zorrilla I, Berrío P, Escudero F, Pérez Y, et al. Coenzyme Q10 improves the in vitro maturation of oocytes exposed to the intrafollicular environment of patients on fertility treatment. JBRA Assisted Reproduction. 2020;**24**:283

[71] Sovernigo T, Adona P, Monzani P, Guemra S, Barros F, Lopes F, et al. Effects of supplementation of medium with different antioxidants during in vitro maturation of bovine oocytes on subsequent embryo production. Reproduction in Domestic Animals. 2017;**52**:561-569

[72] Budani MC, Tiboni GM. Effects of supplementation with natural antioxidants on oocytes and preimplantation embryos. Antioxidants. 2020;**9**:612

[73] Ali A, Bilodeau J, Sirard M. Antioxidant requirements for bovine oocytes varies during in vitro maturation, fertilization and development. Theriogenology. 2003;**59**:939-949

[74] Zullo G, Albero G, Neglia G, De Canditiis C, Bifulco G, Campanile G, et al. L-ergothioneine supplementation during culture improves quality of bovine in vitro–produced embryos. Theriogenology. 2016;**85**:688-697

[75] Gottardi F, Barretto L, Gonçalves F, Perri S, Mingoti G. Effects of Cumulus Cells and Cysteamine during Bovine Oocyte in vitro Maturation on Meiosis Progression and Acquisition of Developmental Competence. Brasil; 2012. pp. 245-252

[76] Sun W-J, Pang Y-W, Liu Y, Hao H-S, Zhao X-M, Qin T, et al. Exogenous glutathione supplementation in culture medium improves the bovine embryo development after in vitro fertilization. Theriogenology. 2015;**84**:716-723

[77] Zhao X-M, Min J-T, Du W-H, Hao H-S, Liu Y, Qin T, et al. Melatonin enhances the in vitro maturation and developmental potential of bovine oocytes denuded of the cumulus oophorus. Zygote. 2015;**23**:525-536

[78] Tian X, Wang F, Zhang L, He C, Ji P, Wang J, et al. Beneficial effects of melatonin on the in vitro maturation of sheep oocytes and its relation to melatonin receptors. International Journal of Molecular Sciences. 2017;**18**:834

[79] Keshavarzi S, Salehi M, Farifteh-Nobijari F, Hosseini T, Hosseini S, Ghazifard A, et al. Melatonin modifies histone acetylation during in vitro maturation of mouse oocytes. Cell Journal (Yakhteh). 2018;**20**:244

[80] Chowdhury M, Choi B-H, Khan I, Lee K-L, Mesalam A, Song S-H, et al. Supplementation of lycopene in maturation media improves bovine embryo quality in vitro. Theriogenology. 2017;**103**:173-184

[81] Patel PA, Chaudhary SS, Puri G, Singh VK, Odedara AB. Effects of β-mercaptoethanol on in vitro maturation and glutathione level of buffalo oocytes. Veterinary World. 2015;**8**:213

[82] Chen N, Liow S-L, Yip W-Y, Tan L-G, Ng S-C. Influence of cysteamine supplementation and culture in portable dry-incubator on the in vitro maturation, fertilization and subsequent development of mouse oocytes. Theriogenology. 2005;**63**:2300-2310

[83] Dalvit G, Llanes S, Descalzo A, Insani M, Beconi M, Cetica P. Effect of alpha-tocopherol and ascorbic acid on bovine oocyte in vitro maturation. Reproduction in Domestic Animals. 2005;**40**:93-97

[84] Tareq K, Akter QS, Mam Y, Tsujii H. Selenium and vitamin E improve the in vitro maturation, fertilization and culture to blastocyst of porcine oocytes. Journal of Reproduction and Development. 2012;**58**:621-628

[85] Wang F, Tian X, Zhang L, He C, Ji P, Li Y, et al. Beneficial effect of resveratrol on bovine oocyte maturation and subsequent embryonic development after in vitro fertilization. Fertility and Sterility. 2014;**101**:577-586

[86] Cao Y, Zhao H, Wang Z, Zhang C, Bian Y, Liu X, et al. Quercetin promotes in vitro maturation of oocytes from humans and aged mice. Cell Death & Disease. 2020;**11**:1-15

[87] Pu Y, Wang Z, Bian Y, Zhang F, Yang P, Li Y, et al. All-trans retinoic acid improves goat oocyte nuclear maturation and reduces apoptotic cumulus cells during in vitro maturation. Animal Science Journal. 2014;**85**:833-839

[88] Saadeldin IM, Swelum AA-A, Elsafadi M, Mahmood A, Yaqoob SH, Alfayez M, et al. Effects of all-trans retinoic acid on the in vitro maturation of camel (Camelus dromedarius) cumulus-oocyte complexes. Journal of Reproduction and Development. 2019:2018-2073

[89] Ma L, Cai L, Hu M, Wang J, Xie J, Xing Y, et al. Coenzyme Q10 supplementation of human oocyte in vitro maturation reduces postmeiotic aneuploidies. Fertility and Sterility. 2020;**114**:331-337

Chapter 13

Dietary Antioxidants and Bioactive Compounds in Food Processing

Veerapandi Loganathan and Lakshmi Mohan

Abstract

The antioxidants available in fresh organic materials could vary significantly from all those we consume through diet, as it has historically been recognized. Plants contain several phytochemicals, which possess strong antioxidant activities. A large variety of phytochemicals have been isolated and characterized from familiar sources, including vegetables, such as onion and broccoli; fruits, such as apples and grapes; spices, such as nutmeg, pepper, and turmeric; and brews, such as green tea, oolong tea, and red wine; which possess strong antioxidant properties. This is typically affected by the usage of thermal and nonthermal food processing methods. This chapter deals with various traditional and unconventional techniques that can be utilized to recover bioactive constituents. Any traditional method's extraction effectiveness is primarily influenced by the solvents utilized. Among the most effective approaches, notably pressurized solvent extraction, supercritical fluid extraction, pressurized low-polarity water extraction, enzyme-assisted extraction, pulsed electric field extraction, ultrasound-assisted extraction, and microwave-assisted extraction were reviewed. The contrasting antioxidant activities of various extraction techniques were emphasized, as well as the processing techniques and industrial applications for unconventional ways of antioxidant extraction. How well this varies throughout absorption, how this impacts gastrointestinal function, and subsequent accumulation into the plasma, but which *in vivo* biological consequences it has on the internal organs all are aspects to consider.

Keywords: antioxidants, dietary antioxidants, bioactive compounds, food industry, food processing, BHT: Butylated hydroxytoluene; BHA: Butylated hydroxy anisole, extraction, microwave-assisted extraction

1. Introduction

Antioxidants are elements, which are derived from natural and chemical substances, which is having the potent ability to scavenge free radicals by losing an electron and neutralize or slowdown the autooxidation process. Several free radicals are unbalanced and extremely reactive. Antioxidants are ready to contribute to an electron either by oxidizing or reducing other molecules [1]. Also, these antioxidants are capable of preventing and inhibiting cell membrane, structural, DNA, Lipids, carbohydrates, and cellular protein damage. During our body's metabolism and diet, it produces lighter and strong antioxidants, such as uric acid, ubiquinol, glutathione micronutrients α-tocopherol, and ascorbic acid. Even though numerous amounts of antioxidants are there in the form of macro and micronutrients, such as vitamin E, Vitamin C, and beta-carotene to scavenge free radicals [2]. Both ionizing processes and nonenzymatic reactions involving oxygen and organic molecules can lead to the form of free radicals. Few organs are internally produced by some free radicals, such as mitochondria, peroxisomes, xanthine oxidase and some pathways arachidonate, phagocytosis, reperfusion injury, and other external factors.

Fruits and vegetables are one of the best sources of antioxidants. Consuming fresh juices, pastes, and canned foods gives an enormous quantity of antioxidants to our body [3, 4]. Whatever, during food processing least number of antioxidants are loosed and hence, might impact the final product to stimulate health properties [5]. During the twentieth century, food industries introduced antioxidants to inhibit the oxidation process of packed and stored foods [6]. While the impact of antioxidants as loss and gains of bioavailability in food processing have been studied before [7]. It is very important to develop augmented approaches for the preservation of food and the development of activity and bioavailability of antioxidants. It is also used to study about significant of the functional elements of food materials that we used in our daily diet and the changes in the composition of food during processing [8]. Especially performing thermal and nonthermal processing, determining the bioavailability of dietary antioxidants level and quality of dietary antioxidants [9–11].

2. Classification of antioxidants

Generally, antioxidants are present in various foods in various forms. Those antioxidants are classified depending on their functions, mode of action, characteristics, and type of nature [12]. The known major antioxidants are natural and synthetic antioxidants (based on the type), dietary, and endogenous and exogenous antioxidants (based on the function). Furtherly it is classified as enzymatic and nonenzymatic antioxidants. The enzymatic antioxidants are catalase, glutathione, and dismutase, and nonenzymatic antioxidants are tocopherols, melatonin, ascorbic acid, vitamin E, and uric acid. These antioxidants play a very crucial role in food processing and preservation [13].

2.1 Endogenous antioxidants

The only antioxidants with the ability to synthesize their own antioxidant compounds are called an endogenous antioxidants. Further, they can be classified based on their structural characteristics as enzymatic and nonenzymatic antioxidants. The body utilizes a variety of endogenous protective mechanisms alongside dietary antioxidants to support and protect against various consequences. Those enzymes utilized nutrient cofactors copper, zinc, selenium, iron, and manganese to react with toxic intermediate oxidative complexes for maximum catalytic activity [12]. The amino acids are glycine, glutamate, and cysteine synthesized glutathione is an essential water-soluble antioxidant.

2.2 Exogenous antioxidants

Vitamins, polyphenols, carotenoids, as well as certain mineral complexes are examples of naturally occurring sources through which exogenous antioxidants could be synthesized [12]. Antioxidants are getting more prominent, particularly in those intended to avoid the anticipated adverse consequences of the existence of reactive oxygen species in the internal organs and the degeneration of additional dietary constituents, such as fats [13].

2.3 Dietary antioxidants

Ascorbate, tocopherols, carotenoids, and bioactive plant phenols are types of dietary antioxidants. The antioxidant vitamins in fruits and vegetables, some of which possess more potent antioxidant properties than others, are mainly accountable for their health benefits [14–16]. Among the most exhaustively researched dietary antioxidants include vitamins C and E, ß-carotene, other carotenoids, and oxycarotenoids, such as lycopene and lutein [13]. Vitamin C is thought to be the most significant water-soluble antioxidant in extracellular fluids. Before lipid per oxidation commences, it has the potential to remove free radicals in the aqueous environment. The most potent chain-breaking antioxidant in the cell membrane, wherever it protects cell wall fatty acids from lipid peroxidation, is vitamin E, a prominent lipid-soluble antioxidant. Vitamin C has allegedly demonstrated the ability to stimulate vitamin E [17].

It is also hypothesized that ß-carotene and certain other pigments protect lipid-rich tissues from damaging free radicals. According to studies, several vitamins and ß-carotene may enhance the other's actions [18]. Although carotenoids seem to function as "pathogen-associated molecular enhancers" in individuals, flavonoids protect plants from either a wide range of environmental stresses. The anti-inflammatory, anti-allergic, antimicrobial, antiaging, and anti-carcinogenic characteristics of flavonoids have been demonstrated [13].

2.4 Natural antioxidants

Those oxidants known as naturally occurring antioxidants could be present in foods, including fruit and vegetables and livestock [19]. All-natural compounds, especially berries, plants, nuts, beans, branches, stems, and barks, possess antioxidant compounds [19]. Vitamin C, E, and A (ascorbic acid, tocopherols, and carotenoids), different polyphenols, comprising quercetin, proanthocyanidins, and lutein, and ubiquitin known as a coenzyme Q_{10}, a type of dietary protein, are among the most abundant vitamins in food products [13]. Plants namely the vitamins as well as other originating molecules in our food create natural antioxidants. The majority of fresh fruit and vegetable include ubiquitin, a specific type of protein, which is a potent antioxidant [20].

Living beings get all these elements mostly through plant-derived substances [11]. The excellent sources of antioxidant substances, comprising vitamins A, C, and E, ß-carotene, and essential minerals, are fruits, vegetables, and medicinal plants [21]. The total amount of phenol in various parts of plants, or even of the same vegetables and fruit varies greatly [22]. Enzymatic antioxidants and nonenzymatic oxidants make up the two main categories of the biological antioxidant system [23].

2.4.1 Enzymatic antioxidants

Both primary and secondary metabolic inhibitors are even further characterized as catalytic antioxidants. The basic protection is composed of three essential enzymes that prevent the production of free radicals or neutralize them: glutathione peroxidase, catalase, and superoxide dismutase [23]. Glutathione reductase and glucose-6-phosphate dehydrogenase are two supplementary metabolic inhibitors [24]. Even though these two enzymes really should not directly counteract free radicals, they might enhance existing endogenous inhibitors in their abilities to achieve this.

2.4.2 Nonenzymatic antioxidants

The production of reactive oxygen species (ROS) and reactive nitrogen species (RNS) are certainly scavengers by nonenzymatic antioxidants, which include proteins (glutathione), vitamins E and C (that also inhibit the oxidative damage of cellular membrane), nitrogenous compounds, including uric acid, which inherently acts as an antioxidant against peroxynitrite in bloodstream, albumin, bilirubin, N-Acetylcysteine (NAC), and melatonin [17, 25, 26].

2.5 Synthetic antioxidants

Antioxidants that are chemically synthesized and added to perishable foods as preserves to contribute to the inhibition of peroxidation are termed synthetic antioxidants, since they cannot appear in nature [27]. Synthetic antioxidants were created in order to provide a consistent catalase activity analysis method to correlate with antioxidant properties and to be incorporated into foods. Such bioactive molecules are included in the food to enhance storability and to assist it to resist alternative treatments and environments. Consequently, synthetic antioxidants are incorporated into essentially all packaged products, which are supposedly acceptable [25]. The two most commonly used synthetic scavengers are butylated hydroxytoluene (BHT) and butylated hydroxyanisole (BHA). Considering the daily allowance and effective dose for the synthesis of various inhibitors, contradictory results were obtained [14]. Moreover, mixed data exist on the influence of antioxidant compounds on people's well-being. BHT, BHA, propyl gallate (PG), dodecyl gallate (DG), and tertiary butylhydroquinone are among the chemical additives currently authorized to be used in foods [2, 27].

3. Sources of antioxidants

The majority of natural antioxidants in use today are derived from plant sources, such as fruits, vegetables, spices, and herbs [26]. These foods are particularly rich in plant secondary metabolites, such as phenolic compounds, terpenoids, alkaloids, vitamins, and carotenoids [28].

The most popular antioxidants are the essential oils extracted from culinary spices and herbs, such as thyme, oregano, marjoram, basil, lavender, and rosemary. They have been reported to be good sources of natural antioxidant-rich molecules, but have limited applications due to their strong aroma and flavor characteristics [29, 30].

Another common source of dietary antioxidants is the brewed tea used around the world. They include non-fermented (green), semi-fermented (Oolong), aged (Pu'er), and fermented (black). Tea is very rich in polyphenols. Fresh green tea leaves have been reported to contain around 36% polyphenols, on a dry-weight basis [26]. Aqueous tea extracts are also good sources of natural antioxidants owing to a large number of metabolites, such as catechins, tannins, and other flavonoids, in a fresh brew. They have the additional advantage of not presenting a strong flavor when compared to essential oils [29].

The polyphenols in green tea have been observed to bring about programmed cell death otherwise known as apoptosis in numerous cancer cells, such as prostate, lymphoma, colon, and lung cancer cells. Black tea, on the other hand, was found to inhibit DNA synthesis while enhancing the apoptosis of benign and malignant tumor cells. The antioxidant activity of green tea catechins is normally in the order of EGCG (epigallocatechin gallate) almost equal to ECG (epicatechin gallate) activity, which is better than EGC (epigallocatechin) and greater than EC (epicatechin), while that of theaflavins of fermented teas are theaflavin digallate (TF-2) greater than theaflavin monogallate (TF-1 A & B) than theaflavin (TF). The antioxidant activity of green tea almost often surpasses that of oxidized black tea and its extracts [31].

Gallic acid is a recognized natural antioxidant that induced fragmentation of DNA in THP-1, HL-60, U-937, and ML-1; four diverse human myelogenous leukemia cell lines, but not in erythroleukemia (K- 562) cell lines and human T-cell leukemia (MOLT-4). Gallic acid was found to induce apoptosis in HL-60 RG cells through ROS (reactive oxygen species) generation, an influx of $Ca2+$ leading to the activation of calmodulin. The primary pigment in turmeric, curcumin, and phenolic compound was found to induce apoptosis in transformed human and rodent cells in culture. Curcumin mediates this chemopreventive action by inhibiting the formation of cyclooxygenase metabolites, which provides a mechanism for the induction of apoptosis. Quercitrin, quercetin, and kaempferol are flavonoids present widely in around 70% of all plants. Flavonoids differ notably in their antioxidative effectiveness, depending on their structure [31].

The most effective dietary antioxidants belong to the family of phenolics and polyphenolics. Phenolic compounds occurring in foods belong to the phenylpropanoid (C6-C3) family and are derivatives of cinnamic acid. These compounds are formed from phenylalanine, and to a lesser extent in some plants from tyrosine, via the action of phenylalanine lyase, or its corresponding tyrosine lyase. Edible oils and oilseeds provide a rich source of unsaponifiable matter that contains a variety of active ingredients that may be used to prevent or control deteriorative processes. The non-triacylglycerol constituents in oils and oilseeds belong primarily to the tocols (tocopherols and tocotrienols) family, phenolics and flavonoids, sterols, phospholipids, carotenoids, and triterpene alcohols as well as the phytic acid family of compounds [27]. Carotenoids play a major role in the prevention of various health disorders, such as cancer, metabolic disease, and cardiovascular diseases [32].

4. Extraction of antioxidants from natural sources

Antioxidants are isolated and purified from different parts of plants, such as roots, stems, leaves, fruits, seeds, and peels. The attributes of antioxidants from natural sources and their antioxidant potential depends not only on the quality of the extract concerning its geographic origin, nutritional aspects, and storage, but also on the methodologies used for their extraction.

The methods for analyzing antioxidants include the estimation of total antioxidant activity by electrochemical or spectrophotometric methods. The specific detection and assessment of different antioxidant molecules are facilitated by various chromatographic—TLC, HPLC, LC, GC, MS, NMR, capillary electrophoresis, and NIR methods. However, before quantification can be done, it is required to extract the different components from the food matrix. This involves technologies such as the use of organic solvents for solvent extraction, subcritical water extraction, supercritical fluids, high hydrostatic pressure, microwave procedures, pulsed electric fields, or ultrasonics.

The yield of antioxidants extracted from the plant material is affected mainly by the environment under which the process of extraction occurs. Every plant material is unique in terms of its structure and composition; therefore, the behavior of the resulting material-solvent system is unpredictable upon combining it with solvents. Assisted techniques using original fluids, which are referred to as nonconventional methods of extraction, such as supercritical fluids, supercritical water, ultrasound-assisted extraction, enzymatic-assisted extraction (EAE), microwave-assisted extraction (MAE), supercritical fluid, and pulsed electric field (PEF) have become more efficient and popular in recent times [33].

4.1 Solvent extraction

Solvent extraction is a technique that involves applying a solvent to extract or separate the desired component, called the solute from solid food material. The separation factor in solvent extraction is the chemical equilibrium that exists between the solid and solvent phases. And the concentration difference of the component between the two phases is the driving force for solvent extraction. An ideal solvent for extraction should have a high affinity for the solute being separated, it should be selective and dissolve the component of interest to a large extent while having a minimum capacity for the other undesirable components. It should be chemically stable, forming no irreversible reactions with contacting components, regenerable, and have low viscosity values for easy pumping and transportation [33].

The most efficient solvents used in extracting anthocyanins, being polar molecules, are aqueous mixtures of methanol, ethanol, and acetone. Among the most frequent solvent extraction methods are the ones that use acidified ethanol or methanol as solvents. The acids in the solvent system rupture the cell membranes and release anthocyanins. As this can cause damage to the anthocyanin structure, it is advised to acidify the solvents with organic acids, such as formic or acetic acid, rather than mineral acids, such as 0.1% HCl, to minimize damage [33].

Alcoholic solvents are used to extract antioxidant phenolic compounds from various sources. Ethanol, a polar solvent has been shown to effectively extract several secondary metabolites, including flavonoids, catechol, glycosides, and tannins, from raw plant materials. It is also to be noted that in food processing industries, ethanol is preferred over methanol due to its inherent toxicity. Lycopene, a fat-soluble antioxidant present in large quantities in tomatoes, is extracted with organic solvents, such as benzene, acetone, petroleum ether, ethanol, hexane, and chloroform.

4.2 Extraction using supercritical fluids

Extraction with the help of supercritical fluids (SCF) has gained popularity in the food processing domain. Similar to conventional solvent extraction, SCF extractions use fluids in their supercritical states, which have desirable transport properties that enhance their potential as solvents for extraction processes [34]. CO_2 is one such example that is nontoxic, noninflammable, and requires only a bare minimum amount of solvent for the process. Extraction is quicker, takes about 10–60 min, is selective, and requires only small quantities of sample and no additional cleanup. An improvement over this method is the use of enhanced solvent extraction, which uses carbon dioxide, organic solvents, or water at high temperatures and pressure. SCF extraction has been used successfully for extracting anthocyanins and polyphenols from grapes, wine, and some herbs [34].

4.3 Ultrasonics

Ultrasonics is one of the commonly used techniques in the food and beverage industry, which enhances the mass-transfer phenomena. It has been successfully applied for extracting anthocyanins, polyphenols, and flavonoids from various plant sources.

4.4 Microwave-assisted extraction (MAE)

Microwave-assisted extraction (MAE) helps reduce the time needed for extraction and the quantity of solvent used. MAE involves extraction under controlled conditions of temperature and pressure with or without the addition of a solvent. It has been reported that using closed vessels cuts down the extraction time and increases the efficiency of extraction. MAE has been used to extract phenolics in a very effective manner [35]. Recent advances in this domain include microwave hydrodiffusion and gravity (MHG) and solvent-free microwave extraction (SFME).

4.5 Subcritical water extraction (SWE)

Subcritical water extraction uses subcritical water or pressurized hot water below the critical pressure of 22 MPa to extract natural compounds from herbs, plants, and food materials, such as pomegranate seed residues, red grapes, potato, and citrus peels [8].

4.6 High hydrostatic pressure (HHP)

High hydrostatic pressure (HHP) works by improving mass transfer rates, thereby increasing cell permeability and secondary metabolite diffusion by changes in phase transitions. HPP has been reported to be utilized in extracting anthocyanins and polyphenols from grapes, red fruits, and grape skins [35].

4.7 Enzyme-assisted extraction (EAE)

Enzyme-assisted extraction (EAE) has been used efficiently to release and recover bioactive molecules from several algal and plant sources, such as lemon balm, red algae, alfalfa, and pumpkins. Enzymes are capable of catalyzing the degradation of plant cell walls, thereby releasing the bioactive compounds stored inside the cells. Examples of enzymes used for this procedure are cellulases, hemicellulases, pectinases, etc. [35].

Other major techniques, such as pulsed electric fields and high voltage electrical discharges, are also gaining popularity as noninvasive techniques to extract secondary metabolites from plant sources.

5. Processing of antioxidants

Despite the knowledge that there are numerous antioxidants in nature, typically just a few amounts of basic ingredients, especially vegetable fatty acids and oils and rosemary leaves, are utilized to synthesize extracts with antioxidant potential [31]. Considering these substances have enough potential to cause serious harm, cytotoxic,

By-products	Amount of phenol
Onion peel	105 g/kg
Orange peel	1.8 g/kg
Lemon peel	13.3 g/kg
Grape peel	13.8 g/kg
Potato peel	7.8 g/kg
Apple peel	2.4 g/kg

Table 1.
Antioxidant amounts in different by-products.

or neurotoxic to people, the desire for bioactive components has resulted in a reduction in their utilization [15]. It is, therefore, argued that synthetic substances, such as BHT, are hazardous for ingestion when used in therapeutics because they could have negative health consequences for humans [34]. The unfavorable effects of antioxidant compounds on well-being have been significantly reduced through investigation.

The amount of production of natural antioxidants from waste vegetables and other fruits has generated a significant amount of attention. Huge quantities of waste products, particularly peels and nuts, are generated during the process of processing fruits, vegetables, and grains [34]. Regulatory constraints mean handling these substances is a challenge that is already complex. As a result, unique perspectives on utilizing these materials as by-products for further utilization on the development of additives or supplement with high amounts of nutrients have drawn increasing attention considering that these are greater commodities and their recovery may be economically feasible. According to the original source, the production of fruit and vegetables and oilseeds generates different quantities of by-product (**Table 1**) [17].

6. Antioxidant composition varies during food processing

Consumption of natural antioxidant compounds from food products that are already abundant in all of these bioactive substances [36]. Although food processing is proven that it has a significant impact on nutritional properties and pharmacological activities [31]. Food processing involves both thermal and nonthermal procedures, including storing, sorting, washing, packaging, and transportation, to produce the desired final product [18]. Antioxidants are lost during the processing of fruits and vegetables, and processed foods have significantly lower bioavailability when compared to fresh foods, which leads to rapid oxidation, enzymatic reaction, and degradation of enzymes due to thermal processing [37]. However, there is significant information that shows food processing might not even necessarily have such a negative influence on the effectiveness of dietary ingredients [33].

6.1 Thermal treatments

The majority of commercially available food processing techniques include one or even more than one thermal process in order to achieve a variety of final products.

The chemical content and nutritive values of the food material could change after the thermal process in addition to the desired consequence because of quantitatively or qualitatively changes in the amount of antioxidant properties, among several other factors. One of the main antioxidants, carotenoids, are widely distributed in tomatoes, watermelons, guava, papaya, and apricots [24]. Carotenoids are degraded if these food products are exposed to various treatments. Many vegetables and fruits contain phenols and phenolic substances. The majority of these food processing technologies include thermal treatments, which are reported that the plants do not have the ability to retain phenolic acids [38]. The outcomes of phenolic acids in food production can be significantly influenced by the product's composition and the processing methods, but the dietary substrate has also been shown to be an even more important factor [7].

6.2 Nonthermal treatments

Cutting, blending, peeling, and crushing, as well as other nonthermal food processing technologies, could all have an influence on the antioxidant characteristics of food products. Additional "emerging" or "progressive" nonthermal food processing techniques have recently been developed, including high pressure, pulsed electric field, and ultrasonic processing [20]. Excessive temperatures could lead to their breakdown or polymerization, and that has negative consequences on some of these bioactive constituents, but they might also assist to extract higher carotenoids from the plant source. Various nonthermal processing technologies were suggested as alternative approaches to yield a product of a higher quality.

7. Changes in antioxidant bioavailability during food processing

Antioxidant compounds must be released from the food material through metabolism in the gastrointestinal tract and thereafter biologically modified into ingestible components in order to demonstrate their nutrition properties or to be active compounds [16]. In order to be used in metabolic processes, substances can then gradually enter the circulatory system and be delivered to the blood circulation, becoming "bioavailable" [39]. "Bioavailability" is a word that describes the transportation and diffusion of active ingredients to specific cells and tissues, enabling those cells and tissues to demonstrate a range of antioxidant actions [40]. Oral bioavailability has frequently been assessed through *in situ* digestive assays. These methodologies mimic digestion in the small intestine and gastrointestinal tract, and in certain cases, Caco-2 cell absorption simulation was achieved initially [41]. The concentration of these molecules, their intermolecular interactions, and the molecular structure of the plant and food products are the characteristics that have a substantial impact on the oral bioavailability and digestibility of natural antioxidant substances. The concentrations of various bioactive constituents in the respective food are influenced by pre and postharvest handling, resulting in a significant impact on plant-based product are composed. As an outcome, processed food products may have varying levels of dietary and possibly bioavailable antioxidant compounds. Furthermore, modifying the molecular structure of the essential constituents during food processing seems to have the chance to have a significant favorable or detrimental effect on availability [40].

Research on the contribution of food processing technologies on the bioavailability of antioxidants is completely lacking overall.

8. Applications of antioxidants

Natural and synthetically derived antioxidants have found wide applications in the food processing sector as food additives in meat, fruits, vegetables, beverage, spices, fats, and oil industries to enhance the appearance, taste, and color, and help prolong the shelf life. The addition of dietary antioxidants to meat and derived products has been observed to be effective in lipid oxidation and metmyoglobin formation. These compounds include plant phenolics as natural antioxidants, for instance, vitamin C—ascorbic acid and vitamin E—α-tocopherol (E306), culinary herbs, and spices, such as oregano, rosemary, basil, thyme, sage, pepper, nutmeg, clove, cinnamon, and extracts from tea and grape seed. The potential applications of natural extracts with antioxidant activity in food are being thoroughly investigated for potential uses, including health paybacks, nutritional profile improvement, and shelf-life extension [1].

Ascorbic acid, E300 is added to cut fruits, beers, jams, dried potato, and other foods to prevent foods from going brown due to oxidation reactions that cause discoloration. It is also added to replace the vitamin C lost during processing.

Rosemary oleoresin has proven to be as successful as polyphosphate and a combination of BHT and BHT-citric acid in automatically deboned poultry meat and sausages made from automatically deboned poultry meat [16, 34] worked on ethanolic extracts of rosemary and demonstrated that it improved the stability of butter and that this effect was concentration-dependent. The research study also assessed the ability of rosemary extract to inhibit copper-catalyzed oxidation and proved that the extract could chelate metal ions.

Pepper nigrum extract isolated using supercritical carbon dioxide extractions was found to be efficient in preventing lipid oxidation in ground pork samples. The potent antioxidant activity of pepper has been credited to piperine and piperine isomers, such as chavicine, isopiperine, isochavicine, and some monoterpenes.

Farag et al. showed that the essential oils of Cuminum cyminum and Thymus vulgaris inhibited the oxidation in butter that was stored at room temperature. At a concentration of 200 ppm, these essential oils were more efficient than Butylated hydroxytoluene in inhibiting the oxidation of lipids.

It is a fact that all emulsified products tend to have a shorter shelf life when compared to edible oils, due to their lesser resistance to microbial spoilage. They are, therefore, stored under refrigerated conditions, so that autoxidation is low and the naturally present tocopherols are stabilized them. Some edible oils, such as sunflower oil, are less resistant due to high polyunsaturation, often requiring the addition of natural or synthetic antioxidants. When it comes to frying oils, the best way to add antioxidants is just before their operation. It has been observed that adding rice bran oil with inherent natural antioxidants enhanced the shelf life of nuts processed in oils, such as soybean or rapeseed [20].

The application of synthetic antioxidants has to be reduced further and replaced by safer alternatives, such as natural or nature-identical antioxidants. Prolongation of the shelf life of highly processed foods has to be accomplished by modifying existing recipes, introducing culinary herbs and spices, which contain a high concentration of inherent antioxidants, using high-oleic edible oils requiring lower added antioxidant levels, and by use of natural protein hydrolysates, which have good synergistic activity.

9. Conclusions

There is increasing evidence to prove that consuming a range of dietary antioxidants available in natural foods reduces the risk of major health issues due to their antioxidant capability through several mechanisms. Care must be taken to choose optimal processing methods to ensure the quality of antioxidants from fresh fruits and vegetables and their products in order to achieve the objectives. The mode of action of these antioxidants in the body needs more research. Due to safety concerns, regarding the use of synthetic antioxidants and natural antioxidants acquired from edible sources, their by-products and coproducts are in the spotlight today. Further studies on the isolation of antioxidant compounds using nondestructive methods and their effects in animal models and human subjects are necessary to evaluate their potential benefits. Additionally, it is mandatory to confirm the bioavailability and lack of toxicity of such compounds. Delivery of isolated antioxidant metabolites as functional food ingredients or dietary supplements will help in promoting good health and reducing the risk of disease. In the last few decades, there has been considerable interest in the food as well as the pharmaceutical industry, for extracting and purifying antioxidants from natural sources. A sensible selection of appropriate food-handling methods right from the farm to the consumer for every type of product will make sure that the health-related benefits of specific antioxidants are maximized.

Author details

Veerapandi Loganathan* and Lakshmi Mohan
Saintgits College of Engineering, Kottayam, Kerala, India

*Address all correspondence to: veerapandi.l@saintgits.org

References

[1] Admassu S, Kebede M. Application of antioxidants in food processing industry: Options to improve the extraction yields and market value of natural products. Advances in Food Technology and Nutrition Sciences. 2019;**5**:38-49

[2] Moure A, Cruz JM, Franco Ruiz DJ, et al. Natural antioxidants from residual sources. Food Chemistry. 2001;**72**:145-171. DOI: 10.1016/S0308-8146(00)00223-5

[3] Gülçin I. Antioxidants and antioxidant methods: An updated overview. Archives of Toxicology. 2020;**94**(3):651-715. DOI: 10.1007/s00204-020-02689-3

[4] Gülçin I. Antioxidant activity of food constituents: An overview. Archives of Toxicology. 2012;**86**(3):345-391. DOI: 10.1007/s00204-011-0774-2

[5] Al-juhaimi F, Ghafoor K, Ozcan MM, Jahurul MHA, Babiker EE, Jinap S, et al. Effect of various food processing and handling methods on preservation of natural antioxidants in fruits and vegetables. Journal of Food Science and Technology. 2018;**55**(10):3872-3880. DOI: 10.1007/s13197-018-3370-0

[6] Kumar S. The importance of antioxidants and their role in pharmaceutical science - a review. Asian Journal of Research in Chemistry and Pharmaceutical Sciences. 2014;**1**(1):27-44

[7] Arfaoui L. Dietary plant polyphenols: Effects of food processing on their content and bioavailability. Molecules. 2021;**26**(10):2959. DOI: 10.3390/molecules26102959

[8] Ratnam DV, Ankola DD, Bhardwaj V, Sahana DK, Kumar MN. Role of antioxidants in prophylaxis and therapy: A pharmaceutical perspective. Journal of Controlled Release. 2006;**113**:189-207. DOI: 10.1016/j.jconrel.2006.04.015

[9] Barba FJ, Mariutti LRB, Bragagnolo N, Mercadante AZ, Barbosa-Canovas GV, Orlien V. Bioaccessibility of bioactive compounds from fruits and vegetables after thermal and nonthermal processing. Trends in Food Science & Technology. 2017;**67**:195-206. DOI: 10.1016/j.tifs.2017.07.006

[10] Ahmed M, Eun J-B. Flavonoids in fruits and vegetables after thermal and nonthermal processing: A review. Critical Reviews in Food Science and Nutrition. 2018;**58**(18):3159-3188. DOI: 10.1080/10408398.2017.1353480

[11] Akbarirad H, Ardabili GA, Kazemeini SM, Khaneghah MA. An overview on some of important sources of natural antioxidants. International Food Research Journal. 2016;**23**(3):928-933

[12] Pérez JAM, Aguilar TAF. Chemistry of natural antioxidants and studies performed with different plants collected in Mexico. In: Morales-González JA, editor. Oxidative Stress and Chronic Degenerative Diseases - a Role for Antioxidants. London, UK: Intech; 2013. pp. 59-81. DOI: 10.5772/52247

[13] Yadav A, Kumar R, Yadav A, et al. Antioxidants and its functions in human body - a review. Research in Environment and Life Sciences. 2016;**9**(11):1328-1331

[14] Pisarikova B, Zraly Z, Kracmar S, Trckova M, Herzig I. The use of amaranth (genus Amaranthus L.) in the diets for broiler chickens. Veterinární Medicína. 2006;**51**(7):399-407. DOI: 10.17221/5560-VETMED

[15] Emmons CL, Peterson DM. Antioxidant activity and phenolic contents of oat groats and hulls. Cereal Chemistry. 1999;**76**(6):902-906. DOI: 10.1094/CCHEM.1999.76.6.902

[16] Barbut S, Josephson DB, Maurer AJ. Antioxidant properties of rosemary oleoresin in Turkey sausage. Journal of Food Science. 1985;**50**:1356-1363

[17] Oreopoulou V, Tzia C. Utilization of plant by-products for the recovery of prteins, dietery fibers, antioxidants and colorants. In: Oreopoulou V, Russ W, editors. Utilization of by-Products and Treatment of Waste in the Food Industry. New York, USA: Springer; 2007. pp. 209-232. DOI: 10.1007/978-0-387-35766-9_11

[18] Kiokias S, Varzakas T, Oreopoulou V. In vitro activity of vitamins, flavonoids, and natural phenolic antioxidants against the oxidative deterioration of oil-based systems. Critical Reviews in Food Science and Nutrition. 2008;**48**(1):78-93

[19] Grozea MBAI. Antioxidant (antiradical) compounds. Journal of Bioequivalence & Bioavailability. 2012;**4**(6). DOI: 10.4172/jbb.10000e18

[20] Anbudhasan P, Surendraraj A, Karkuzhali S, Sathishkumaran P. Natural antioxidants and its benefits. International Journal of Food and Nutritional Sciences. 2014;**3**(6):225-232

[21] Sies H, Stahl W, Sundquist AR. Antioxidant functions of vitamins, vitamins E and C, beta-carotene, and other carotenoids. Annals of the New York Academy of Sciences. 1992;**669**:7-20

[22] Mohdali AAA. Evaluation of some Food Processing by-Products as Sources for Natural Antioxidants [Thesis]. Chicago, IL, USA: Technical University of Berlin; 2010

[23] Ramos L, Kristenson EM, Brinkman UT. Current use of pressurised liquid extraction and subcritical water extraction in environmental analysis. Journal of Chromatography A. 2002;**975**(1):3-29

[24] Badin EE, Quevedo-Leon R, Ibarz A, Ribotta PD, Lespinard AR. Kinetic modeling of thermal degradation of color, lycopene, and ascorbic acid in crushed tomato. Food and Bioprocess Technology. 2021;**14**(2):324-333. DOI: 10.1007/s11947-021-02579-1

[25] Cermak R, Durazzo A, Maiani G, B¨ohm V, Kammerer D. R, Carle R, Galensa R. The influence of postharvest processing and storage of foodstuffs on the bioavailability of flavonoids and phenolic acids. Molecular Nutrition & Food Research. 2009;**53**(S2):S184-S193. DOI: 10.1002/mnfr.200700444

[26] Brodowska KM. Natural flavonoids: Classification, potential role, and application of flavonoid analogues. European Journal of Biological Research. 2017;7:109-110

[27] Shahidi F, Ambigaipalan P. Phenolics and polyphenolics in foods, beverages and spices: Antioxidant activity and health effects–a review. Journal of Functional Foods. 2015;**18**:820-897

[28] Tajkarimi M, Ibrahim S, Cliver D. Antimicrobial herb and spice compounds in food. Food Control. 2010;**21**:1199-1218

[29] Tanemura N, Machii Y, Urushihara H. The first survey of gap between the actual labelling and efficacy information of functional substances in food under the regulatory processes in Japan. Journal of Functional Foods. 2020;**72**:104047. DOI: 10.1016/j.jff.2020.104047

[30] Embuscado ME. Spices and herbs: Natural sources of antioxidants—A mini

review. Journal of Functional Foods. 2015;**18**:811-819

[31] Shahidi F, Naczk M. Food Phenolics: Sources, Chemistry, Effects and Applications. Lancaster, PA: Technomic Publishing Co.; 1995

[32] Kamiloglu S, Boyacioglu D, Capanoglu E. The effect of food processing on bioavailability of tomato antioxidants. Journal of Berry Research. 2013;**3**:65-77. DOI: 10.3233/JBR-130051

[33] Yin J, Becker EM, Andersen ML, Skibsted LH. Green tea extract as a food antioxidant. Synergism and antagonism with α-tocopherol in vegetable oils and their colloidal systems. Food Chemistry. 2012;**135**:2195-2202

[34] Zegarska Z, Amarowicz R, Karmac M, Rafalowski R. Antioxidative effect of rosemary ethanolic extract on butter. Milchwissenschaft. 1996;**51**:195-198

[35] Ballard TS, Mallikarjunan P, Zhou K, O'Keefe S. Microwave-assisted extraction of phenolic antioxidant compounds from peanut skins. Food Chemistry. 2010;**120**(4):1185-1192

[36] Burton-Freeman BM, Sesso HD. Whole food versus supplement: Comparing the clinical evidence of tomato intake and lycopene supplementation on cardiovascular risk factors. Advances in Nutrition. 2014;**5**(5):457-485. DOI: 10.3945/an.114.005231

[37] Boz Z, Koelsch Sand C. A systematic analysis of the overall nutritional contribution of food loss and waste in tomatoes, spinach, and kidney beans as a function of processing. Journal of Food Process Engineering. 2020;**43**(11):e13509. DOI: 10.1111/jfpe.13509

[38] Garzoli S, Cairone F, Carradori S, Mocan A, Menghini L, Paolicelli P, et al. Effects of processing on polyphenolic and volatile composition and fruit quality of Clery strawberries. Antioxidants. 2020;**9**(7):632. DOI: 10.3390/antiox9070632

[39] Sikora E, Cieslik E, Topolska K. The sources of natural antioxidants. Acta Scientiarum Polonorum. Technologia Alimentaria. 2008;7:5-17

[40] Carocho M, Ferreira IC. A review on antioxidants, prooxidants and related controversy: Natural and synthetic compounds, screening and analysis methodologies and future perspectives. Food and Chemical Toxicology. 2013;**51**:15-25. DOI: 10.1016/j.fct.2012.09.021

[41] Dimitrios B. Sources of natural phenolic antioxidants. Trendsin Food Science & Technology. 2006;**17**(9):505-512. DOI: 10.1016/j.tifs.2006.04.004